The World of Aromatherapy

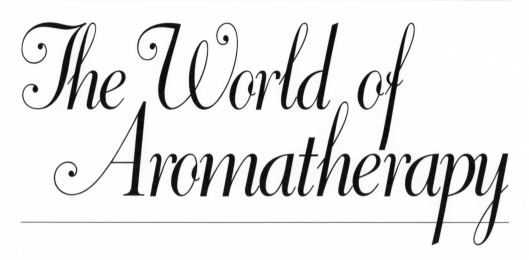

The World of Aromatherapy

An Anthology of Aromatic History,
Ideas, Concepts and Case Histories

by The NAHA Women of Aromatherapy
National Association for Holistic Aromatherapy

Edited by

Jeanne Rose *&* Susan Earle

Frog, Ltd
Berkeley, California

The World of Aromatherapy

Copyright © 1996 by Jeanne Rose and Susan Earle. All rights
reserved. No portion of this book, except for brief review, may be
reproduced in any form without written permission of the publisher.
For information contact Frog, Ltd. c/o North Atlantic Books.

Published by Frog, Ltd.

Frog, Ltd. books are distributed by
North Atlantic Books
P.O. Box 12327
Berkeley, CA 94712

Cover and book design by Leigh McLellan
Printed in the United States of America

Library of Congress Cataloging-in-Publication Data

Rose, Jeanne, 1940–
      The world of aromatherapy / Jeanne Rose and Susan Earle.
          p.   cm.
      Includes bibliographical references.
      ISBN 1-883319-49-8
      1. Aromatherapy. I. Earle, Susan. II. Title.
RM666.A68R67   1996
615'.321—dc20   95-48253
                                                            CIP

      2   3   4   5   6   7   8   9 / 98

Dedication

To Barbara Bobo,
a tireless promoter of the fragrant life,
a dear friend and confidante, and fellow
lover of a good bath. Never has anyone
worked with such enthusiasm, grace,
and joy to bring the life of pleasurable luxury
to the masses. May she continue to prosper
in good health for the benefit of all.

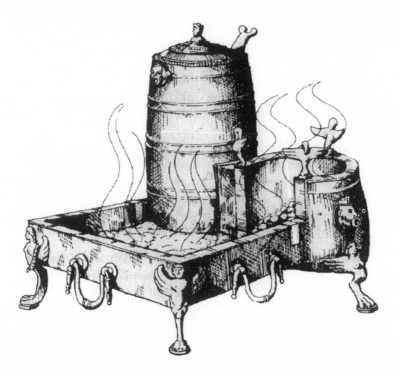

Acknowledgements

Permission for the Cover Art, *Fumée d'Amber Gris*, 1880 by John Singer Sargent, Oil on canvas, 54 3/4 ×35 11/16 in, Sterling and Francine Clark Art Institute, Williamstown, Massachusetts.

The editors would like to thank the following for their gracious permission for use of their material:

The Aromatherapy Quarterly, 5, Ranelagh Ave., Barnes, London SW13 OBY, UK Fax: (011 44) 181 392 1691 for "A Healing Partnership: Oils & Crystals" by Tricia Davis; Summer 1993, No. 33; "Benzoin" by Shirley Whitton; Autumn 1994, No. 44; "Scent Soul & Psyche" by Julia Lawless as edited by Séza Eccles; Autumn 1994, No. 44; "A Day in the Life of an Egyptian Embalmer" by Wanda Sellar; Winter 1994, No. 43.

HarperCollins Publishers Limited, 77-85 Fullham Palace Road, Hammersmith, London W6 8JB, UK, for the use of "Scent Soul & Psyche" from *Aromatherapy and the Mind* by Julia Lawless.

Jeanne Rose, 219 Carl Street, San Francisco, CA 94117 for use of "Synthetic versus Natural;" "The Culinary Aromatherapy Chart;" and "A Fragrant Dinner Menu from Around the World."

The Aromatherapist, Training Department, Shirley Price Aromatherapy Ltd., Essentia House, Upper Bond Street, Hinckley, Leicester, LE10 1RS, UK for use of "Aromatherapy in the Theatre" by Lucy Scott. February 1995, Vol. 2, No. 1.

Llewellyn Publications, P.O. Box 64383-120, St. Paul, MN 55164, for the use of "Performing a Consultation" by Ann Berwick from *Holistic Aromatherapy*.

Alexandra Avery for the use of "Aromatherapy Then and Now," an excerpt from her book *Aromatherapy and You: A Guide to Natural Skin Care.*

Professor Massimo Maffei, Department of Plant Biology, University of Turin, Italy, who supplied the abaxial epidermis pictures of Mentha piperita L.

The Editors would also like to acknowledge:

All who contributed submissions.

Séza Eccles of *The Aromatherapy Quarterly*, for serving as liaison between the editors and *Aromatherapy Quarterly* writers, and for her time and effort in helping us with the obtaining of permissions from English publishers.

We received numerous articles, in a variety of forms, from around the world.

Thank you to Ginger Ashworth for taking the faxes, phone messages, disks in all programs for all computers, handwritten notes, and typed pages unaccompanied by disk and compiling them in a manageable format on three Macintosh-readable disks.

Table of Contents

Editor's Note   xi

Introduction   xiii

Preface   xvii

I Background

1   Aromatherapy Then and Now, *by Alexandra Avery*   3

2   A Day in the Life of an Egyptian Embalmer, by Wanda Sellar   9

3   Essential Oil Distillation: Profiles of Four Distillers in the
    1990s, *by Sara Hindman*   14

4   Two Products of Distillation, *by Jeanne Rose*   26

5   Are Synthetic and Natural Oils Identical?
    An Anthrophosophical Approach, *by Victoria Edwards*   32

    Synthetic versus Natural   37

6   The Science of Essential Oils and Their Toxicity,
    by Maria Lis-Balchin   39

II Self Care

7   An Exquisite Aromatherapy Skin Care Treatment,
    by Joni Loughran   53

8   Aromatic Inspirations, *by Zia Wesley-Hosford*   65

9   Bathing in the Souls of Flowers, *by Barbara Bobo*   70

10 Your Medicine Tin of Five Essential Oils, *by Candace Welsh*   83

11 Nurturing During Pregnancy with Aromatherapy,
    by Ixchel Susan Leigh   94

12 Aromatherapy for Pregnancy and Birth, *by Susan Earle* 100

III A Scentual Mix

13 Magic at Our Fingertips, *by Emilee Stewart*   113

14 Scent, Soul, and Psyche, *by Julia Lawless*   116

15 Goddess Traditions and Aromatherapy, *by Leila Castle* 125

16 A Healing Partnership: Oils and Crystals, *by Tricia Davis* 131

17 Perfumery with Rare Essences, *by Christine Malcolm*   140

18 Essential Oil Blends to Perfume Your Body, *by Jeanne Rose* 147

19 Culinary Aromatherapy, *by Mindy Green,*   152

    Culinary Aromatherapy Chart   164

    A Fragrant Dinner from Around the World   165

IV The Oils

20 Benzoin, *by Shirley Whitton*   169

21 The Women's Oils, *by Victoria Edwards*   177

22 Mints Are Not Just for After Dinner, *by Linda Hein*   192

23 Essential Botany, *by Jeanne Rose*   200

V Case Studies

24 Planting Aromatherapy Seeds, *by Elizabeth Jones*   219

25 Aromatherapy and Health in the Theatre, *by Lucy Scott* 227

26 Doctor Predicts Human Eggplant . . .
But Essential Oils Save the Day!! *by Sheryll Ryan*   240

27 Aromatherapy Institute Case Studies,
by Maria Dolores Gonzales   242

28 Memory Loss and Alzheimer's Disease, *by Deanna Wolf*   247

29 Parkinson's Disease Project: Is Aromatherapy an Effective
Treatment for Parkinson's Disease? *by Shirley Price*   250

VI Business and Research

30 Bringing Credibility to the Aromatherapy Industry,
by Marianne Griffeth   265

31 Endometriosis, Infertility, and Aromatherapy,
by Valerie Ann Worwood   277

32 Integration of Botanical Remedies and Kinesiology,
by Anne Hall   282

33 Percutaneous Confusion or the Evidence on Cutaneous
Absorption of Essential Oils, *by Sylla Sheppard-Hanger*   288

34 Scientific Research Validates Psychological Benefits of
Fragrance, *by Annette Green*   298

35 Performing a Consultation, *by Ann Berwick*   303

VII A Student's Project

36 Aromatherapy: Making Sense of Scents, *by Meg Seiter*   313

A List of Essential Oils and Their Correct Latin Binomials 332

Sources For Everything 336

Bibliography 340

The National Association for Holistic Aromatherapy (NAHA) 348

KEEP ESSENTIAL OILS OUT OF YOUR EYES	DILUTE ESSENTIAL OILS BEFORE USE	IDENTIFY YOUR ESSENTIAL OILS BY THEIR LATIN BINOMIALS, part of plant, variety and chemical type	ALWAYS CHECK ESSENTIAL OILS FOR COLOR & SCENT before purchase

ESSENTIAL OILS ARE CONCENTRATED AND VOLATILE. . .
Do not use candles and essential oils together because of this flammable quality.

Editors' Note

All plants and their essential oils, like all medicines, may be harmful and dangerous if used improperly—if they are taken internally when prescribed for external use, if they are taken in excess, or if they are taken for too long a time. Allergic reactions and unpredictable sensitivities or illness may develop. There are other factors to consider as well—since the strength of wild herbs and various essential oils varies, knowledge of their growing conditions and distillation methods is helpful. Be sure your herbs are fresh and whole and your essential oils are not contaminated with foreign objects like melting rubber stoppers. Keep conditions of use as sterile as possible.

We do not advocate, endorse or guarantee the curative effects of any of the substances in this book. We have made every effort to see that any botanical that is dangerous or potentially dangerous has been noted as such. When you use plants and their essential oils, recognize their potency and use them with care. Medical consultation is recommended.

The botanical names listed under each herb and essential oil do not always refer to one species only, but also to others which have been recognized as substitutes in herbal medicine.

Please note, in this book, names of plants and their essential oils that are used therapeutically in herbalism or aromatherapy are capitalized, which follows ancient tradition.

Introduction

While they may look smooth, though possibly a bit veiny, the leaves and petals of aromatic plants are a landscape of structures. Among the dips and bubbles are glands filled with numerous chemical components which form a highly aromatic fluid, known as an essential oil. As sunlight touches the leaves of the plant, the glands burst, and the aromatic fluid contained within them is quickly evaporated and diffused, turning from liquid to gas with millions of droplets spreading into the atmosphere from areas of higher to lower concentration. This tendency to evaporate quickly is known as volatility, and essential oils are considered volatile substances. Perhaps a number of molecules are inhaled by a human being, traveling the olfactory path into the limbic system to bring a smile, calm the mind. Perhaps a molecule finds its way to the ocean, another to a cloud. Who knows how far and how long the molecules travel, who and what they affect on their journey.

The use of essential oils for health and well being is considered both a science and an art. Consider the steam distillation of plants, a process by which plants and water are passed through a still to produce an essential oil and a hydrosol, both of which are used in the practice of aromatherapy. Distillation is based on principles of science: the transformation of liquid to vapor, water to steam when heat is introduced, and the subsequent return of vapor to liquid and steam to water when the substances are cooled; the principle of diffusion in which molecules move from an area of greater concentration to lesser concentration; and others. Yet, distillation is an art as well as a science. The distiller must have "the nose," that delicate sense of smell that determines when the heat is too much and distillation is occurring too rapidly, or the precise moment when the final drop of top quality essential oil has been distilled and it is time to stop the process in order to avoid spoiling the integrity of the essential oil.

Consider the essential oils themselves. They are made of numerous chemical components which can be identified in a laboratory setting. Yet, when scientists synthesize each individual component of a specific oil, then put those components together in the same way as they appear in the oil from the plant, the synthetic oil not only smells different from the pure essential oil, it also lacks the therapeutic capability of the botanically produced essential oil. Perhaps there are minuscule amounts of components which are unidentifiable by scientific means. Perhaps Nature has artfully created the oils in a way which is impossible for humans to reproduce.

The world of aromatherapy is enlivened by the synergy of art and science. Any attempt to understand the scientific nature of aromatherapy—chemical components of oils, plant production, the physiological affects of essential oils—will eventually lead to its art, to the mysteries of Nature, to that which cannot be understood or defined in limited, unchanging terms. And any extended use of aromatherapy as an artistic practice whether in ritual use, natural perfumery, massage, or the healing arts, brings the practitioner back to science. Not only are essential oils volatile, the practice of aromatherapy is itself a highly volatile science-artform, the distances traveled dependent only upon the atmospheric limits created by the practitioner. As we explore the world of aromatherapy, art and science combine in a never-ending process of further discovery and exploration.

This book is a collection of works by women who find their pleasure, their livelihood, their inspiration, in exploring the volatile world of aromatherapy. Guided by their hearts, their minds, and their vision, they perform an unpredictable dance between art and science, their steps often traveling even beyond their own expectations. They do not merely practice aromatherapy, they participate in its continual creative expansion and re-creation.

It is a pleasure to have worked with some of the most highly respected and well known writers, teachers, and practitioners in the history of aromatherapy as we know it. Many of these women are directly responsible for the transformation of aromatherapy from an eclectic hobby practiced by few to the (still eclectic) healing art, big business, and hobby practiced by many that it has become. It is equally joyful to participate in presenting aromatherapy authors who had yet to be published and whose valuable experience may have otherwise escaped our embrace.

The opportunity to work with Jeanne Rose has been an inexpressible honor. She is a true master at living in the world of aromatherapy, a world in which dividing lines between art and science, mind, body, and spirit, scent and sight, and other such limits, are continually questioned and easily discarded. More than a leader, she is a Visionary whose practical and creative contributions span the fields of herbalism and aromatherapy and well beyond. Their implications for the well-being of people and planet alike will surely be realized for decades to come.

Susan Earle
San Francisco
1996

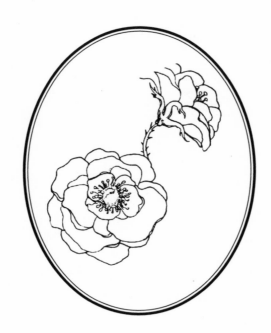

Preface

There are an increasing number of books available about aromatherapy, some are general, while others are specific to a special interest such as women, health care practitioners, or massage therapists. There are books by magnificent authors, each of which presents the writer's own particular perspective to a widely appealing art.

The National Association for Holistic Aromatherapy (NAHA) is a nonprofit organization dedicated to high standards of aromatherapy education and practice. As an educational organization, our desire was to publish a single informative volume that would accurately present a wide variety of approaches to the use of essential oils and hydrosols. As a diverse, member-run organization, our aim was to expose the reader to the perspectives of real people who practice, study, research, and live in the world of aromatherapy.

Women have been the backbone of all aspects of aromatherapy practice. NAHA's membership is ninety percent women, and the organization's administrative board and regional and district directors, all of which are volunteer positions, are women. *The World of Aromatherapy*, a collection of works written by The NAHA Women of Aromatherapy, is a tribute to those women who have dedicated themselves and their valuable time to the development of aromatherapy as a viable healing art. One of those women is my co-editor Susan Earle. This book is in large part an expression of the dedication and joy she brings to her work.

Jeanne Rose
San Francisco
1996

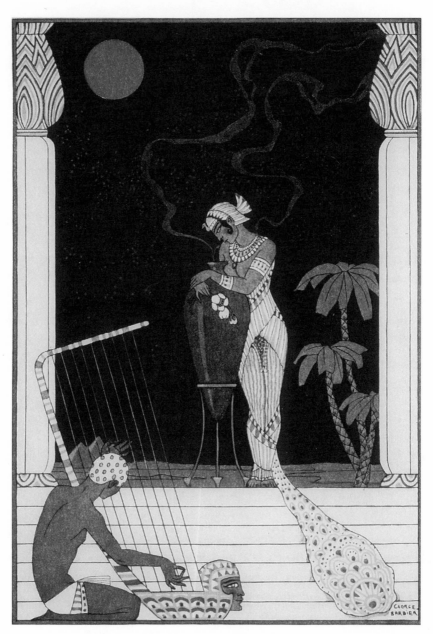

Egypt, by George Barbier

I

Background

1

Aromatherapy Then and Now

Alexandra Avery

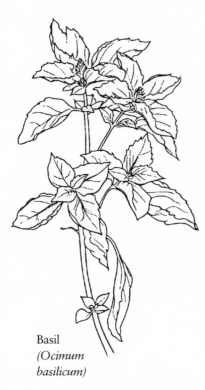

Basil
*(Ocimum
basilicum)*

Alexandra Avery grew up among the tropical blooms of Hawaii. As a child, her favorite play was hosting flower feasts in tree forts along the beach. Preparations for such feasts were made in the jungle thickets of beach-side plantings. Red Hibiscus flowers became petal salad, served on the perfectly round plates of the Sea Grape tree. Honeysuckle blossoms became delicate honey-cup desserts. She festooned the branches with Jasmine, a fragrant canopy under which she dreamed up new flower dishes. What began as child-play grew into Alexandra's research and practice of aromatherapy.

Involved in aromatherapy since 1976, she is a researcher, writer, speaker, and manufacturer of her own aromatherapy and herbal formulas. Her line of natural body-care products has received several awards for its purity and efficacy. Ms. Avery's company was one of six small businesses to be awarded "honor roll" in the Council on Economic Priorities book, *Shopping for a Better World.*

Ms. Avery has developed aromatherapy programs for spas and salons, and currently operates a Hawaiian health retreat that specializes in Hawaiian and aromatherapy body treatments.

*T*he art of aromatherapy is not new to the world. The use of plants and their oils has been used to heal and beautify the body for tens of thousands of years. Whether ingested, absorbed through the skin, or simply inhaled, plant aromas are known to have a powerful effect on the body, mind, and emotions. Today, the study of aromas has been elevated to a science that employs the balancing and beautifying properties of pure herbal and floral essences to enhance the condition of the skin, body, hair, mind and, indeed, even the environment.

Treatments with essential oils take many different forms. For centuries, aromatherapy has been a part of Ayurvedic medicine, an Indian system that focuses on restoring balance within the body, thereby promoting a healthful state of being. Since its first recorded use some five thousand years ago, Ayurvedic medicine has been incorporating the healing powers of plants and their essences in candles, incense, and massage oils. Today, Ayurvedic doctors continue this practice with plant-infused oils and essential oils to soothe the skin and mind as well as to balance glandular functions.

In Egypt, infused flower oils were mixed with charcoal and ground herbs and pressed into small cone shapes that were worn inside men and women's hairpieces to both scent the hairpiece and relax the mind. It was the Egyptian priestesses and priests who extended the medicinal use of plant-infused oils to the cosmetic use, creating a synthesis of inner and outer health and beauty. One of the Egyptian's most valuable contributions was the development of embalming techniques, using the very same oils for embalming that had been used to rejuvenate and soften the skin. Herbs were also infused in vinegar, then drunk, as they still are today, to maintain and improve health.

Many Roman and French leaders left legends of the prodigious use of aromatics for both healing and pleasurable purposes. In ancient Rome, streets were lined with Rose petals to celebrate the arrival of certain leaders. Feasting halls were often scented with hammocks of flower petals that rained on the diners throughout the feast.

In 1100 A.D. the art of perfumery was pioneered by an Arabian doctor named Avicenna. His discovery of plant distillation led to the opening of the perfume market in the Middle East. At the same time, the Chinese were practicing with many aromatics, combining aroma-therapy treatments with acupuncture.

During the plague years of the Middle Ages, lockets containing aromatic restoratives were worn by women and men. Only much later did Western medical practitioners begin to realize the antiseptic potency of essential oils. Many herbalists who relied on infused oils to keep their health intact were later burned at the stake for sharing this information.

In France, Louis XIV, who became known as the "sweetest smelling monarch," ordered the water in Versailles' fountains replaced with flower waters for special occasions. His successor, Louis XV, had a different scent designated for each day of the year, and the cost of scents used by his mistress, Madame de Pompadour, constituted the largest item of household expense. Napoleon was a lover of Spanish Jasmine, splashing himself with over sixty flasks a month. He is known to have emptied entire bottles over his head to revitalize himself on the battlefield. We now know through modern scientific research that Jasmine is indeed a restorative and a stimulant.

The person who coined the term "aromatherapy" was the French chemist René Maurice Gattefossé, who experimented intensively with flower essences and their medicinal uses. He was particularly instrumental in the development of our understanding of the antiseptic uses of oils. It was Gattefossé who discovered the healing effects of Lavender essential oil. A 1910 laboratory explosion left him severely burned; gas gangrene sores rapidly developed. He rinsed his hands with terpene-free Lavender oil. The healing was remarkably quick.

Aromatherapists—people employing the healing and beautifying properties of aromas—may work with over four hundred essential oils. These oils are extracted from the roots, leaves, resins, bark, flowers, seeds, or the rinds of fruits.

Each person may react differently to the same aroma, especially in dealing with conditions of the mind. Robert B. Tisserand, author of *The Art of Aromatherapy*, explains: "Each essence has its own personality, its own set of attributes, and this can be used to bring out certain qualities in us, helping us to see ourselves more clearly, to understand our faults, and to let the beauty and joy of our souls breathe a fresh, summery fragrance through our minds." Many essential oils enhance relaxation so that one is able to concentrate in a more perceptive and positive mode.

Aromatherapy deals with the mind and emotions as well as the skin and body. The molecular composition of the essences allows them to easily penetrate the skin, helping to stimulate circulation, lymph flow, and the detoxification and revitalization of the cells.

The heating and cooling powers of essential oils assist in regulating the proper circulation to and from cell tissues. First, cells receive an increased supply of oxygen and nutrition essential to cell function. Second, the return circulation is improved, cleansing the cell of wastes created during cell metabolism. This oxygenating and detoxifying power of essential oils aids in hydrating the tissues and maintaining optimal capillary action and vitality in the tissue.

The molecules of essential oils are small enough to penetrate the skin's outer layers. This allows for rapid penetration into the skin and makes essential oils efficient carriers for other ingredients in natural cosmetics. How deep into the lower layers they penetrate is the subject of current research.

Research is proving that the natural preservative properties of essential oils have a life-extending effect on skin cells. Most essential oils have strong bactericidal and fungicidal properties, without the weakening and depleting side effects of synthetic antibiotics. It has been demonstrated over the years that essential oils are effective against almost all pathogenic bacteria occurring in infectious diseases. Rather than weakening the immune system as do many conventional drugs, aromatherapy has the ability to stimulate and strengthen the immune system.

Most people are surprised to learn that our sense of smell is ten thousand times more sensitive than our sense of taste. Our olfactory system may even contain more receptor cells than the eyes. Of all the five senses, the sense of smell has the most direct and expedient connection to the brain.

When inhaling a flower or an essential oil, scent molecules are received immediately within the brain via the smell receptors or olfactory nerves at the back of the nasal cavity. The scent is then registered within the limbic system, the most primitive part of the brain. Here lies the seat of our emotions, our memory, the base of our learning ability, and the regulator of sensory motor activities. Humans appear to have a physiological response to odor.

Olfactory science, the study of smell, is a rising star in the field of human research. There are an estimated five hundred thousand scents to distinguish on our planet, each described mainly through associations with something else. We have, interestingly enough, a very limited vocabulary when it comes to describing odors. Unlike sight and sound, it is difficult to measure smell. In vision one can refer to a rainbow of color; in sound, one relates to sound frequencies. The sense of smell has no spectrum to which to refer.

The study of scent is receiving increased scientific support. Many academic centers such as Columbia and Duke have conducted tests to show that certain odors produce mood changes, a belief that has been held by aromatherapy practitioners for centuries. In such studies, EEG machines measured the effects of a variety of odors on a specific type of brain-wave activity very sensitive to changes in mood. These objective measurements were studied along with psychological mood-mapping techniques that rely on the person's subjective evaluation of scents.

Psycho-aromatherapy is opening up new understanding for the human mind. A Duke University Medical School experiment determined that the sense of smell is responsible for triggering the rise of a natural biochemical called histamine when a person smells a food to which she or he has a known allergy. Related studies have worked with cancer patients, using positively associated scents to counteract negative associations with chemotherapy treatments.

Research is showing that women have a greater proclivity toward scent identification and association than do men. Tests have shown that, although the scent-color association appears to be a learned response, women have an easier time drawing connections between scent and color (such as the smell of Lemon to the color yellow).

It is now known that some diseases, such as Alzheimer's, are associated with a decreased ability to sense. In this time of immune-deficiency disorders, some doctors and researchers are aligning the sense of smell with the immune system. "There is some belief that the sense of smell is the external version of the immune system, that by smelling certain things there is actually a connection to the immune system that produces the necessary reactive antibodies to counter it." (Dr. Tom Orofino, William H. Wheeler Center for Odor Research, Chattanooga, Tennessee.)

Research companies are each seeking to protect their piece of the fragrance pie. After a study found that muscle tension and blood pressure were lowered after inhaling an Apple-spice blend containing Nutmeg oil, IFF (International Flavor & Fragrances) sought and received a patent on the use of Nutmeg as a stress-reducing odorant. Could that have been the secret in mom's good old-fashioned Apple pie?

By the end of this decade, the psychological effects of scents may be setting the mood in many unexpected places. Imagine an environmental system diffusing relaxing aromas in city subways and mind-alerting aromas in truckers' cabs. These research efforts are being applied in state and private ventures around the world. A calming forest scent effuses through a large public rest stop on a Japanese highway; this same system is now operating in some U.S. hotels.

Calming fragrances are also being used in many work places with beneficial results. In a Japanese study, a soothing Lemon fragrance was wafted throughout a factory of video-terminal operators for one month, and the worker's error rate dropped in half. Researchers theorized that the calming scent helped to diffuse a high-tension environment.

Will mood-altering scents become the Muzak of the nineties, improving lives by enhancing alertness, productivity, relaxation? In an era in which perfume and fragrances have been sold for personal aesthetics alone, we are now discovering a new and even more valuable aspect of fragrance—its functional and therapeutic benefits. This is not entirely surprising to those who remember the days of smelling salts (an ammonia compound that stimulates the trigeminal nerve, relieving a fainting spell).

Environment may serve as an important ally or adversary of our sense of smell. Almost all of the products we use in the bathroom, kitchen, office, and household in general are heavily perfumed. There are many odors that can be perceived even when diluted billions and trillions of times. Our olfactory sense is almost continually barraged with a myriad of odors. Olfactory desensitization can occur with an over-stimulation of scent.

There are few who have not experienced the onslaught of an overly scented environment. Most cosmetics have fragrances that consist of fifty to one-hundred-fifty chemicals. The average person uses about twelve different cosmetic products daily. That amounts to a large arsenal of chemicals barraging the skin and senses on a daily basis.

Many essences in cosmetic formulations are derived from natural sources but are broken down and processed to such an extent that they end up with few or no signs of the original beneficial properties. One of the most important distinctions in aromatherapy is that the essences used must be of natural origin to be of complete benefit to the body and mind. That is, the essences must be from plants rather than synthetically reproduced. It is easier for the body to absorb and utilize aromatics when they are pure, natural substances that are inhaled, worn, or ingested.

It is the desire of most aromatherapists to nourish bodies, minds, and spirits in a vital, restorative way. The benefits inspire celebration of our own essence and its unique rhythm with nature. This natural rhythm embodies compassion and appreciation for all of life. One can live as the flowers do, in a most creative expression of beauty.

2

A Day in the Life of an Egyptian Embalmer

Wanda Sellar

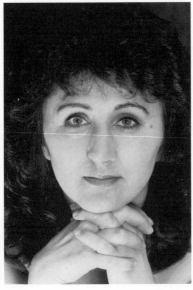

Chris Harris

In England, *Wanda Sellar* has worked in the healing field for twenty years. For the first ten years she was a journalist with the *Daily Mirror* newspaper and assistant and advisor to "agony aunt" Marjorie Proops. Ms. Sellar has ten years of experience as an aromatherapist in private practice, also working in Hoolloway Prison. She has a diploma in psychology and counseling from London University. She is the author of *The Directory of Essential Oils* .

Wanda Sellar gives an imaginative evocation of a trade that could have been the fore-runner of the aromatherapist's.

I awake to the smell of Juniper and Cinnamon, which my wife burns to fumigate the house. The sunshine pours in and opens my eyes onto another day. From my balcony, I see the black buffalo bathing in the cool waters of the Nile, and in the Acacia tree below, a nightingale still sings. For a few moments, I savour the peace before the growing noise of commerce springs the city awake.

Here in the City of the Dead, on the West Bank of Thebes, I live and work. On the east side of the Nile, the populace not involved with the embalming process reside in the City of the Living.

Thebes took over from Memphis as the capital some time back in the 11th Dynasty (2133–1991 B.C.). The change was quite simply due to economics—not much changes in this world of ours! Thebes controls many of the lucrative trade routes to the gold mines in the Nubian mountains, and much of this gold is used in funeral ornamentation. From the Land of Punt we obtain the precious oils of Myrrh, Frankincense, and Cinnamon that are indispensable to our work.

Our houses are made of mud bricks and clay, and almost everyone complains of overcrowding. Not only do we share the space with quarrymen, carvers, and draughtsmen—those whose professions are directly involved with mummification—but also vermin and insects, which are plentiful in this hot climate.

My wife, Khuni, brings me breakfast of oats and fruit, as she's done for many years past. I know she wishes I had another trade, but what else can I do in these days of high unemployment? In any event, it is a family tradition, since it was my father's work and his father's before him. It is a peaceful occupation, and my clients never complain.

I kiss my wife good-bye and watch her hurry back into the house to wake the children, five-year-old Lei and Kheri, my son, who is now ten. I'm proud to say that he is showing great interest in my work, though it does make me worry about his future. His wife, too, may not like being married to an embalmer.

Personally, I think it is a noble profession, preparing the dead for their future life. Yet ironically, people despise the embalmers on the lower scale, like my late father-in-law. My wife remembers only too well the jibes and sneers from the neighbours. Since the poorer families have little money, the lower-class embalmers use cheaper preservatives. There is also a dreadful rumour going around that they even abuse the corpses! It's no wonder that some families don't release the bodies

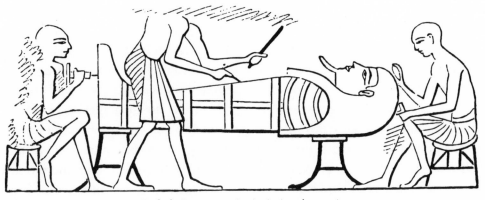

Embalming mummies (painting the case)

immediately, waiting at least three days after death before handing them over for mummification.

Not everyone, however, can be an embalmer for the upper classes and royalty. They keep us gainfully employed, since life expectancy in their world of intrigue is somewhat short. High-ranking dignitaries, sacred crocodiles and cats all pass through our hands. Obviously, embalming is available to all, except criminals and slaves, and it is incumbent upon the priests in the Temples to provide it.

In our hot climate, putrefaction sets in quickly, so we have to get to work immediately after the mourning rituals are over. It's a process that takes many weeks of preparation, almost two months for a king. First, the bodies are washed, then the brain and viscera are removed and preserved in Cedarwood oil. They are placed in several canopic jars, which accompany the mummified body in the tomb. The entrails have to be removed; otherwise the bodies will rot. Our embalming tools, consisting of forceps, knife, and hook, are made from copper and bronze.

Embalming prevents the body from decay, since we believe that the Soul—we call it Ka—only leaves the body temporarily and will return one day. It cannot do so if there is no body. Some people say the Soul takes up temporary residence in a bird, but my wife laughs at the notion. That's heresy, of course, and I tell her to keep quiet.

Some of our neighbours, particularly the Sumerians, say we are too preoccupied with the dead. Our tombs are more splendid than our homes, they say. This is true, but I think we Egyptians are misunderstood. We mummify because we love life, and the whole process of embalming is to make sure that we have a body to inhabit again.

We give great respect to what, after all, is the vessel of the Soul. The body is cleansed by washing it from excess salt with Nile water, and by hooking the brain through the nostrils and the viscera through an incision in the flank; then the inside is flushed out with Palm wine and herbs of Galbanum, Chamomile, and Mastick. This is cleansing and anointing. Then the stomach is filled with Myrrh, Cassia, Cinnamon, and other aromatic essences. A sacred amulet now occupies the place of the heart, and the body is closed by stitching across the gut. The body has to be dried, which helps with the preservation process, and is, therefore, immersed in a powder called Natron (a chemical containing sodium/aluminium). It is then anointed with Juniper and Cedarwood and rubbed with the costly Mum and infusions containing precious oils of Myrrh and Cinnamon, which are strong preservatives. Mum, incidentally, is from the Arabic word for Bitumen—a black pitch-like substance that acts as a consolidant.

We work to the chant of the mortuary priests, hired by the deceased families. The richer the family, the more priests, and the louder the incantation. The prayers are to Anubis, the jackal-headed god who guards the bodies in their last resting place. But mainly, the priests, after anointing the head, recite so that the deceased may pass on to the next world. The ritual aspect is very important in this whole ceremony, and Frankincense is burnt in censors since it has such strong powers of evocation. It is useful for fumigation purposes too, since it helps to ward off the fleas and rodents.

Dying is a costly business and keeps many people employed. Embalmers, priests, engravers, painters, carpenters, sculptors and jewellers are all involved. Golden amulets, rings, and bracelets are put into the folds of the wrappings, which are often around twenty yards long. The body is swathed in the finest linen, obtained from the royal looms. The cosmeticians paint the face, lips, nails, palms of the hands and soles of the feet. As fashion changes, so does the appearance of the corpse. They once had elaborate coiffeurs, but now they are totally shaved for the sake of hygiene, since elaborate hair pieces became repositories for insects. The richer the family, the more colourful the Mummy and sarcophagus. We have quite a few "Mummy models" for them to choose from, so they know what they are going to get in advance.

We work a long day, though we do have half an hour's break for lunch, which is mostly Garlic, Radishes, Olives, Onions, and Barley bread. Sometimes, my wife packs a cake made from the Dom fruits, since stomach ailments are not uncommon, and usually occur if we have not had access to fresh water for some time. I finish off my meal by chewing Cardamom seeds, to help keep my teeth white.

Final arrangements for the Mummy include placing a collar of ornamental plants around its neck. These include beads, dried fruits, Olive, Celery, and Mint leaves. They also provide a form of insecticide, since mite infestation of Mummies is common. Sometimes, we use Peppercorns secreted in the nostrils and abdomen, or Onions in the ears, pelvis, or thorax as repellents against snakes. When the body is ready, finally coated with a resin solution, we hand it back to the relatives, who make the funeral arrangements.

The funeral procession consists of a long line of servants carrying articles of tomb furniture and chests of clothes, and dragging the canopied shrine containing the Mummy. This shrine is often made from Cedarwood, which is imperishable, and we believe that it will preserve forever the body within. Garlands of flowers and wreathes are placed in the tombs, consisting of Poppies and Cornflowers, as well as the blue and white Lotus, symbolic of new life. Bouquets, sometimes in the shape of the Ankh, a symbol of eternal life, are presented to the deceased relatives. The main component of the shrine is often Papyrus stems, with their feathery flowers, since they symbolize the resurrection of the deceased.

The hillside facing the river contains the tombs of the nobles and high-ranking officials. The kings are buried in an isolated valley on the western side of the mountain, known as The Gate of Kings. The poor servants only have the desert for their resting place.

In the days of the great pyramids, many of the king's servants and family were buried with him. Though we might see it as a barbaric practice now, they were, in fact, generally happy to die with their master, as they deemed it a great honour. Things have changed now, of course, and we wait to die naturally before we are buried!

After a hard day's work, I spend the evening with my family. Supper is usually of dried fish, milk, Dates, and honey, which we eat by the light of a lamp lit by Olive oil. Sometimes we visit our neighbours and discuss our work. For nearly 2,000 years now the Theban hills have entombed the bodies of high-class Egyptians. What does the future hold? I wonder.

3

Essential Oil Distillation

Profiles of Four Distillers in the 1990s

Sara Hindman

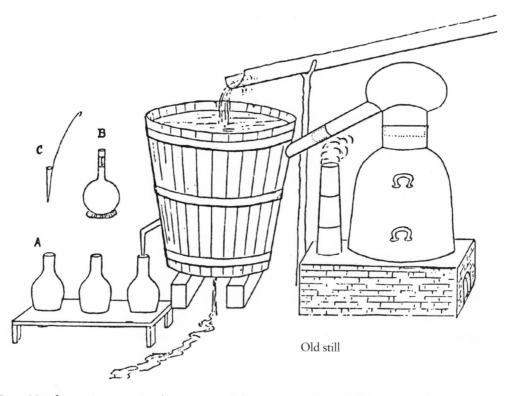

Old still

Sara Hindman is an aromatherapist and flower-essence practitioner. She is very interested in research and educational aspects of natural medicines, currently serving as secretary for the National Association for Holistic Aromatherapy. She is also editor of NAHA's quarterly newsletter, *Scensitivity*. She lives in northern California with her husband and two dogs.

*T*his book has been written to honor the contributions made by women in the field of aromatherapy. Why would the editors wish to include an article about essential oil distillation and four men currently involved in this work? Simply because without the distillation process, many essential oils would not exist.

Do you ever wonder about the transformative journey this fluid took to become an essential oil? How does it proceed from the branch, leaf, root, or blossom to become that rich, fragrant, magical liquid with wondrous qualities? As you hold that little bottle of precious oil in your hand, think about how it was created. Essential oil molecules are contained within a plant's cellular walls, and the majority of essential oils are obtained through the means of hydro- or steam distillation.

Centuries ago, the sweet fragrance of flowers was originally "trapped" in various aromatic gums, such as Myrrh or Frankincense, or in natural oils that could contain the plant's fragrance. Ancient Egyptians were known to create and use perfumes and they are credited with developing the first crude distillation unit, the solar still.

Alchemy is the basis of distillation, and all distillation techniques originate from ancient alchemical principles. This art is considered one of the magical arts and always takes place in three stages: separation, purification, and recombination. Paracelsus, the father of modern pharmacy, a sixteenth-century doctor and theorist, contributed enormously to our modern understanding of alchemical principles. He described alchemy as the "voluntary action of man in harmony with the involuntary action of nature." A modern alchemist, Frater Albertus, described alchemy as the "raising of vibrations." In their never-ending search for the elixir of life, alchemists turned to experimenting with herbs, flowers, and other plants, and essential oil distillation was born.

Alchemy in the Western world was mostly based upon ancient Egyptian tradition. In the Western world, this hermetic art was practiced under the supervision of kings and queens and was taught exclusively through oral traditions. It was against the law to divulge secrets of their alchemic arts. Alchemy was a venerable technology found in ancient Egypt and China, and alchemical preparations were part of Indian Ayurvedic medicine. Such preparations also contributed to the medicines of ancient Greece.

During the Crusades, the Arabs were responsible for bringing theoretical and practical alchemy to the Europeans, who combined it with the Christian tradition. The alchemists of the second and third centuries perfected the alembic still, a small Arabian device brought to Europe during this time.

An alembic still consists of three parts, originally made entirely of glass: a heating vessel, a vapor-collecting and condensing head with a long beak-shaped neck, and a receiving vessel. Alembic stills are distinguished by their unusual shapes. The head of the vapor container is usually quite large, in order to allow maximum expansion of gases before condensation. Traditionally, stills were made of copper with a tin lining. Other materials, such as aluminum, plastic, or wood, have been used without success. Stainless steel is a popular choice today because it does not react with the oils being processed. Many of the old "moonshine" stills are examples of alembic stills. Coils of copper tubing allow the vapors of fermented mash to be passed through them, condensed, cooled, and collected in a receptacle.

Distillation is the most common method used to extract essential oils from plants. Other methods used to obtain essential oils include carbon dioxide extraction, enfleurage (a method used especially in the manufacture of perfumes in which essential oils are extracted into fats, where they can be removed with alcohols), cold pressing of the oils, or employing chemical solvents. The type of plant material and its composition often determine what method of extraction is best.

Distillation is the physical process used to produce, purify, or isolate a substance. A substance can exist in one of three different states: gas, liquid, or solid. A well-known example is water, which has three common states: steam, fluid, or ice. In his treatise on essential oil, Ernest Guenther defines distillation as "the separation of the components of a mixture of two or more liquids by virtue of the difference in their vapor pressures." When the flowers or other plant material are combined in a container with water and heated, steam is created and the essential oils contained within the plant cell wall are vaporized. This mixture of water vapors (steam) and essential oil gases rises and escapes into the condenser, is cooled and reliquifies. The resulting oil and water mixture flows into a receptacle where they are separated, and both have valuable qualities and uses. The cooled water, known as the hydrosol, can be used because it contains minute essential oil droplets and the water-soluble parts of the plant.

This process of collecting aromatic oils from plants and flowers through the use of hydro-distillation is one of the most effective and least expensive means of gathering essential oils. It also has the distinct economical advantage of field utilization, in which portable stills can be used immediately after plants are harvested.

Water Distillation

There are three basic types of essential oil hydro-distillation. The first is the simple and ancient method of water distillation. The equipment used for this method is simple, economical, and easily transportable to the field. However, water distillation is the least economical of the three types. It requires more experience, expertise, care and knowledge than any other form of distillation. This method of essential oil distillation is used in large-scale commercial production only when the plant materials cannot be processed by any other means.

The plant material is placed in the body of the still and covered with water, and the whole contents of the still are brought to a boil, usually by direct fire. The temperature within the still is about 100°C. Care must be taken not to burn the plant materials through contact with the still walls, and vaporized water must be continually replaced. Water distillation is good for production of the highest quality oils because the low temperature and low pressure can be easily established and controlled. This method is employed today for oils with heat-sensitive properties, such as Rose and Orange blossom.

Water and Steam Distillation

The second method of distillation utilizes both water and steam. Plants and water are again placed within the still chamber. In this case, the plant materials are placed on a grill and separated from the water below. Steam from a separate apparatus is pumped through the still. Even though water is heated within the still body, the idea is that only steam from the boiling water, or that being pumped into the unit, comes in contact with the plants. The water-steam method of distillation is best suited for leafy, herbal materials. It works well for seed, root, and woody materials also. Although this type of still is more complicated and expensive than the water-only still, it can easily be transported and installed near the harvest field. In fact, this method of distillation is especially suited for field work in small- or medium-sized stills. The quality of the oil produced is usually good, and the yield will be satisfactory if the steam is able to evenly penetrate the plant materials. Cumin seed, some types of Eucalyptus, Angelica, and Carrot oils are examples of essential oils produced in this manner.

Steam Distillation

The third basic type of distillation is direct steam distillation. Steam distillation is the most cost effective form of hydro-distillation and has the highest rate and capacity of production. In this method, the plant material is placed in the chamber of the still. Steam is generated from a nearby source and pumped into the chamber containing the plant materials. This steam may be saturated (wet, with lower temperature and pressure) or super-heated (dry, with higher temperature and pressure, and larger volume). The steam separates the volatile oils from the plant cells when the boiling point is reached.

Steam distillation is done rapidly and, if done correctly, produces a high quality product. While high-temperature distillation results in a greater yield, it may prevent the plant materials from releasing their more subtle properties. Steam distillation is used almost exclusively for the industrial production of essential oils. Peppermint oil is an example of an essential oil produced this way.

Although each plant requires its own particular type of distillation, the method employed to extract the essential oil is usually a personal choice of the distiller. A delicate balance of distiller skill and experience, along with the proper temperature, technique, and time spent in the still are imperative to produce a high quality oil. It is very easy to destroy volatile molecules and subtle components of a plant, ruining the essential oil.

The distillation of essential oils at the close of the twentieth century is not much different than it was at its beginning. Of course, there are great advances in technology regarding essential oils: gas chromatography, mass spectroscopy, delineation of oil chemotypes, genetic and biological research. However, the distillation process continues to consist of a heat source, a chamber to hold the plant material, access to heat, a condenser, an oil-water separator, and a container to hold the oils and water, just as it did in ancient times.

Distillation in the 1990s

Who are today's distillers? What makes a person choose to become involved in this art? What is each person's contribution to the art of distillation? Is it a love for nature and the plant kingdom? Is it a desire to help fellow farmers create a better life for themselves during these economically challenging times? Could it be the experimentation with wild plants and concerned protection of endangered species?

Perhaps it is an understanding of how all life is intimately connected, be it from the animal, mineral, or plant kingdom. Or could it be their finely tuned and developed senses that enable them to know exactly when the distilled oil is perfect?

In order to learn more about this process, I talked to four men currently distilling essential oils. They were approached with a full-page questionnaire about distillation and their involvement with essential oil production. Three live on the West Coast of the United States, and one lives in the Midwest. They range from a farmer-engineer to a research scientist, an alchemist, and a cognac distiller. I hoped to learn about the "man behind the still" and how each personalizes the process of distillation.

There is something that drives these men to produce essential oils. It has to be more than just the pursuit of monetary worth. I wanted to know about each man and his interpretation of the distillation process. Gathering information for this article was frustrating. I did not learn as much as I wanted to about the personal side of a distiller. I do know that each one of them uses only organic, often wild-crafted, plants to produce his essential oils. The highest standards are maintained, and the resulting oils are of exquisite quality. I recently learned that I own a pint of oil produced by one of these men. At the time I received this oil, I did not know its origin, only that it was unlike any other essential oil I had ever experienced.

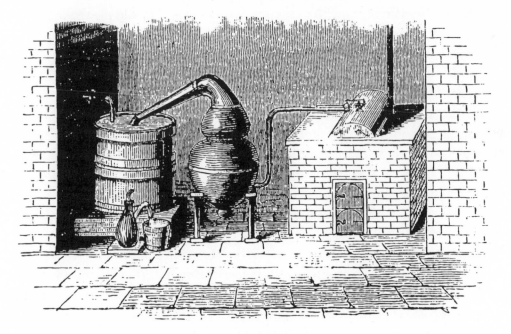

Lavender still

While gracious and friendly (for the most part) to a neophyte without distillation experience, these men were not very forthcoming with information. The essential oil industry is a $20 billion-a-year business, and much of their work is of a proprietary nature. One man even stopped the interview in the middle of our discussion, without explanation. He was a fascinating person, and it was unfortunate that he decided not to continue the interview. I did not learn much about each one's methods and the equipment used in distilling oils. I did not wish to invade or infringe upon the proprietary nature of this work, but it was very disappointing to continually run up against the secretive mind-set that pervades the entire aromatherapy industry. I was, however, able to gain some insight into the art of distillation in the 1990s, and those special individuals so dedicated to the continuation of this alchemical process.

The Geneticist

George Sturtz lives in Oregon, where he does research as a plant breeder-geneticist. Growing up on a farm in the Texas Panhandle, he was constantly out in the pasture, fascinated by science, exploring plant life, and learning about nature. His formal training was in genetics, plant breeding, and agronomy. For the past sixteen years, he has been involved with new crop development. He told me that he "enjoys distilling new plants I have found or developed to see what nature has produced. Every plant is different, and the possible genetic combinations are virtually endless. The thrill of discovery is a big part of it. It is part of the overall process of science, the pursuit of knowledge, and contributing to our understanding of nature."

Sturtz began distilling and extracting essential oils in 1981, while working on a graduate degree in Mint breeding. He learned the art of distillation on his own, observing how others did it, reading and experimenting until his technique was refined. He built his first still with junkyard parts and the help of a local glassblower. He uses steam distillation only, in a small "research pot still." Because his emphasis is on research, he only produces about one-half pound of essential oil at one time. He has distilled over "a hundred different species of plants as well as several hundred chemotypes within the species." He has done extensive work with Mints, and has studied various native plants throughout the Pacific Northwest, mainly in the Carrot and Daisy families. He evaluates native species of plants for potential use as crops for the flavor, fragrance, and pharmaceutical industries. He uses sophisticated techniques and equipment to determine the quality and composition of the oils he produces, and works with research databases in various universities to determine the composition of his distilled oils. Gas chromatography and mass spectroscopy is used to identify the essential oil components.

George Sturtz is very excited and enthusiastic about his work. He still enjoys going out into nature, just as he did as a child on his Texas farm. He goes out into the wild, searching for native plants that might produce valuable essential oils. Even though he has "gone down several blind alleys in the past, I find the biggest bottleneck to new essential oil products is the conservatism of the flavor and fragrance industry."

One of his goals is to develop new specialty crops that could help small farmers. Crops for essential oil production have the potential for higher earnings than Wheat, Corn, or Beans, so farms with small acreages could benefit from his research. It takes about ten years to develop a new crop, and Sturtz recently released a new patented Mint into commerce. He has several new essential oil plants in late stages of development. He told me that he feels "fortunate to be able to do the work that I do. . . . The process is so exciting, collecting in the wild. . . . The work is so interesting and rewarding."

The Engineer

Herb Bartel lives in Missouri on a 160 acre farm. During 1993–94, he was employed as a consulting engineer for Boeing in Seattle. While living in Washington state, he had the opportunity to visit an alternative crop program in Vancouver, British Columbia. He was intrigued by this program, and felt that some of the essential oil crops being raised might be valuable for the farmers in the Midwest. Research is now in progress to determine what crops are suitable, and a comparative base for testing has been established.

It took Bartel about a year to set everything into place. His original still design came from Russia. With information gained from studying the laboratory still in Vancouver, he modified the original Russian design. He built a stainless steel still that is set up for multiple uses. He learned the art of essential oil distillation through the time honored process of trial-and-error, and feels that he is still on the learning curve.

Bartel's initial distilling efforts took place in Idaho using evergreens: Junipers, Cedars, and Scotch Pines. His work with the evergreen oils has been very interesting. Initial experiments were with Cedar leaves, of which six hundred pounds of leaves produced one quart of a "thin oil that didn't separate very well." Six hundred pounds of cedar shavings resulted in a two percent yield. His continuing efforts have paid off handsomely. His still now produces about one-half to three-fourths of a gallon of high quality essential oil per run. Jeanne Rose reported that his leaf and bark essential oil from the *Juniperus virginiana* tree was "absolutely divine! It smells like it came right off the tree!"

Bartel is interested in setting up a cooperative program with neighboring farmers to produce essential oil crops. The farmers with whom he has discussed this program are very enthusiastic, although local governmental agencies seem to be lukewarm to the idea at the present time. In the meantime, Bartel has made arrangements with three neighboring farms to grow Tansy, Yarrow, and Melissa crops. They intend to produce oils and collect the hydrosols from these plants during the fall harvest. His plans include mounting his portable still onto a trailer and going wild-crafting throughout the Pacific Northwest next year.

As an engineer, his original focus was purely on the technical and mechanical aspects of essential oil distillation—how to best build a still, analyzing each component carefully, maintaining high standards for safety factors, scouting the best location to build a still with a plentiful cold water source. With the knowledge he has gained, he intends to market custom made stills. In addition to this upcoming venture, he has received a precious gift—a new appreciation for the plant kingdom, as well as a love affair with Nature. His new found fascination with plants now shares equal time with his love of design and mechanics.

The Cognac Distiller

Hubert Germain-Robin is a third-generation distiller from France. He now lives in Northern California, where he distills fine cognacs, fruit brandies, and sherries that are shipped around the world. While visiting the United States in 1982, he discovered that no one was distilling brandies in California, so he and a partner went into business. His first distillation took place in 1983. He had an old alembic still dismantled and shipped from France, and built everything, finishing a small distillery in the mid-1980s.

As his company expands, Germain-Robin has begun exploring the distillation of essential oils. He is so excited about this venture that he has established a new company, Cyranose, to distill oils and hydrosols for the culinary and cosmetic industry. He uses an alembic still for production of essential oils. This still processes one hundred pounds of plant materials at a time. He experiments with various locally grown plants. His initial experiments with local Lavender resulted in an oil high in camphor and borneol, due to the particular Lavender chosen and to the growing conditions, not distillation techniques. (See "The Lavender Project," *Scentsitivity,* Winter 1994–95.) Germain-Robin feels there is a great opportunity for essential oil production in California, and he is very excited about using French distilling techniques in his adopted land. "This is a new country; the potential is unbelievable."

His distillation methods are simple and traditional. He went back to France and learned essential oil techniques from the Lavender distillers. He feels that California offers a tremendous opportunity for growing and producing a great Lavender oil. Since California and France have similar climatic and growing conditions, he is very enthusiastic about creating a Lavender oil industry in this state. Germain-Robin has the gift of a "nose," that wonderful ability to discern through his sense of smell exactly when the essential oil is perfect. "When the 'flavors' are weak, you stop." His techniques are steeped in tradition, his approach is slow and conservative, and everything is done by hand (and nose) so that a great product is created. "Experience is everything." With this slow approach, he says it is "hard to mess it up."

He loves his work, and is always excited about it. He is working with different varietals to see how the various soil and climate conditions during plant growth affect the essential oils. The quality of plants used for distillation is of utmost importance: "no chemicals; everything must be very natural." He is very enthusiastic about his experiments with distilling essential oils for the food industry. He is exploring herbs, and producing oils made from Rosemary, Tarragon, Oregano, Thyme, Marjoram, and Lemon Verbena. "Imagine what the chef could do with a few drops of Rosemary oil in Olive oil. . . ."

The Alchemist

The fourth distiller interviewed for this article is Carl Lee, an alchemist living in Northern California. He began his hermetic studies in 1972, and studied alchemy with Frater Albertus for twelve years in Utah. Continuing the alchemical tradition, Lee was very secretive about his work. The only information he would share about his still was that he built it himself and that it "gives a copper note."

His wife told me that during the installation of the still, a precious sapphire ring was lost in the earth under the equipment. Perhaps this is the secret of his wonderful oils. . . . He considers the design of the still to be of utmost importance, because he believes that the "shape of the vessel will affect distillation." He explained that the shape and materials used give the "still note," which in turn, affects the odor and taste of the essential oil. He has designed the curve of the glass to match the shape of the rising vapors in order to produce a more "natural oil."

Lee considers his methods of producing essential oils to be part of a sacred art. He shapes his distillation techniques in accordance with the laws of nature and laws of organics. Everything is done according to natural methods. "Plants grow in nature; therefore the natural laws must be observed." Planting cycles, seasonal conditions, planetary influences, and the type of equipment used are the foundations of his work. Lee believes that *when* essential oils are distilled is just as important as when the seeds are planted or the plants are harvested.

He distills oils with the help of his wife, Jahna Lee. Their roles in the art of distillation are based completely on the "old world, the old way." They have very high standards, with continuous, constant attention to details. During the distillation process, someone carefully tends the still at all times. For the Lees, this careful and complete attention is a way of life, an example of what they consider to be the sacredness of their work.

Native, local plants are harvested on the ridge near their home. They are careful not to overharvest and deplete the supply, which restricts their annual production. They distill small amounts of oil each year. Only about fifteen ounces of each essential oil are produced annually. They produce essential oils of Sweet Fennel *(Foeniculum vulgare)*, Mugwort *(Artemisia vulgaris)*, Mountain Sage *(Artemisia californica)*, Black Sage *(Salvia mellifera)*, German Chamomile *(Matricaria recutita)*, and White Yarrow *(Achillea millefolium)*.

The Lees have been experimenting with a unique product they call "co-distillates." So far, this "marriage within the still" has produced two co-distillates, Chamomile and Lavender, a sky-blue oil, and Rose and Lavender. They are both very excited about these essential combinations. They also produce hydrosols of Rose, Lavender, and Chamomile. Lee's future plans include teaching distillation workshops from the standpoint of the home cook. He would like to show students how they could distill "their own Lavender oil in a stainless steel pot."

The Home Distillery

Until Carl Lee begins teaching people how to distill their own oils using equipment from the second-hand store, you may have to experiment on your own. It is very easy to set up a home still. All you need is a teapot, plastic tubing, a stove, water to cool the oil-water mixture, and a bowl to collect the results. A close friend is going to help me attempt to distill some Pine Geranium oil from my garden next week in my copper cooking pots. I am hoping it will turn out better than some of my high-school chemistry experiments.

The Aromatherapy Book: Applications and Inhalations, by Jeanne Rose, provides basic instructions. The aromatherapy chapter (Chapter 32) of Rose's *Herbal Studies Course* also includes articles on simple stills that can be built in the kitchen. Texts on alchemy will provide additional information on stills and basic distillation procedures.

Just as Mother Nature writes her signature across the face of every blossom, each distiller adds a personal imprint to the essential oil created. The time, experience, and love of the craft add a distinctive component to the finished oils, as much a gift to us as the flowers' essence in the completed elixir. Learning about the journey that each magical liquid has traveled on its way to become the aromatherapist's partner makes one even more appreciative of this healing art.

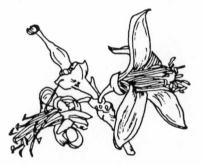

Lemon *(Citrus medica limon)*

4

Two Products of Distillation

Jeanne Rose

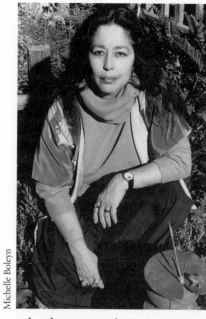

Michelle Boleyn

Jeanne Rose, a California native daughter, is a leading pioneer in the revival of herbal and natural remedies and aromatherapy to maintain good health. She is also an international authority on the therapeutic uses of herbs, both medicinal and cosmetic, and a well-known teacher of aromatherapy since 1972.

The author of fourteen herbal books including the *Herbal Studies Course*™ and *Aromatherapy Studies Course*™ by correspondence, Jeanne Rose has a rich background in plant use. Her latest accomplishment is *Herbs & Aromatherapy for the Reproductive System,* the first in a series of books addressing herbal and aromatic therapies for personal health. Jeanne is an 'academic enthusiast', refining her work on the medicinal uses of herbs and therapeutic values of essential oils through relentless research. Jeanne Rose has been the national spokesperson for Bath & Body-Works Aromatherapy. She was aromatic consultant for The Donatello Hotel in San Francisco, Toto of Japan and regularly designs original aromatics for her clients. Her aromatic garden is world-famous and has appeared in *Herb Companion, Country Gardening,* and the Japanese publication *Herb.* She is the current president of NAHA.

romatherapy is often defined as the use of essential oils for mental and physical well-being. Yet a recent development in the field of aromatherapy expands the very definition of this deliciously sensual healing art. Hydrosols, the aromatic water resulting from the steam distillation of plant materials, were often thought of as a "secondary" product of essential oil distillation. Yet, as their availability and use becomes more widespread, hydrosols are quickly becoming a partner in aromatherapy with essential oils.

When the word "aromatic hydrosol" is mentioned, the first response of many people is, "Oh, yes, yes. . . a mister, right?" WRONG. Although a hydrosol is often marketed in a spritz-type bottle, a "mister" is not always a hydrosol. The key is to read the ingredients. If it says some variation of "essential oil in water," it is just that, and not a hydrosol. If it says "hydrosol" or "hydrolate," then it is a hydrosol.

So what, exactly IS a hydrosol? What we must always remember is that essential oils come from plants. They are an intimate part of the plant; they are the fragrant essence of a plant. A few molecules of essential oil are stored in a cell, and each fragrant plant has many of these cells. When steam or boiling water comes in contact with the cells that contain the fragrant essential oil, these cells are heated up and the cell wall bursts, allowing the essential oil to escape, to be vaporized as a gas and to continue through the distillation equipment with the water vapor. This water—spring water, in most cases—has been heated until it turns to steam, which is forced into the still, softening and then bursting the cell walls and taking along with it the essential oil as vapor.

The steam and vapor go to the head of the still and flow down the neck into the condenser. The condenser has cold circulating water around it, which cools the steam and vapor so that they again become water and essential oil. At this point the water is called the hydrosol (hydro = water and sol = solution), or water solution. Since the hydrosol sometimes has a milky color, it has also been called a hydrolate. The hydrosol has dissolved within it micro-molecules of water-soluble plant components, as well as enough molecules of essential oil to give scent and substance to the hydrosol. The micro-molecules of healing, water-soluble plant components, and tiny amounts of water-soluble essential oil as scent are what makes the hydrosol therapeutic.

The process of distillation which creates the essential oil and hydrosol is an alchemical one. As Christoph Streicher states, "During the distillation process, the ascending steam dissolves the essential oil contained in the plant, temporarily associating with it in a highly aromatic ethereal oneness of opposite values: water and oil, which normally do not associate . . . in recent times it has become more and more evident that the hydrosols are also exceptional carriers of intelligent vibrational impulses of plant life."

Hydrosols can come from *any* plant that is distilled such as Bay Laurel water from the leaves of the Bay Laurel tree; Eucalyptus water from the Eucalyptus distillation and herbal hydrosols such as Melissa (Lemon Balm) water, Peppermint waters, Rosemary water, Lemon Verbena water and Thyme water. Hydrosols can be floral waters *if* they have been distilled from flowers such as Lavender, Orange Petal, or Rose.

Aromatherapy uses of hydrosols. As do essential oils, the uses of hydrosols benefit mind, body, and spirit and are only limited by the imagination. Hydrosols represent the highest benefits of the combination of herbal-therapy and aromatherapy.

"Synergy" is a term often used in aromatherapy and means two factors have united to create a new result which is greater than the sum of its parts. Essential oils and hydrosols can be used together, synergistically.

The body. Water is a vital component for healthy skin tissue, and hydrosols are water with power! Hydrosols are useful in all manner of skin and body care. Hydrosols are a powerful therapeutic agent in their own right and are valuable for skin and health particularly for babies, invalids, elderly persons, and people with sensitive skin. They are cooling, anti-inflammatory, stimulating or relaxing, gentle, and selective antiseptics with qualities that can be uplifting, soothing to irritated skin, gentle, and balancing. They can be used as nasal douches, vaginal douches, a facial spritz, aftershave, make up freshener, toners for all sorts and types of skin, revitalizers for devitalized skin, toning and strengthening. Hydrosols are nearly free of irritating components such as the terpene hydrocarbons and are extremely well-suited for very sensitive skin.

Hydrosols are a valuable ingredient in all body care products: creams, lotions, shampoos, face masks. Use them with essential oils for a truly remarkable product.

The mind and emotions. One spritz for freshening-up and one instantly recognizes that hydrosols have more than surface value. Since hydrosols contain micromolecules of essential oil, their effects on the mind and emotions are the same as those of both aroma- and herbal therapy. Yet, while you would never spray a bottle of Lavender essential oil in your face, Lavender hydrosol is delicate enough to do just that! It tones the skin and the emotions! Hydrosols have become a favorite tool for reducing stress and depression and calming tempers. They can wake you up or put you to sleep.

The spirit. The elixir of life infused with the spirit of a plant. Anoint, bathe, spritz, enjoy, breathe.

Culinary uses. Hydrosols are a delightful culinary addition. Use them diluted where ever you would use water—soups, cakes, pies, cookies, teas, cocktail hour, steamed veggies.

Watch out for impostors. . . . Demand quality. Hydrosols are aromatic, and are from the living tissue of plants including flowers and leaves. As a true and naturally made substance from the distillation process a hydrosol CANNOT be made synthetically. As mentioned previously, the only product that is a pure, aromatic hydrosol is one that says "100% hydrosol" on the label. Always look at the ingredients.

The best hydrosol is a fresh hydrosol. As a plant product, hydrosols do have a shelf life. At home, any hydrosol not in use should be kept in the fridge. Buy 16 oz., keep 8 oz. in your bag and 8 oz. in the fridge. Many hydrosols are produced overseas, and this can be problematic if you want a hydrosol that has not spoiled and turned rancid. Many imported hydrosols sit on hot ships and in stuffy warehouses for months before they even make it to the store shelf, where they may sit another month or so before you buy them. These are not fresh hydrosols! Always look for domestically grown, organic hydrosols.

The only problem that I see with using European hydrosols is that hydrosols are fragile and break down after a while, just as milk or other perishable products do. Often the hydrosols from Europe are old and smelly because of the long time in transit from European fields via ship to the US, and then on to the consumer. Make sure that you request only the freshest and sweet-smelling of these various hydrosols. AND, if the hydrosol has added preservatives, do not use it at all for culinary or therapeutic purpose. It can only be used as an addition to the daily toilette routine, in the bath, or spritzed to refresh the air or your skin when you are driving.

Now that you know what floral waters and hydrosols are and how they are used, it is also helpful to know where they may be obtained. See the Source List for California-grown, California-distilled hydrosols.

Consult the chart below for uses of hydrosols.

Uses of Floral Water and Hydrosols

Floral Hydrosols (Waters)	Skin Care	Mental Care	Culinary
Chamomile, German	anti-inflammatory for soothing, irritated skin	emotionally calming	***
Chamomile, Roman	anti-inflammatory for dry, inflamed, sensitive skin	psychic soother	***
Jasmine	true hydrosol does not exist		***
Lavender	gentle, balancing, cooling, all skin types, universal toner, cools burned skin, hydrating, for oily or impure skin, for sensitive skin, balancing, bathing	relaxing, revitalizing, eases mental stress, reduces mental fatigue, for jet lag	can be added to mineral water or all dessert foods
Lavandin	bathing, toner	relaxing, revitalizing	add to mineral water
Lavandin CT, Borneol, Camphor	acne or herpes	stimulating	add to desserts or jellies
Orange Blossom	hydrating to dry skin, for bathing	aphrodisiac, uplifting	1 tsp. in cup of coffee eliminates jitters
Rose	toner for all skin types, aftershave, after-bath splash	aphrodisiac, eases nervousness and mental strain	add to desserts or jellies

Herbal Hydrosols	Skin Care	Mental Care	Culinary
Bay Laurel	toning, aftershave	uplifting	good with meat foods, sprinkle on steamed veggies
Eucalyptus	helpful for blemishes & acne, regenerative	purifies the air	* * *
Everlast (Helichrysum)	heals and soothes irritations, depleted and inflamed conditions, helpful in reducing scarring when used on fresh wounds	detoxifying, soothes the heart	can be added to mineral water or wherever a honey scent is desired
Lemon Balm (Melissa)	herpes, for bathing	calming, sedating, insomnia, mental stress	in water, for cooking lamb, in fruit punch
Lemon Verbena	revitalizing to normal skin types, balancing	stimulating	as a sleep aid
Linden	very soothing	relaxing, relieves anxiety, depression, insomnia, euphoric	in mineral water, as a sleep aid
Peppermint	relieves itching, redness, inflammation and acne, cooling, for bathing	uplifting, energizing, cooling, for hot flashes	taken by itself to soothe digestion
Rose Geranium	for bathing, cellular regenerative, balances oil glands, oily or dry skin, cleans up doggy odor	stimulates adrenal cortex, antidepressant, cooling, for hot flashes	in water, jellies, fruit desserts
Rosemary	revitalizes skin, for bathing	restores energy, alertness, for tired feet	meat dishes, sprinkle on steamed veggies
Thyme	acne, dermatitis, eczema, insect bites	stimulating, increases circulation, revitalizes	for lamb or non-sweet cookies, for veggies

5

Are Synthetic and Natural Oils Identical?

An Anthroposophical Approach

Victoria Edwards

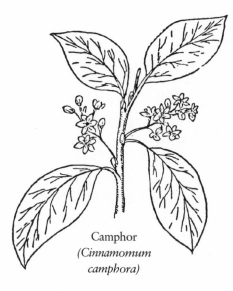

Camphor
*(Cinnamomum
camphora)*

Victoria Edwards began her research and study of herbs and massage arts at Berkeley in the late 1960s. Continuing to follow her interest in nature led her to biodynamic gardening techniques and making her own massage and body oils from the flowers and herbs she grew and wild-crafted. Jeanne Rose first introduced her to aromatherapy in 1976. Since that time she has been formulating personal blends for thousands of clients and created Leydet Aromatics, a mail order business specializing in the finest quality essences.

Ms. Edwards has worked with international leaders of aromatherapy, and has published articles in numerous journals. She was the founding president of the first American Aromatherapy Assocation from 1987–1991. Lecturing in three countries and holding classes in herb identification, making lotions and potions, color and aromas, massage arts including Jin Shin Jyutsu, and many facets of aromatherapy, she has taught aromatherapy seminars throughout America, Canada, and Japan.

Ms. Edwards is currently working on a book she started writing ten years ago.

I will be presenting a brief overview of some basic elements found in the plant world, and contrasting this to the developments in modern chemistry that have resulted in the production of synthetic substances. Goethean (pronounced "Gert-ian") spiritual science can help shed light on the subject. Although Goethe's work was done more than a century ago, his insights into life's deeper laws transcend many of those found in modern-day science. Materialists may deny this, but it sometimes takes centuries to understand genius.

The Chemistry of Life

Starch, sugar, and cellulose, the most characteristic plant materials, are carbohydrates. When subjected to oxidation (heat) all three break down into carbon and water. The elements that compose these substances are carbon, hydrogen, and oxygen. These elements are known as the breakdown products.

Carbon has the unusual property of being able to combine not only with hydrogen and other atoms but also with itself. Carbon is the main component of several million known compounds, and has a tremendous capacity for organizing and structuring matter.

Hydrogen, in contrast to carbon, is the Earth's lightest substance. (Hydrogen content increases in the upper stratosphere.) Hydrogen is also connected with warmth, having one of the hottest of all flames. Warmth plays a role in the process whereby starch changes into sugar and sugar into subtler substances, observable when summer's heat causes the plant to pour itself out into the universe as fragrance and colour. When summer takes over, its sublimating warmth brings forth the ethereal marvel of the blossom. Scent rises sunward and streams out into the endless reaches of the universe.

Oxygen constitutes twenty percent of our atmosphere. Our longing for oxygen is really a longing for life, which oxygen supports. Water, being composed of eighty-nine percent oxygen, is the source of life for the Earth's vegetation. Plants consist mainly of water, as can be seen by the difference in weight between fresh and dried plants.

Oxygen is the antithesis of hydrogen. While hydrogen is the bearer of the being or idea of plants, the element that carries them out into the cosmos, according to Goethe, oxygen is the bearer of forces whereby "being" becomes "appearance."

The Plant's Life Cycle

When nature stirs again in spring, the idea of the plant begins incarnating, reaching a peak of embodiment at midsummer when it blossoms and sets its fruit. It has then spent itself as to appearance. As it fades away and withers, leaving nothing but seeds, the being of the plant withdraws again from manifestation. It uses the seed as an anchorhold for further reappearance in the following season. This marvelous rhythm of being and appearance, of blossoming and germinating, expanding and contracting, is the primal phenomenon described in Goethe's doctrine of metamorphosis. The rhythm uses the activity of fire-force (hydro-gen) and oxygen as tools.

The sugar produced from starch when hydrogen acts upon it has a tendency to go towards etherealization. Flower scents known to chemists as etheric or ethereal oils all contain a great deal of hydrogen. That they have similar characteristics in nature to this substance is obvious in their great volatility—they "fly away" and are highly flammable. It is also a familiar experience to find these aromatic substances becoming increasingly fragrant as they follow the law of their own being: etherealization.

Coal-Tar Chemistry

Coal, which was formed in very ancient times, is a result of layers of mummified plant materials. When coal is coked (heated in air-tight ovens), coke becomes the byproduct of gas manufacture. Another byproduct of the coal and gas industry is coal tar. Originally a nuisance, it has become the mainstay of modern chemical industry.

Fractional distillation of tar produces solids and distillates. Paraffin is the chief product of lignite tar, whereas coal tar is composed almost wholly of cyclo-parafins. Chemical analysis shows their components to be carbon and hydrogen (hydrocarbons). Carbon's capacity for reorganization makes for a huge number of possible combinations. Mineral oils have a composition similar to lignite tar. Fractional distillation yields products of the paraffin group: benzene petroleum, paraffin, and paraffin oil.

The reason for the neglect of coal tar until 1846 was its resistance to chemical and oxidizing agents. Coal-tar derivatives do not burn easily, and cannot be used to fuel internal-combustion engines. The deadlock was broken with the discovery that a combination of sulphuric and nitric acids could break down the cyclo-paraffins.

Treatment of benzene with this mixture yields nitro-benzene, known as false oil of Bitter Almonds. This very aromatic substance was used to scent floor wax and shoe polish.

The use of very complicated processes to achieve the fixation of nitrogen led to the first synthetic coal-tar dyes. Perkin put the first aniline dye on the market in 1856. Baeyer made a synthetic indigo that could be factory produced. Soon followed the endanthren dyes and the whole range of other dyes now commercially available.

The Birth of Synthetics

Between 1858 and 1865 Kekulé, a German chemist laid the groundwork for the modern theory of structure in organic chemistry. According to anecdotal legend, Kekulé fell asleep and dreamed that carbon atoms joined hands and danced around him in a circle. It was this dream that inspired the creation of his structural chemistry. Soon, substances were discovered that had an effect on the human organism. The era of synthetic drugs had arrived.

Salicylic-acid preparations such as aspirin were produced from phenol. There were sweet-tasting substances as well among these intermediate products of dye manufacture. The sweetest were at once synthesized and put into production. This was the origin of saccharine, dulcin, and other such sweeteners.

Nitro-benzol, the primary substance of this whole development, is aromatic in character. Here too, ingenious synthesizing yielded an abundance of other artificial scents. This led to the development of the whole synthetic perfume industry with its immense variety of compounds, each imitating a different plant fragrance.

No one can dispute that this expansion of coal-tar chemistry is a triumph of the human mind. But what was behind it spiritually, and how are these substances related to the cosmic whole? The illustration above demonstrates how natural substances born of starch are etherealized in the exhaling of the cosmic breath, and change into sugars, blossom colours, scents, honey, etheric oils, and healing substances of plant origin.

Downwards from the middle zone there is a gradual densifying and mineralizing, via cellulose, until a biological zero is reached in the form of carbon, or coal tar. Here, human ingenuity takes hold and brings forth a synthetic mirror-image of the natural world: synthetic colours, scents and flavors, drugs, pesticides, fertilizers, etc.

Matter is the most spiritual in the perfume of the plant. —Rudolf Steiner

Heaven and Earth

Contrasting the two realms, we get the impression that the upper one is the realm of dynamic biological reality, the scene of cosmic activities between Heaven and Earth an endless metamorphosis. The underworld of coal-tar chemistry, in which humans have descended deeply into the Earth to excavate and it is like a ghostly reflection of the dynamic creativity of the cosmos. Here the static world of atoms and calculable results takes the place of nature's dynamics. In plant preparations a rather large complex of substances is generally used (aqueous, alcoholic extract, volatile oil distillate, oil extract, etc.), and under some circumstances two or more plants are combined to form a new therapeutic whole. The use of isolated alkaloids, glycosides, hormones, etc. was recommended by Rudolf Steiner only in exceptional cases; still less often did he advise the use of synthetic products such as the customary chemotherapeutic agents, most of which completely lack any genuine relation to the human organism, in the sense of humanity mirroring the macrocosm.

Synthetic versus Natural

Natural

The industry has many definitions for the word "natural," and not all of them can be considered *natural*. In the world today, flavors and fragrance have a market of about 5–10 billion U.S. dollars. The products that incorporate scented flavors and fragrance, both "natural" and "artificial," are found in our everyday lives in foods, snacks, drinks of all kinds, for body care and daily care. "Natural" is defined by the industry as follows:

1. **Natural** from the plant or botanical.
   Example: Strawberry extract made only from pure Strawberry fruit.
   Example: Peppermint essential oil distilled only from Peppermint plants.

2. **Natural Flavor** but not from the named botanical.
   Example: Black Currant flavor comes from a plant called the Buchu *(Barosma betulina)*, and generally not from Black Currants or Black Currant leaves. Yes, it *is* a natural ingredient, but just not from the named plant.

3. **Natural with Other Natural Flavors** (WONF)
   Example: Lemon flavor comes from a combination of Lemon oil *(Citrus limonum)* and Orange oil *(Citrus sinensis)* and *Litsea cubeba.*

Synthetic

4. **Nature-Identical** flavorings and scents are chemical synthetics, which are structurally the same as those found in nature.
   Example: Using L-Carvone when the scent and flavor of Spearmint is desired.

5. **Artificial** flavorings are not yet identified or declared as occurring in nature.
   Example: Using ethyl methyl phenyl glycidate as artificial strawberry flavor when the flavor of Strawberry is desired.

It is obvious from the above that the industrial world has a different concept of natural than most of us do. In the world of herbalism or aromatherapy, *only* the first (#1) definition of natural is what we use as *natural*. So beware when reading labels, and make sure you are getting exactly what you want.

Many people claim to have "environmental illness," stating that they are allergic to scents and super-sensitive to aromas. For many of these people, a sample whiff of a light, pure essential-oil blend will prove that what they are allergic to is *synthetics.* When you first mention to these people that what they may be allergic to is synthetics, they may swear that they have also experienced sensitivity to natural scents. **But remember:** much of what most of us have been told is *"natural"* is really *synthetic!* When you ask them what natural oils they have experienced sensitivity to, they will invariably mention the amber, synthetic patchouli, and China Rain synthetic oils that are often marketed as natural but are actually blends of synthetic oils.

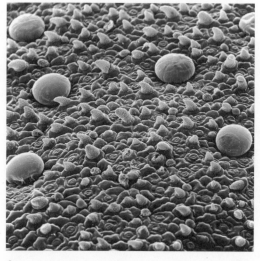

a

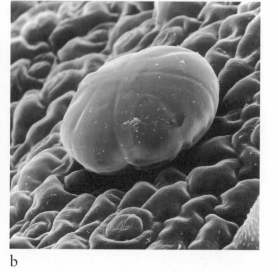

b

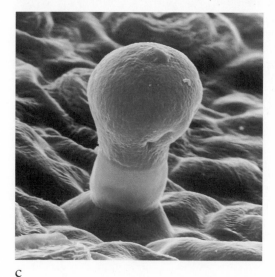

c

Essential oil glands:

a. *Thymus vulgaris* surface of leaf

b. *Thymus vulgaris* one gland enlarged

c. Three cell *Mentha spicata*

photos courtesy of Professor Massimo Maffei, Department of Plant Biology, University of Turin, Italy

6

The Science of Essential Oils and their Toxicity

Maria Lis-Balchin

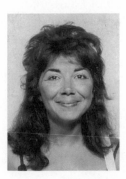

Maria Lis-Balchin, Ph.D, graduated from London University with a B.Sc. Honours Degree in biochemistry and zoology. After many years in medical research investigating the biochemical aspects of neuropsychiatry and neurological diseases, she began doctoral research as a toxicologist, later continuing her studies as a biochemist at Westminster Hospital Medical School. Lis-Balchin is currently a senior lecturer at the South Bank University, where she has pioneered a new unit at degree and master's level in the science of essential oils and aromatherapy.

*E*ssential oils produced commercially are often subjected to a number of chemical processes which benefit the main commercial users—the food, cosmetic and perfumery industries (99.8%). The object of these changes is to make the products either more water-soluble (hydrophilic) or alcohol-soluble, to extend their shelf-life, to make them more consistent from the olfactory angle, or to make them more commercially attractive to both the producer and buyer. These chemical processes can involve simply removing some components, such as the terpenes to make them more hydrophyllic, or even downright adulteration to keep the cost down.

Rectification

The term "rectification" encompasses a large number of changes that can be made to an oil, such as the process of removing some components of the oil in order to make the oil more soluble in alcohol and longer-lasting. Deterpenation, for example, involves the removal of terpenes (all "head" fractions). Deterpenation is used frequently for citrus oils.

Rectification can also include certain adulterations. Many pure or truly organic essential oils which are very expensive, such as that of Melissa, are very rarely sold. When seen on the market, these oils have often been subjected to chemical adulterations in order to reduce the cost of such precious oils.

Vacuum distillation is used for most rectification, and this involves fractional distillation under reduced pressure at a certain temperature (depending on what is to be removed).

Rectification primarily removes residual water and very light fractions from the "heads" and heavy sesquiterpenes and waxes of high boiling point from the "tails" of oils. Citrus oils are often de-sesquiterpenized.

Rectification can make different essential oils very similar.

Differential solubility is also used for separating the more valuable oxygenated components from terpenes, as used for citrus oils industrially. This method involves cold temperatures and is based on the varying solubility of the fractions in a particular solvent, such as aqueous alcohol. Centrifuges and counter-current extractors are also used.

Chromatography, using columns filled with silica gel, etc., is used to separate off terpenes or other components.

Cutting

This is a means of making the original essential oil go further using a number of alternatives:

Nature identicals are volatile oils made up of components obtained solely from plant sources. These components can be from the same species, or even from a completely different plant source.

Synthetics are composed of entirely synthetic components, such as chemicals made in the laboratory from various starting materials including plant components. Some are very cheap and nasty, whilst others are so similar to the natural product that most people cannot distinguish between them. Most expensive perfumes contain about 50-100 ingredients, of which a high percentage are synthetics.

Substitutions are often done using cheaper plant essential oils, such as the use of Petitgrain for Neroli or Ajowan for Thyme.

Dilutions can be done using many chemicals and plant components to make a larger profit for the supplier. Dilutions are done with DPG (dipropyl glycol), turpentine fractions, or fixed oils.

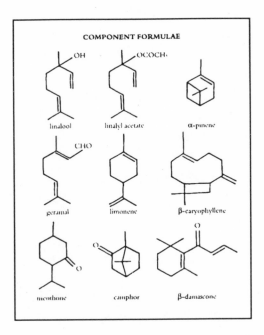

COMPONENT FORMULAE

linalool   linalyl acetate   α-pinene

geranial   limonene   β-caryophyllene

menthone   camphor   β-damascone

Folding involves mixing batches of the same essential oil, which can be stored for about two years and could then be processed further to terpeneless or sesquiterpeneless stages if required.

Essential Oil Composition

Each essential oil is composed of 100-300 components, each of which has its own odour and physical/chemical characteristics. Most of the components called "terpenoids" are very similar, and all arise from Acetyl (CH_3 COO) units via either a five-carbon unit called isoprene or via the shikimic pathway from amino acids.

The terpenoids have either a ten-carbon structure and are known as monoterpenoids, or a fifteen-carbon structure, called sesquiterpenoids. Each of these can be oxygenated, giving rise to a number of derivatives, such as alcohols, aldehydes, phenols, etc. Many of these components are very active due to their innate chemical structure, and these components are often responsible for bioactivity. Cinnamaldehyde in Cinnamon is a very potent bactericide as is eugenol in Clove and thymol in Thyme.

Essential Oil Analysis

The best separation techniques are gas chromatography with the addition of detectors utilizing mass spectroscopy (MS), nuclear magnetic resonance (NMR) or ultra-violet (UV) spectroscopy, etc. The use of specialized capillary columns with numerous stationary phases allows for the separation and quantitization of most components in essential oils. However, only very specialized techniques using cyclodextrins can show adulteration by synthetics. These involve the detection of stereo-isomers, which often differ in proportion in natural and synthetic essential oils. Lavender adulterated with synthetic linalool or linalyl acetate, for instance, has high racemic mixtures, whereas pure Lavender has a different composition of enantiomers. The proportion of enantiomers makes a great deal of difference in the medicinal properties of the essential oil.

Gas Chromatography

This simply involves a long column packed with an absorbent or coated with a non-volatile liquid. The essential oil, which is vaporized at the entry point, passes through the column with the help of a carrier gas, which is usually helium or hydrogen. The column is located in an oven in order to enable a change in temperature to be established, perhaps from 70°C to 250°C at a given rate, such as 3°C per minute, depending on the separation required and the particular essential oil.

The mixture of different chemical components will pass through the column at different speeds, depending on their individual solubility between the stationary phase and combining with the carrier gas. The least soluble components (in the stationary phase) pass through faster, and therefore have a low retention time. The components are detected as they pass out of the column, and appear on the chromatogram as a series of peaks.

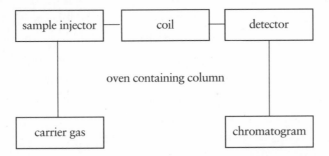

The chromatogram represents the "fingerprint" of an essential oil. Each peak represents one component, provided the conditions have been perfected. Each peak has an area determined by its height multiplied by 1/2 base, or the area of the triangle.

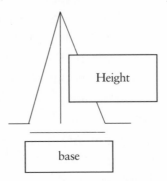

The individual peak areas are then added up to a total, and each peak area is calculated as a percent of this total. This gives the basis for comparison with standard published data (ISO). For example:

Lavender *(Lavandula angustifolia):*   linalyl acetate   min.   30%
                                        linalool   min.   25%

Usually the main peaks are compared, but sometimes minor peaks are especially important in showing adulteration. For example:

Rose oil *(Rosa damascena)* (Turkish): approx. 0.59% cis. Rose oxide
0.2% trans. Rose oxide

These, together with 200 other components, make up pure Rose oil. Cheap Rose oil can be made by using synthetic citronellol 30%, geraniol 25%, nerol 10% and phenylethylalcohol 3% + linalool 1%. The synthetic Rose oil costs about 1/1000th as much as pure Rose oil!

The chromatogram of an essential oil can look completely different if a different gas chromatography apparatus is used, if the column is changed or simply the running conditions are altered. Even experts have problems identifying components on their own chromatograms; therefore it is unlikely that chromatograms are meaningful to non-chemists. Often chromatograms are supplied by manufacturers in order to authenticate the essential oil sold, but each batch of oil must be accompanied by a chromatogram in order to make this claim worthwhile. The cost of each analysis is at least fifty dollars, and it is therefore unlikely that each batch of essential oil has been analysed by small retailers!

Chemotypes and Other Variations in Essential Oils

Chemotypes

Some species, such as Thyme *(Thymus vulgaris)* have a tendency to produce seedlings that when grown have variable chemical composition. This results in chemical variation in the oils produced by the different plants, giving rise to the term "chemotypes." Different chemotypes can grow specifically in different areas, or else they can have a narrow distribution in one field. Trees like Tea Tree show very great variability; adjacent trees can give rise to leaves producing essential oils of very different composition. Plants raised by micro-propagation often display great variability and the only way to prevent changes in the chemical composition of the essential oil that comes from such plants is by taking cuttings, rooting these cuttings separately and distilling the mature plants.

Species differences

There are many "groups" of essential oils that contain a number of different species under the same name, such as:

Chamomile
There are three main commercial Chamomile oils, which originate from three different species of the same family (Compositae):

German *(Matricaria recutita)*

English (Roman) *(Chamamaelum nobile)*

Moroccan *(Chamamaelum mixta)*

Each of these oils has a different smell, which is reflected in the different chemical compositions. The use of one instead of another is therefore rather unscientific!

Eucalyptus
There are over 200 oil-producing Eucalyptus trees. The three main commercial Eucalyptus oils are:

E. globulus

E. citriodora

E. radiata

The odour and chemical composition of these three are again different.

Other Variations
The essential oil composition can vary in the same plant due to physico-chemical variations including temperature, humidity, seasonal changes, water, fertility of the soil, hours of sunlight, fertilizers applied, etc. There is also a change in composition during the development of the leaves, as in the case of Geranium. There are also diurnal and nocturnal changes. The latter is the scientific basis for picking Jasmine flowers early in the morning, when the essential oils are at their best.

ISO
The International Standardization Organization of essential oils was largely set up for the food and cosmetics industries, in order to establish criteria to ensure similarity of products.

However, as the composition of essential oils differs from season to season and batch to batch, "blending" must often take place to ensure constancy in the product. "Blending" may be done with different batches of the same essential oil, other essential oils or their components, as in the case of "nature identicals," or simply and most cheaply by the addition of synthetic components. The ISO may therefore inadvertently encourage adulteration.

Bioactivity

Scientific studies on bioactivity of essential oils have largely been centred round *in vitro* tests. These are largely concerned with their anti-microbial and anti-fungal activity, with some pharmacological and biochemical evaluations. Prior to 1994, most of these tests were carried out on essential oil samples which were not finger-printed using GC or GC/MS; therefore, one can only assume the oils were pure and unadulterated. However, a survey carried out by the author indicated that many commercial oils were very much adulterated, and that there was an enormous variation in biological activity as well as chemical composition in the same "named" oil. Sixteen Geranium oil samples showed a variation in activity ranging from three to sixteen micro-organisms affected, and this is not related to the major components.

Toxicity

Toxicity is defined as an adverse effect of a compound. This can vary from feeling sick to vomiting; from a slight headache to a raging migraine; from tinnitus to vertigo; from aggressive to maniacal or homicidal feelings; from having a depression to feeling suicidal. It can cause dermatitis or spots in a particular area or all over the body. Such spots could be small and insignificant or large, very itchy exudating ones. Other symptoms can include feeling faint, having palpitations or blackouts, raised or lowered blood pressure, etc.

Most toxicity manifestations are, however, studied in animals like rats, who not only cannot express themselves about their feelings and tell us about headaches, etc. but also have a different physiology and metabolism. They cannot vomit, and cannot convert many compounds into the same metabolites as we do. The only toxicity criteria measurable in the rat (or mouse) are: dermatitis (but this is difficult unless the fur is shaven off!) and some central nervous system aberrations, such as falling over or lying upside down.

LD50: The main toxicological evaluation is just concerned with the death of the animal. The LD50 standard measurement is defined as the 'Lethal Dose that kills fifty percent of the animals'. It is a number of grams of a substance (or mg., or μg.) which is related to the body weight of the animal, that is gm./kg., body weight. This dosage can then be extrapolated to humans directly: 10 gm./kg. is equivalent to 700 gm. per the 70 kg. average human. This is equivalent to eating 700 gm. of sugar (which is considered non-toxic) in one sitting! Nobody could do this without vomiting and, if pumped directly into the stomach, this dose of sugar would probably kill the person due to its hyper-osmotic effect, which would cause severe dehydration leading to collapse.

Any LD50 value over 5 gm./kg. is considered to be non-toxic; and values of 1-5 gm./kg. are relatively safe. The LD50 is, however, only a relative value of toxicity, and it does not indicate long-term toxicity, teratogenicity or carcinogenicity.

Long-term effects can manifest themselves one to thirty years after a person has been subjected to small doses of chemicals. This is due to an accumulation of the chemical over a long period, usually in a target organ or in fat deposits throughout the body. Stress initiated by bereavement, divorce or weight loss can mobilise the chemical in large doses and cause toxic manifestations.

Teratogenic effects are seen only in the next generation, the mother or father having had no toxic symptoms after exposure to the chemical. The offspring, however, can be born deformed or limbless, or with defective internal organs that have not fully developed, as in the case of thalidomide taken by expectant mothers during the first few months of pregnancy.

Carcinogenetic effects are often seen as part of long-term usage of chemicals. It may be due to direct mutation of some cells, or the production of a carcinogenic effect via co-carcinogen.

Dermal and Oral Toxicity: There can be two effects of dermal application of chemicals, (1) local skin effects, such as reddening or dermatitis; or (2) systemic effect in other parts of the body. The chemicals can be absorbed almost directly into the bloodstream and are therefore largely unchanged (unmetabolised). This is in contrast to an oral intake, where the chemical is "digested" and therefore converted (metabolised) into many derivatives, some of which may be more or less toxic than the original chemical. These new chemicals enter the bloodstream and can attack target organs or tissues.

Because of the difference in the uptake of the chemical by the oral and dermal route, two LD50 values are often given. The dermal LD50 is usually ascertained in the rabbit, which has a more sensitive skin than the rat.

Note of Caution: Although both the oral and dermal LD50 are often quoted, the values for the essential oils generally used are non-toxic. However, there is a possibility that the volatile oils could exert a toxic effect directly through intake into the respiratory tract. There is only a one-cell thickness to traverse from the alveoli in the lungs into the blood system; therefore, like respiratory gases, the volatile lipophilic essential oils are taken up very rapidly. There should therefore be some concern to both patient and aromatherapist (but especially the latter, who is using essential oils all the time).

Absorption of essential oils through the respiratory tract can have a local or systemic effect (as for dermal absorption). The local effect could be an asthma attack, breathlessness, wheezing or hyperventilation.

Sensitisation: This can be affected by the intake of the chemical via any route, oral, dermal, or respiratory. Sensitisation involves the immune system. There may be a long period of time between the first impact of the chemical and a sensitisation reaction. The initial manifestation of the reaction is usually dermatitis or a local swelling. For instance, almonds taken by sensitised people cause swelling of the larynx and this causes inability to breathe. The sensitisation reaction can be very violent including anaphylactic shock, which causes a general collapse of breathing and blood pressure, and can be fatal within minutes.

Note of caution: Once a person is sensitised allergic by a chemical, even a distantly-related chemical can cause a reaction. This is relevant to essential oils, as many oils contain similar components. This aspect of toxicity has not been studied.

Irritation: In the case of dermal toxicity, irritation refers to the effect of a substance on the skin. Irritation is an indication that the chemical has been absorbed, and that the cells are reacting against it. The two main irritation manifestations are reddening and swelling. This is usually studied using a "patch test" whereby a constant amount of chemical is applied to a one inch square area of skin, which is then covered for twenty-four hours. The exposed area is then evaluated for reddening and swelling. **Note:** The most sensitive areas of "skin" in the body are those with soft mucus membranes, such as the eyes, nose, and vagina. Essential oils should not be applied to these places unless highly diluted.

Phototoxicity refers to the effect of UV light on a chemical that may have already combined with a natural body compound. Sunlight or artificial UV light can have the same effect, and it is unwise to use sunbeds after aromatherapy massage, especially if the essential oil blend had citrus oils in it. The phototoxic effect is similar to severe sunburn, which can redden and burn the skin and cause desquamation. There is also a "tanning" effect on the skin, which may become blotched with brown pigmentation.

All essential oils, bar a very few, have been studied for toxicity using animal studies. There is no reason to believe that organic oils are less toxic than any other, nor that they have never been tested on animals! The problem, however, remains that many oils are adulterated, and therefore their toxicity is unknown.

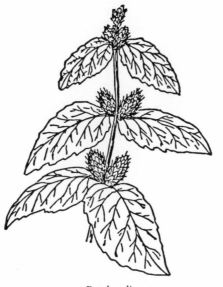

Patchouli
(Pogostemon cablin)

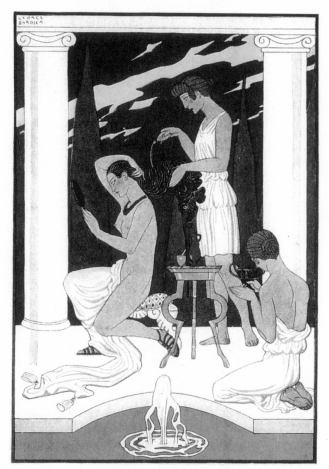

Ancient Rome, by Georges Barbier

II

Self Care

7

An Exquisite Aromatherapy Skin Care Treatment

Joni Loughran

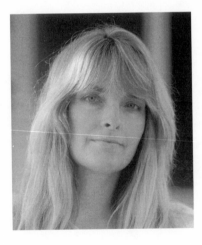

Joni Loughran, L.C., Ph.D., is a licensed cosmetologist and cosmetology instructor. She has a doctoral degree in health sciences, and is a graduate of the highly regarded Dr. Hauschka method of skin care. Joni currently has a private skin care practice, and serves as a consultant to natural cosmetic manufacturers. Her articles appear regularly in national health magazines and trade journals. She is on the Personal Care Advisory Board for *Let's Live* magazine and she is the author of *A Lifetime of Beauty: The Definite All-Natural Guide to Skin & Hair Care* and *Joni Loughran's Natural Skin Care: Alternative & Traditional Techniques.*

*T*he following is a detailed description of a meticulously composed aromatherapy skin care treatment that is offered by The Facial Room at Petaluma
Natural Foods in Petaluma, California, where women of all ages have experienced the pleasure of aromatherapy at its best. This very special treatment has
been described by recipients as a "journey," a "vacation," and an "escape." Indeed,
it is all that and more, for the strength and presence of aromatherapy combined with
the human touch is quite powerful. Though this two-hour treatment truly is a comprehensive "skin care treatment," most people know or soon realize that it is also
something else. It is an uplifting and rejuvenating offering that relieves stress and
pampers the spirit. It is an occasion to feel the grace of living communicated through
the senses. It is an opportunity to know simple elegance at the core. It is a gift.

It is my hope that the ensuing description will serve the reader as "how-to"
instructions if the reader is an æsthetician (skin care professional), as an enticement
for the lay person to "experience the pleasure," or as an invitation to learn more
about aromatherapy and treat friends and family to the gift of the aromatherapeutic touch.

The Environment

The room, the space, the environment, the setting—their influences enhance an
aromatherapy treatment, so it is important that they are created by thoughtful
design and that they are just right. The Facial Room is tucked away in the back of
a popular natural-food store located in the historic section of downtown Petaluma. This site was chosen because the natural food store has a friendly ambiance
and attracts people who care about health and well-being. This aromatherapy skin
care treatment caters to these principles. But, most importantly, the location was
chosen because the store smells good. Facial rooms are usually found in salons,
and salon odors from chemical treatments are terribly offensive—not a good setting for an aromatherapy treatment. Here in the health-food store the aromas are
earthy and real—fresh fruits and vegetables, herbs and spices, flowers and essences. They are the welcoming committee to The Facial Room.

Because we, as human beings, are nurtured and nourished through our senses,
this treatment lovingly caters to each one of them—sight, touch taste, hearing, and
smell. By the time you leave, each sense will have been attended. Sight: the color of
the room, the art, the flowers, the pleasant surroundings. Touch: the massage, the
treatment's steps. Taste: the elixir that is offered at the end of the session. Hearing:
the sound of beautiful music. Smell: the aroma of the essential oils.

The Facial Room is comfortable and peaceful as well as neat and clean. Your treatment begins as soon as you step in the door and encounter an environment designed to relax. *Relax.* The lighting is soft and low. The walls are painted a lovely shade of pink-peach that is specific to "soothing the savage beast." Soft, gentle music envelops you,[1] and diffused essential oils fill the air with a serene bouquet— the first encounter with the charm of aromatherapy.[2]

Tending the Feet

After changing into a facial gown, you are comfortably seated with your feet immersed in an aromatherapy foot bath. The warmth of the water and the essential oils combine to create a soothing hydrotherapy and aromatherapy moment.[3] During the time your feet are soaking, you are consulted about your skin care habits and lifestyle. These factors will determine the approach to your individual aromatherapy skin care treatment—which products will be used, which oils will be chosen, or what areas will need the most attention. After fifteen or twenty minutes, your feet are patted dry, and then you are reclined and covered with a sheet and a warm flannel blanket. In warm weather the sheet may be enough, but because the temperature of the body drops during relaxation, an additional blanket is often more comfortable.

While reclined, your feet are held for a moment. This is a polarity-therapy technique that is both comforting and grounding. Then the feet are slowly massaged. The massage continues the flow of relaxation that began when you first entered the room, and is an excellent opportunity to employ an aromatherapy massage oil.[4] Massage is often considered the most effective way of benefiting from essential oils. They are quickly absorbed into the skin and into the body, delivering the unique characteristics of that particular oil. During this step, benefits are reaped not only from the qualities of the essential oils but also from the energy and healing qualities of the human touch. Reflexology techniques[5] can be used during this step to complement the treatment, and for additional benefits.

Presence

After your feet have been mindfully attended, the æsthetician (referred to as a female but men can do this, too) positions herself behind you at your head. This is a very important time for the æsthetician to prepare herself to begin the heart of the aromatherapy treatment and to be in a truly positive state to work with you. Up to this point, you and the æsthetician may be chatting, but from here on, it is preferable to have no talking. Chances are that you will both want to be quiet anyway.

Whether you are an æsthetician or a lay person giving this treatment, follow these steps:

1. Close your eyes.
2. Center and ground yourself.
3. Clear out and let go of any negative energy or feelings.
4. Stretch your hands, palms, and fingers as far as possible for a few moments and then rub them together briskly. This will bring up the energy in the hands. In Chinese medicine, this is called "putting chi on the palm."
5. Lastly, you should deep breathe—dropping the breath well into the body— and expand your vision by disengaging your focus so perception is broadened and more can be brought into the treatment.

This five-step preparation is very important to maximize the benefits when doing "hands-on" work. Together, these steps take about thirty seconds to do. If you are prone to absorbing other people's energy, it is also important to establish a protective barrier so that you can "give" without being drained or taking on any problems that are not your own.

Analysis

After the æsthetician has prepared herself to work with you, the treatment resumes. A headband is used to hold the hair away from your face, and then your skin will be looked at closely, touched, and sensed. Sometimes this will be under a bright light, with your eyes covered by goggles. The color, overall appearance, and texture of your skin will be checked. The pigmentation, pore size, general condition, and elasticity will be analyzed. This input, combined with the information from the earlier consultation (while your feet were soaking) will determine the treatment design, which products will be used, and which essential oils will be best for your skin.

Facial Compresses

For many, this next step is the favorite—warm water, a soft cloth infused with heavenly essential oils, and gentle pressure from guided hands—what could be more pampering?! Facial compresses are a pre-cleansing step that warms and relaxes the skin. The æsthetician fills the basin with warm water (the degree of warmth depends on the type of skin), and four drops of the gentlest essential oils are added and then stirred in briskly before dipping the compress cloth. Lavender, Rose, Chamomile, and Neroli are good choices. If there is concern about "hot spots" of essential oils (because oil and water do not mix), the essential oils can first be mixed with a small amount of vodka or vinegar, which will enable them to diffuse in the water. There are also commercial aromatherapy products available that are formulated for this purpose and are mentioned in the Source List.

After the essential oil is added, a soft cloth is dipped in the water (a new cloth baby diaper works great), and the excess water is wrung out. Then the cloth is applied to the face, cupped around the chin and brought over the cheeks with the ends laid on the forehead. The nose should not be covered, so breathing is kept free. Gentle pressure from the æsthetician's hand holds the moist, fragrant warmth next to your skin until the warmth dissipates. This is repeated at least ten times.

Cleansing and Steaming

After the facial compresses have softened the soil on the face, your skin is ready to be thoroughly and gently cleansed. The cleanser for your skin type is chosen and applied. Cleansing is done with the hands (not a machine) using a soft, slow circular motion combined with hugging and pressing techniques. After the entire face has been cleansed the cleanser is removed with soft, damp sponges. Your skin is then toned with a misting of a hydrosol,[6] and your lips and eyelids are protected with a balm for steaming. Both of these specific areas have skin that is thin and fragile, so it should be protected from the heat of the steam. Steaming will also help to activate the conditioning qualities of the balm.

Steaming is a hydrotherapy treatment. It is good for the skin because it enhances the body's natural cleansing process and helps to clean the pores from the inside out. Steaming also superhydrates the skin with moisture, and softens dead skin cells on the surface so they can be easily cleansed away. The warmth and moisture of the steam relaxes the facial muscles and soften oils and dirt that may have become clogged in the pores. Steaming increases circulation that brings vital nutrients and encourages cellular rejuvenation.

The amount of steaming time and the distance of the steamer depend on the type of skin. Oily, less delicate skin can be steamed for longer periods at a closer distance. Sensitive or aging skin should be steamed for shorter periods at a greater distance. Some professional steamers are designed to incorporate essential oils into the steam, combining the valuable attributes of aromatherapy. The æsthetician should be certain the steamer is checked before adding essential oils, because if it is not designed for their use it could damage the machine. After steaming, your skin is blotted with clean, warm sponges and then sprayed again with a hydrosol.

Facial Mask #1: To Cleanse

Facial masks designed for deep cleansing are formulated with clay. There are a variety of facial quality clays available. Rose and green clay are good choices. Commercial clay masks are also available, and are listed in the Source List. Clay has remarkable detoxifying qualities and can be used for just about everyone. Depending on your skin type, the clay is mixed with other ingredients to cleanse and condition.[7] After the mask is prepared, it is applied with a soft brush in long, smooth strokes, avoiding the eye area. The mask remains on the skin for about ten minutes. A clay mask should not be allowed to dry completely or it can begin to pull moisture *from* the skin. If the mask begins to dry too fast, moisten it with a hydrosol misting. When the time is up, the mask is moistened well with a hydrosol for easy removal and then wiped off with warm, damp sponges.

Massage

While the mask is on your face, your upper chest and shoulders are massaged with an aromatherapy massage oil. The essential oil of preference is Rose. Rose is the perfect essential oil to massage over the heart. After all, Rose is for love and works on the heart chakra to harmonize the spirit and instill peace and happiness. True essential oil of Rose is one of the most elegant and exquisite oils that you will ever encounter.

The method and character of the massage lies in the hands of the æsthetician. The strokes should be long and smooth. The touch should be firm and definite but gentle. Acupressure points can be used to further relaxation. The massage continues for ten minutes, working in synchronicity with the music and the rhythms of the breath.

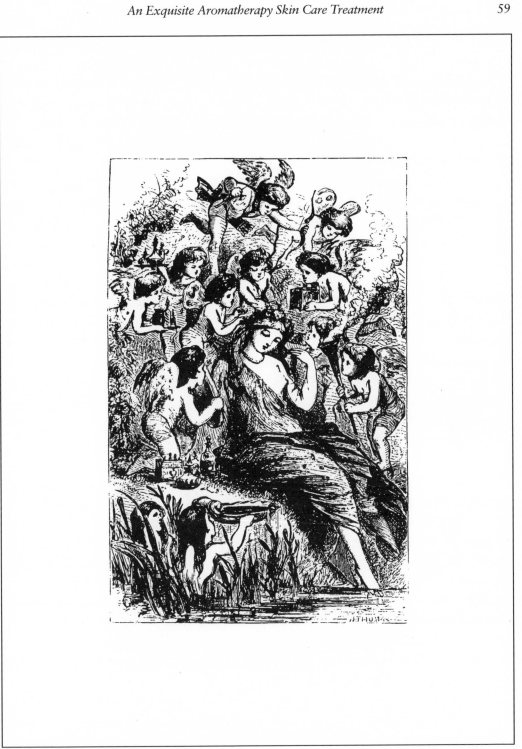

Venus toilet

Facial Mask #2: To Condition

Aromatherapy facial oils used as a mask are excellent to deeply condition the skin. A finely tuned and formulated facial oil is chosen for your skin.[8] The æsthetician warms and energizes the oil in her hands and then lays her hands on your face— pressing and holding and then changing position until all of the skin has been anointed with the nourishment and etheric essence of the blend. Warm compresses are applied over the oil and gently held in place until the heat dissipates. The cloth is warmed again and reapplied. This is repeated several times. The last cloth is allowed to rest on the face to cool.

Balancing

The treatment is nearing completion. At this time the æsthetician returns to your feet and holds them. Her warm hands are in contact with pulse points and your feet will be held until energy returns there. Because so much attention is given to the upper body during this entire aromatherapy treatment, a subtle energetic imbalance can occur. Holding the feet at the end of the treatment is a polarity-therapy technique that helps to correct such an imbalance. A silky aromatherapy body powder[9] is smoothed over your feet as they are gently but briskly massaged. Further stimulating techniques are used to help bring you out of deep relaxation.

The Final Touches

The æsthetician returns to the head area, removes the now-cool compress and gently wipes your skin to remove any unabsorbed oil. The upper chest and shoulders are also wiped to remove excess massage oil.

The compress is rinsed well, dipped in a basin of cool (not cold) water, and applied to your skin. Three to five compresses are used. Cool water has a bracing effect on the skin and is quite refreshing. It also aids in bringing you out of deep relaxation. If you are giving this treatment, it is thoughtful to let the person know that the cool compress is about to be applied, so that it does not shock them. Just say softly to them, "This is a cool compress."

Your face and upper chest are misted with a fragrant hydrosol. The headband is removed, the ear lobes are massaged and your head is held in the cradle of the æsthetician's hands for a while. This cradling is another polarity-therapy technique and is exceptionally comforting. A prayer is offered for your well-being. The æsthetician will let you know it is time to sit up, and the back of the chair is lifted into an upright position. You are given a cool drink of water or a special elixir (see Source List). Some people drift far away during this treatment and need assistance to "come back." It can be very helpful to sniff a few drops of Basil, Rosemary, or Peppermint on a tissue, if this is your experience.

The time directly after the treatment is wonderful for a few enjoyable moments alone. Indulge yourself and savor the inner silence. When the æsthetician returns she will review your skincare program and make suggestions for any skin care problems you may be having. Literature, brochures, and information sheets are given for your education, and samples of cosmetics are offered for you to try. This concludes the treatment. Breathe deeply, appreciate the spirit of grace and beauty, and remember to be kind to your skin with quality products, a gentle touch, and pure essential oils.

Summary of How Aromatherapy Is Used in This Skin Care Treatment

1. Essential oils diffused in the room prior to entering.
2. Essential oils used in the foot bath.
3. Essential oils used in a massage blend for the feet and for the shoulders and upper chest.
4. Essential oils used in the facial compresses.
5. Hydrosols used to tone the skin, wet the skin, or moisten a mask.
6. Essential oils used in a cleansing clay facial mask.
7. Essential oils in a facial oil used as a conditioning mask.
8. Essential oils used in the body powder.
9. Essential oils sniffed to help bring out of relaxation.

The Most Commonly Used Cosmetic Essential Oils

Lavender *(Lavandula angustifolia):* versatile, balancing, soothing
Carrot seed *(Daucus carota):* nutritious, rejuvenating
Chamomile *(Chamamaelum nobile):* soothing, anti-inflammatory
Geranium *(Pelargonium graveolens):* balancing
Lemon *(Citrus limon):* cleansing, refreshing

Rose *(Rosa damascena):* harmonizing, anti-inflammatory, rejuvenating
Sandalwood *(Santalum album):* soothing
Tea Tree *(Melaleuca alternifolia):* antiseptic
Ylang-Ylang *(Cananga odorata):* balancing
Frankincense *(Boswellia carterii):* rejuvenating
Jasmine *(Jasminum officinale):* soothing, toning
Neroli *(Citrus aurantium):* rejuvenating
Rosemary *(Rosmarinus officinalis):* stimulating

Endnotes

1. Music is one of the most powerful mood enhancers. The music should be carefully chosen. The tempo should be even and relaxing, but not so "transporting" that it affects the concentration and focus of the æsthetician's work.

2. The essential oils should be diffused in the room ten minutes prior to the arrival of the person who is receiving the treatment. It is best not to leave the diffusor on while giving the treatment because it can be overpowering to the person getting the treatment as well as the person giving it. However, a few drops of Lavender or a relaxing blend can be given on a tissue to be sniffed periodically, at the recipient's discretion.

   Oils can be diffused into the air with a diffusor that has a glass-expansion chamber, with one of the new quieter designs, or by using an aromatherapy lamp. If you do not have any of these, you can put the essential oil or blend in an atomizer with water (50 drops in 4 ounces of water). Shake the container and mist the room just before the person receiving the treatment arrives.

   Favorite blends are:
   * Lavender, 5 drops. Bergamot, 2 drops. Clary Sage, 1 drop.
   * Clary Sage, 6 drops. Lavender, 2 drops. Ylang-Ylang, 1 drop.
   * Bergamot, 5 drops. Ylang-Ylang, 2 drops. Clary Sage, 2 drops.
   * Roman Chamomile, 3 drops. Lavender, 3 drops. Mandarin, 3 drops.

   Remember, the attraction or repulsion of any specific oil or blend is entirely subjective and personal. So powerful is this message that if the aroma displeases it may not be beneficial. It is important to take the time to experiment with essential oils and discover the ones that please you.

3. The foot bath is the second aromatherapy application. The bath should be in either a glass or stainless steel container, as plastic does not lend in itself therapeutically to aromatherapy applications. Fill the container with warm water and add one of the following:

    a.   An aromatherapy mineral bath salt. (See Source List or make your own: combine 1 cup sea salt, 2 cups Epsom salt, and 1 cup baking soda in a jar with a tight-fitting lid. Add 30 drops of your favorite essential oil(s) and shake well).

    b.   An aromatherapy bath concentrate (see Source List).

    c.   Four drops of a single essential oil mixed with a small amount of vodka. The alcohol is used as a solvent to dilute the essential oils so they will evenly disperse in the water. This prevents "hot spots" in the foot bath that might irritate the skin. Any single oil or "relaxing blend" can be used in the foot bath. Lavender, Geranium, Bergamot, or Clary Sage are good choices.

4.   You can make your own aromatherapy massage oils by mixing 25 drops of a single essential oil, or a blend of essential oils, into 2 ounces of a carrier oil. At this point in the treatment, it is good to use relaxing oils. Try this recipe: Blend 2 ounces Sweet Almond oil with 10 drops Lavender, 2 Drops of Marjoram, 3 drops of Bergamot, 4 drops of Chamomile, 1 drop of Ylang-Ylang, and 5 drops of Orange (or see Source List).

5.   Reflexology is a technique that uses finger and hand pressure applied to specific areas (reflex points) on the feet and hands. These points correspond to an organ, a gland, or an area of the body. The pressure stimulates the reflex area and is believed to beneficially affect the corresponding body part. This encourages the body's natural ability to heal itself, bringing about better health and increased well-being.

6.   Hydrosols are a by-product of the distillation of essential oils. In the distillation process, the water and oil separate. The water that is left is the hydrosol. Though much less potent than essential oils, hydrosols have a unique, gentle quality and therapeutic value of their own and are perfect as toners and misters.

7.   Suggested guidelines for cleansing masks for each skin type:

    Normal: 1 heaping tablespoon green or rose clay, 1 teaspoon honey, 2 drops Geranium oil, enough water or aloe vera juice to make a paste.

    Dry: 1 level tablespoon rose clay, 1/2 tablespoon instant oatmeal or finely ground regular oatmeal, 1 teaspoon honey, 1 teaspoon Olive oil, enough water to make a paste. Add 1 drop Rose oil and 1 drop Lavender oil.

    Oily: 1 heaping tablespoon Green Clay, 1 teaspoon Aloe Vera juice, 1/2 teaspoon vegetable oil or Jojoba oil, enough water to make a paste. Add 1 drop Bergamot oil and 1 drop Lavender oil.

    Sensitive: 1 heaping tablespoon Rose Clay, 1 teaspoon Avocado oil, enough water to make a paste, 1 drop Rose oil, and 1 drop Roman Chamomile oil.

    Mature: 1 level tablespoon Rose Clay, 1/2 tablespoon instant Oatmeal or finely ground regular Oatmeal, 1 teaspoon honey, 1 teaspoon Avocado or Olive oil, enough water to make a paste, add 1 drop Frankincense and 1 drop Rose, Neroli, or Lavender oil.

8. Aromatherapy facial oils consist of a blend of two parts. The first part is the base oil, which can be a singular plant oil or a blend of plant oils. The most popular oils for this purpose are: Apricot kernel, Almond, Hazelnut, Jojoba, Olive, Kukui nut, Macadamia nut, Squalane, Flax seed, and Calendula. These oils are emollient and rich in nutrients, and are well-suited for skin care. The second part is the chosen essential oil or blend of essential oils. The general proportions are 25 drops of essential oils to 2 ounces of base oil. This can be adjusted to suit the purpose.

Suggestions for Facial Oils

Normal: 1/4 ounce Jojoba oil, 3/4 ounce Sweet Almond oil, 8 drops Lavender, 4 drops Roman Chamomile.

Oily: 1 ounce Jojoba oil or Hazelnut oil, 8 drops Lavender, 2 drops Ylang-Ylang, 2 drops Lemongrass.

Dry: 3/4 ounce Apricot kernel oil, 1/4 ounce Avocado oil, 1 teaspoon Hazelnut oil, 8 drops Sandalwood, 4 drops Lavender.

Sensitive: 1/2 ounce Jojoba oil, 1/2 ounce Olive oil, 3 drops Rose, 3 drops Chamomile, 3 drops Neroli.

Blemished: 5 drops Tea Tree, 10 drops Lavender, 3 drops Chamomile, 1 drop Sandalwood. Mix essential oils into 2 ounces of Aloe Vera juice. Shake vigorously before applying to the blemished areas.

Mature: 1/2 ounce Jojoba oil, 1/2 ounce Hazelnut oil, 1 teaspoon Squalane, contents of one capsule of vitamin E, 8 drops Lavender, 2 drops Frankincense, 2 drops Helichrysum, 2 drops Carrot.

9. Aromatherapy body powder is commercially available (see Source List), or it can be easily made at home. To make a body powder especially for the feet, mix 1 cup cornstarch with 1 tablespoon baking soda (to neutralize odors) in a jar with a tight-fitting lid. Add 10 to 15 drops of your favorite essential oil(s) and shake well.

8

Aromatic Inspirations

Zia Wesley-Hosford

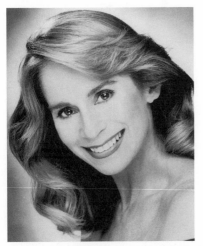

Zia Wesley-Hosford is a licensed skin care instructor, æsthetician, cosmetologist, and certified aromatherapist. She became involved in the cosmetics field twenty years ago when she was attempting to solve some of her own skin problems. She was introduced to European cosmetics made with botanicals, and was encouraged to investigate the link between skin problems and nutrition.

　　She graduated from the Vidal Sassoon Academy in San Francisco, opened a small salon, and began to create her own line of high-quality, natural cosmetics. She has written several best-selling books including her most recent title, *Fifty and Fabulous: Zia's Definitive Guide to Anti-Aging—Naturally.* In addition to heading Zia Cosmetics, Zia maintains her role as a skin care educator and evaluator of skin care products.

　　Currently living in San Francisco, Zia has been a regular guest on KGO Radio's "Ronn Owens Show" for ten years and has appeared as the resident skin-care expert on Seattle's "Northwest Afternoon" and Portland's "a.m. Northwest" television talk shows.

*M*y infatuation with the power and promise of aromatherapy began with a case of adult acne twenty years ago. After endless rounds of dermatologists and æstheticians, I met a woman in Beverly Hills who introduced me to a line of European cosmetics based on botanicals. For the very first time, I saw improvement in the condition of my skin. I was encouraged to explore further and began to study the interrelationship of herbs and nutrition, natural cosmetics, and personal health. Excited by the results of this holistic approach to skin care, I decided to pursue a career as a cosmetologist.

Not until I opened my own small salon, four years later, did I realize how few high-quality natural products were available. Many of my clients' skin problems were actually exacerbated by the commercial preparations being used, most of which commanded extremely high prices. I was enraged by what seemed to be a major consumer rip-off.

The most logical response was to translate my anger into advocacy and information, so over the next five years I wrote three books filled with skin- and body-care tips. I became a licensed skin-care instructor, teaching at a school in San Francisco and tracking the progress of my students' skin over time. As I discovered patterns and developed solutions, I tried them on my clients—with remarkable results. The homemade "recipes" I shared were the humble beginnings of Zia Cosmetics, now a thriving company offering more than thirty-two natural skin and make-up products based primarily on essential oils.

The Appeal of Ylang-Ylang

The very first product I formulated using essential oils was an aloe-based skin toner. I actually did this before having more than a strong interest in and attraction to essential oils and aromatherapy. Cypress oil, a vasoconstrictor with great restorative powers, was a primary ingredient in this toner from the beginning; its effect on broken capillaries is unsurpassed. However, I wanted the product to smell as wonderful as possible. In blending and testing over a hundred essential oils, I kept returning to Ylang-Ylang, which was ultimately my final choice. Several years later, after I had become quite proficient in the area of aromatherapy, I learned that Ylang-Ylang is regarded as a powerful aphrodisiac. Blended with Seaweed extract it makes a wonderful toner for the skin. A similar version for dry and aging skin can be made by adding Rose water, the classic rejuvenator.

Botanical Healing

Because they are able to penetrate the skin quickly and completely, essential oils can address the source of a problem, providing an effective response to dryness, oiliness, irritation, inflammation, or even simple aches and pains. This makes them an invaluable component of therapeutic skin solutions, effective for a variety of problems.

For instance, camphor has traditionally been used to constrict capillaries, calm oil glands, and promote healing; with this in mind, I developed a camphor treatment mask designed to soothe problem skin and spot-treat blemishes. Toxins are rapidly eliminated without dryness to the skin, which only encourages excess oil production.

A good moisturizing mask would contain a blend of Geranium, Lavender, and Matricaria. These are hydrating essential oils that help the skin retain moisture. As the mask is drawn into the skin, circulation and moisture content increase, plumping the skin and diminishing the appearance of fine lines.

For daily use, Chamomile, Lemon, Sandalwood, Geranium, and Lavender essential oils are added to an ultra-rich nourishing cream, to plump up the skin and stimulate circulation. This can be designed to be used day or night, as a nonocclusive moisturizer. It deals with both types of dryness—lack of oil and lack of water. Unlike heavier creams that might contain lanolin, such a mixture penetrates deeply to reverse the signs of aging and restore hydration. Each essential oil plays a role: Chamomile, a powerful healing ingredient, soothes dry, sensitive skin; Lemon brightens dull color and balances the pH; Lavender promotes healing by reducing scars and stimulating the growth of new cells while it helps to balance the skin's moisture content; Geranium controls sebum production, making it valuable for *all* skin types; and Sandalwood is a soothing antiseptic that encourages the skin to trap moisture. Together, these essential oils combine to create a powerful weapon against aging skin.

Moisturizers that contain essential oils penetrate the skin without clogging pores or leaving a greasy occlusive film. In this way, they provide a faster revitalization of damaged tissue. Zia Cosmetics' concentrated moisturizer includes liposomes as well as a nourishing combination of four essential oils guaranteed to heal. Carrot seed oil, which boosts cell production and restores elasticity, has been added to a blend of Chamomile, Lavender, and Ylang-Ylang to create a corrective deep treatment for dry and damaged skin. This particular formulation of essential oils combined with natural liposomes derived from Marigolds helps cells to regenerate quickly, creating a youthful, supple appearance in the skin.

Aromatherapy

The scent-ual quality of botanicals has provided another important ingredient for my cosmetics. The self-tanning creme began as an unscented product. Unfortunately, the natural odor of the tanning ingredient, dehydroxyacetone (DHA), was quite unpleasant. Reluctant to incorporate an artificial fragrance, or to use a fragrance-masking agent, we decided to combine the oils of Cedarwood, Lavandin, and Spearmint to create a pleasant natural scent.

The body moisturizer uses Geranium oil, Sandalwood, Palmarosa, and Ylang-Ylang for the same purpose.

And, as always, the inclusion of essential oils provides an additional bonus: only a very light preservative system needs to be used, as essential oils are potent enough to act as natural bactericides.

User-Friendly Combinations

By developing products to address specific conditions, Zia Cosmetics has tried to take a "user-friendly" approach to essential oils. Rather than marketing "neat" individual oils and suggesting combinations or blends, we have chosen to package pre-mixed formulations, hopefully eliminating some of the consumer's costs and guesswork in the process.

Aromatherapy Treatment Oils are a trio of essential oil blends, each designating a specific skin condition. Aromatherapy Treatment Oils for Hydration, for instance, is a deep therapeutic treatment for water-poor skin. Medicinal grade Geranium oil, Palmarosa, Lavender, Sandalwood, and Matricaria are combined in a base of cold-pressed safflower oil and squalene. Once again, no preservatives are needed. The oils are worked into the skin using a small amount of toner, and within fifteen minutes they penetrate the surface completely. Problems are addressed at a deep cellular level, restoring moisture and enhancing the skin's ability to retain it.

Remember that essential oils are a plant's immune system. In fact, as you probably already know, they are not really "oils" at all, but rather highly volatile fluids that evaporate quickly when exposed to heat or light. In the plant, the oils are located between cell walls and only utilized when the plant is in trouble—too dry, too wet, injured, or too hot. Under such circumstances, the cell walls allow penetration of the healing oils; once they have done their job, the cell walls close, returning to their former position. The particular way in which the oils function for the plant also dictates the proper way for humans to use them: to address a specific problem and quickly resolve it. After this initial treatment period, therapeutic dosages of oils should only be used on an as-needed basis or to treat the problem again, should it arise.

In this way, a teenager with acne could find long-term benefit from a week or two's use of Aromatherapy Treatment Oils for Oil Control. Morning applications of this product help to reduce the secretions of overly active oil glands, which can cause clogged or enlarged pores and breakouts. Extracts of Cajeput, Lemongrass, Lavender, Lemon Thyme, and Sage help to gently regulate internal oil production without drying the skin.

Those who suffer from oil-poor skin can find relief with nightly use of Aromatherapy Treatment Oils for Dry Skin. The stimulating extracts of Basil, Lemon, Rosewood, Vetiver, and Sage *(Salvia lavandulifolia)* activate the skin's oil glands to promote its own natural lubrication. Dry, papery skin with a chalky look begins to normalize; dull, dry skin is revitalized.

By marketing treatment-specific formulations, Zia Cosmetics hopes to broaden public understanding and increase consumer use of essential oils. Many consider aromatherapy a new-age phenomenon, but it is really a modern name for a type of botanical healing the oldest form of medicine.

See the Source List for the address of Zia Cosmetics products.

9

Bathing in the Souls of Flowers

Barbara Bobo

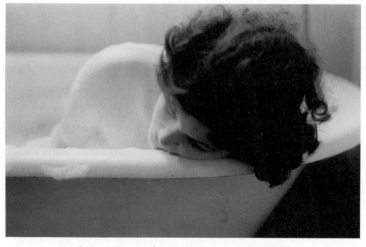

© Jane Grossenbacher, *Woman in the Bath*

Completing course work at Ohio Northern University, Dominion Herbal College, Wild Rose College of Natural Healing, and Original Swiss Aromatics, *Barbara Bobo* has studied the works of notable teachers and authors in the realms of both the Herbal and the Aromatic.

Barbara began selling her handmade soaps as Woodspirits Ltd. Inc. in 1988. Today, Woodspirits products are sold internationally and Woodspirits Ltd. Inc. employs five families including Barbara's, making 4,000 bars of soap weekly at each facility in the U.S. The families operate as independent contractors, running their own businesses from their farms.

Barbara loves to travel and is always interested in building bridges between various people and ideas. Barbara hopes to see a day when more essential oils are produced in America, on the small farms that seem to be vanishing today.

*P*aul Lee, a philosophical herbalist living on the West Coast, once said to me that if he could live his life over again, he would like to be illiterate. A shocking statement to hear from a Harvard Ph.D., but in the context of our conversation at the time—of how we had missed so much of life by being educated in closed classrooms with our noses pressed down onto the printed page—I understood perfectly. My education as an herbalist had been quite the same, reading stacks of books and papers and trying crude experiments with the rudimentary skills I had gleaned from my background in cooking and gardening.

I had no background in the practical use of herbal medicine. Ella Birzneck, my teacher from Dominion Herbal College in British Columbia, had grown up at the hem of her midwife/herbalist/bone-setter grandmother in Latvia. My grandmothers were totally devoted to allopathic medicine. Juliette Levy lived with the Gypsy bands and nomadic Bedouins! This was an adventure I could only read about in books.

Even Jeanne Rose lived near the epicenter of sixties hippie culture, Haight Ashbury. I stood under that famous street sign in 1989, and remarked to the passing throng, "Here I am, twenty years too late!" A voice from the crowd echoed, "No lady, you are just in time!" Well, the voice was prophetic, because in 1989 I was in San Francisco doing something useful and creative, and in 1969 I would have been a runaway, contributing nothing to society, only a burden for it to bear. In 1989 I had something beautiful and useful, and ecological as well.

Getting There

It was only after years of study and experiments that the adventure revealed itself to me. What I could do for herbal medicine was made clear. I realized that we all make our own history, our own adventure. Life is how we perceive it, and what we do with what we are given. I realized that I did not have to travel to Machu Picchu to become a spiritual person, that I did not have to live with the Gypsies to become an herbalist, that I could do something different and yet common, something plain, and yet exquisite.

Turning Point

After completing my work with Dominion Herbal College, I continued to operate my small herb shop, administer to the medical and dietary needs of my family and my farm animals with the herbal medicine that I had learned. But I also began to venture forth on wider business pursuits. My husband, pressed by our eldest son's imminent entry into college, saw the need to increase our income and suggested that I get a "real job." So I began to look for alternatives.

I started a business called "Herbalviews," publishing full-length interviews of herbalists. I had written articles for various newsletters, and thought perhaps there might be a need for this service. I had heard of an aromatherapy conference to be held in Santa Rosa, California, hosted by a now defunct group of aromatherapy enthusiasts. I contacted several editors of botanical newsletters, and they supported Herbalview's business plan. Upon arrival at the event, I ran into an herbalist friend who enthusiastically greeted me with, "Barbara, I just bought some of your soap in San Francisco, and it is really nice." I, disgracefully, it seems, now that I recall the incident, asked her not to make such a big deal over it because I wanted to be known as a writer and not a soap-maker.

As happens many times in life, one utters the most amazing revelations about one's inner thoughts and feelings. I was certainly surprised by my reaction for, as I began to think of it, the skin is surely the largest organ of the body, and the health of the skin is therefore inherently important to one's overall wellness. There it was, an adventure to be embarked upon. I could bring herbal medicine into everyone's daily ritual in small, wonderful delivery systems called soap.

History

This same trip was divided between attending the conference and introducing my soaps to a few large San Francisco health-food stores. This project began months before, when I had returned to San Francisco from a retreat in Oregon with Jeanne Rose and given her several bars of my soap. She had been my mentor for many years, and I was surprised when she walked into the room holding the bar of soap I had given her to her nose. She then told me this was very nice soap indeed, and if I were looking for a way to make money in the realm of herbs, I should sell this soap. Of course I did not take the recommendation lightly, coming as it was from someone who had been in the herbal products field for years.

Upon my return to San Francisco for the spring conference, I brought a satchel of soap with me to see what others thought of the product. Ms. Rose had given me a list of the stores she felt would be interested. Luckily, knowing very little about how to approach the stores was in my favor. Had I thought about it, I would probably have made appointments and, no doubt, never made it through what I now know can be an almost impenetrable web of red tape. I just brazenly marched in, wearing my jumper and flats and looking like the frazzled mother I am. I suppose they could spot me a mile away as a complete Midwestern bumpkin, so they knew it was a new product, and they liked what they saw and smelled.

And I sold! I only visited five stores on that trip, but three of them placed orders, and I was picking up some very good vibes. I reported back to Jeanne, and she chuckled about her predictions. I returned to Ohio thinking, "If they liked me in San Francisco, that means I have something hip, in, and hot!" So, even though I already had a lot of energy, it seemed to become supercharged with that trip.

What had begun in a kitchen with an enameled preserving kettle and the help of my friend and present accountant Sharon Hanlin, who had been making soap for a couple of years, had now grown into a business and a "real job." In reality, it has grown into a lot of "real jobs" for several families.

Soap touches thousands with its incredible alchemy with water, every day and every night, in the most intimate way possible. How many things does one rub all over one's body when completely naked?! I had brought herbal medicine into a daily ritual. We made it possible for the "great unwashed" to experience the plants we loved. Within the ancient realm of bathing, we brought our aromatherapy soaps to the altar of modern daily life!

The Bath as an Experience

One of my customers confided in me that we are "bath whores," and we laughed about it, but knew it was quite true—we will give anything for a bath! We will assemble an incredible array of objects, candles, potions, and paraphernalia tub-side. To spend an inordinate amount of time soaking and sluicing about is quite normal for us. No soap or bubble bath from the dime or discount store would touch our tender parts! We are *collectors*, exhibiting the most discriminating taste in bathtub accoutrements!

Anything French seems to pass the test, at least at first, until one discovers that some of the greatest adulterators in history have been French! We seek out the most obscure mixtures—for example, a peat moss bath that looks like we're step-ping into a swamp pool in darkest Louisiana. The search for the perfect bathing sauces and utensils is never ending. We know we will never accomplish the task because the "bath whores" who concoct this sea of nostrums are just as avid in seeking to create the perfect mix as we are in finding it! As a "bath whore" I have been refining my craft over the years, and you may enjoy a glimpse into my watery world of "The Bath."

I have been designing a relaxing living area in the rear garden of my Ohio countryside home, complete with a hanging bed draped with quilts, and crowned with mosquito netting, for afternoon naps and serious sleeping as well. I have also been working on a new "pool" garden: a limestone terrace surrounding a large pool for koi and various ornamental fish, as well as interesting aquatic botanicals. This pond is surrounded with ferns and flowering plants, mainly in pinks and fuchsia colors, with an occasional sunflower that my wild birds have planted. I also raise African ringneck doves for their beautiful ashy-mauve feathers and restful cooing. These doves are released into my garden once they are fledged, and add to the serene movement of the garden.

The garden is walled, and two of the walls form the sides of a low building where I manufacture my fine soaps. The structure is a typical Ohio farm building built in the early forties, now painted deep red with a green metal roof. The rain on the tin roof adds a soothing sound as well. Jasmine, in a large pot that can be taken indoors, still at the head of the hanging bed, adds to the scent of the garden along with Tuberoses, Dr. Van Fleet Roses, Lavenders, Mints, and Lemon Verbena. I may add other scented plants according to the season and what my travels and reading may glean from nature's perfumes. Brushing against the Mint that overhangs the flagstone path on the way to my bath yields a wonderful welcoming scent.

The low building I have described is in the shape of an "L," and in the inside corner of the "L" is my outdoor tub. Made from a black plastic livestock watering tub, it will comfortably hold two people, but a single bather is usually the case, that one being me, after working in my vegetable gardens, milking my goats, or making 2,000 bars of soap with my family on soap-making night. The hot water is supplied from the same in-line continuous water heater we use inside the building to generate the hot water in our soapworks.

The tub is oval-shaped, and if one sits in the bottom, the water can reach nearly up to one's chin! I have installed a "bench" in the center, which is simply a 2" x 6" board resting on the inner contours of the sides of the tub. The original drain is made to connect to a garden hose, but I had my handyman connect it to the septic system with a regular drain in the bottom, like an indoor tub. The tub is set into an unpainted Cedarwood surround, with recessed lights for very soft lighting at night. Part of the surround extends along the wall to form a bench for dressing and resting. Decorative tin hooks in the form of black stars are attached to the wall above the bench to hold towels.

To the right of the front of the tub is a lovely locust tree, its fern-like foliage shimmering and rustling in the softest breeze. From one of its branches I have hung a special wind chime that imitates the bells of Westminster Abbey in London. I have friends living there, and this reminds me of them. I have also planted a few plants in the garden that I first saw in their gardens.

I often incorporate special botanicals as mental and emotional bookmarks in my garden. Cosmos, with their hot pink blooms, remind me of my mother's garden in the flourescent sixties, and wild Geraniums are a reminder of the garden at the house at Hither Green, where we stayed with my friends Liz and Karen in London while setting up our British franchise. My franchisee, Nickki, joked that the only thing she ever grew was Moss on the windowsill of her flat, and the sight of Moss now reminds me of her as well. To see or smell a flower causes thoughts and emotions to turn! I have placed a small rustic cabinet on the wall above the tub to hold related objects—razors, soaps, the tub stopper—but the area around my outdoor tub soon became cluttered with other more aesthetic accoutrements to the bath. This is where I test my Scented Salt Scrubs, an exfoliating mixture of salt, food-grade vegetable oil, pigments, and essential oils designed to match my soaps.

I have begun to affix special bottles to the masonry portion of the wall as well. I am always finding something pretty wherever I go, and cannot resist anything that might be a container for a lotion or a shampoo! Perfume bottles, some still containing their contents, and even the unusual mineral bottle all remind me of pleasant trips and friends. In front of the tub rests a large flat rock, a comfortable place to stand to disrobe. Even though the lighting is diffused, I generally use a variety of flickering beeswax candles to make my scene more genial. A large clump of Bamboo stands in front of the corner tub to shield it from the direct view of my back porch outdoor bedroom. Its interesting leaves and stems provide an undulating screen for privacy. At the base of this Bamboo screen is a large dome of a rock, like a low stool, with an antique incense burner on its summit. If the night is still, the smoke from the incense is a wonderful fantasy of smoke-shapes and ribbons. I realized, while watching this smoke once, that my earlier habit of cigarette smoking was probably induced by the hypnotic effect of watching my grandfather's cigars and my father's pipe smoke!

Planted near the tub is another favorite plant, the Scouring Rush, or *Equisetum hyemale*. Its long primitive green stems are evocative of the serpent, and every garden should have a serpent! Moreover, it reminds me once again of water and the trips to a beautiful garden near the Atlantic Coast in South Carolina, Brookgreen Gardens, where my family spent many happy hours meandering the paths and enjoying the sculpture gardens and poetry of that lovely place. The *Equisetum* at Brookgreen inhabits the central pool, which is raised to around four feet and consists of old mossy bricks, dripping with water and further cooling the air. In the center of this large circular pool is a nearly life-size stylized sculpture of a man wrestling an alligator! In boxes near the edge stands the thick green bristling tufts of *Equisetum*, a beautiful frame for this exotic scene. So I have brought this common pond-side "water feed" to my own garden as a reminder of the beautiful places I've visited! When the stand becomes thick enough, I will place lighting near the ground, shining up into the eaves of the soapworks.

Under these eaves I have begun to hang some of my favorite "water art." So far my collection only includes posters of *The Bath* by Jean-Leon Gerome, which hangs in The Fine Arts Museum of San Francisco, and *La Naissance de Venus* by William Bouguereau, currently hanging in the Musée d'Orsay in Paris. As this little art gallery is outside, attached to a wooden wall, under the protective eaves of my soapworks, I am using museum posters that I have laminated and stapled to the wall. Very inexpensive, as far as art goes, but quite a nice addition to my garden bathing area. I intend to track down other worthy bathing and water art for my work-in-progress. Much of this art is contained in a most interesting book titled *Taking the Waters* by Alev Lytle Croutier.

Elsewhere in the garden, a "traveling exhibit" until I find the perfect spot, is my four-foot limestone fish sculpture, a twenty-fifth anniversary present from my husband, Alan. "The Fish" forever surfs upon a limestone river. He was carved by my artist friend Chris Berti, whom I met through my artist niece Laura O'Donnell.

So it is in this lovely garden that I occasionally bathe in the quiet seasons of Ohio evenings. Amidst warm water and soft chiming cathedral bells, incense, candles, and cooing doves I bathe, with my own soaps and interesting new products in-testing. In the summer, spring, and fall, there are waving green plants, cooing birds, and frog-song issuing from the koi pond. In winter, clouds of steam and icicles from the overhanging eaves provide a refreshing contrast and remind me of the summer Alan and I sat in a heated pool in the Canadian Rockies while an icy mist laced our damp hair!

Yes, winter is a special time because the little Cedarwood sauna serves as a late night or early evening spot for relaxation, where rubbing snow on our sweating limbs and face is most invigorating. I have not introduced essential oils into my sauna, as I enjoy the fresh scent of the Cedarwood itself. As age dilutes its scent, I will undoubtedly begin anointing the wood with Cedarwood oil. It is to me a more pleasing smell for this area of the world than the more often used Eucalyptus. Inside the sauna I hang pages from interesting calendars. Currently there are pictures of lovely old barns that remind me of our vanishing architecture. My ancestors lived in Switzerland, and their houses and barns are still standing today, monuments of efficiency and beauty. When our Midwestern barns are gone, we will understand why we should have saved them, but many are now left to rot or are sold for their hardwood timbers.

Working

For me, the most exciting thing about working with the essential oils of plants is its similarity to working with the plants themselves. They are indeed subtle and surprising. When you work with a living plant you are aware of its fragility, its beauty, and its strength. With an essential oil, you can only experience its character, or soul if you will, like someone you have only met on the telephone, yet someone who has called you with very personal news. It is a very sensual experience at times, and other experiences bring on bright, pleasant thoughts, like an old friend calling. Never is it a wrong number or unpleasant. Even Galbanum *(Ferula galbaniflua)* stirs up an emotion of fresh, warm earth and adventure.

When I sign my business correspondence I sometimes print under my name the title "Formulator"—I love the sound of that! But honestly, I think the word "concoctor" fits more appropriately. I have amassed quite an array of scents in my little "cellar of scents" by now, but I think what truly guides my choice is a host of ethereal spirits—well, yes—the *woodspirits*. Did I hear some of my teachers moaning, "Didn't she learn anything from all of our words and books?" Yes, I did, but after all of the studying, as in Paul Lee's wish, I practice being illiterate.

Once, as a student of art in my college days, one of my professors was complaining that no one was drawing enough plans before they began their painting. So I tacked at least fifty sketches onto the walls of my studio until that same professor, who might have thought I was mocking him, walked in one day and said, "Okay, already, *paint!*" I must admit it was one of my better works—and it is true that a lot of work goes on before the gears start to turn. Life is always a work in progress and, luckily age was a valued asset in the family I grew up in. With a foundation of study in herbs and their essential oils, now I paint!

I remember when I first started to see the potential in essential oils and aromatherapy. In my small herb shop, and in lectures and classes, I had extolled the

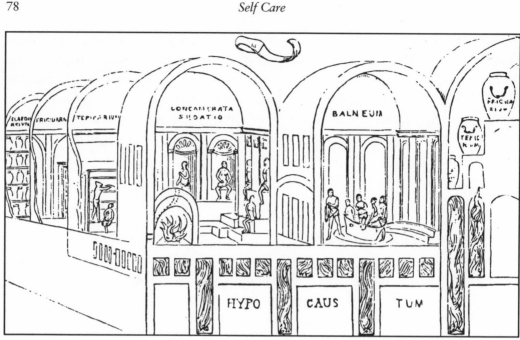

Roman baths

many amazing qualities of simple herbal remedies, and had sold a quantity of teas, salves, and capsules. It always struck me as odd that people would ponder long and hard before swallowing a tea or capsule—but would rub onto their skins, or sniff deeply, anything I offered them in a bottle or jar. They did not appreciate the medical fact that the fastest route to the blood stream is not to inject, but to inhale!

Customers would protest that they only wanted cheap synthetic fragrance oils because they were going to make potpourri for Christmas gifts, and that it did not have to be an expensive essential oil. What an interesting concept! At the most important gift-giving time of year they would combine their precious flowers they had sweated over all spring and summer, only to pollute their labors and the air with toxic, unknown synthetic imitators—well, clearly there had to be another way.

Another event galvanized my thinking on the term "natural product." A neighboring farmer had helped my sons unload a truckload of straw, and as a "thank you" I offered to show him our little soapworks and gave him a few bars of soap. As I was loading him down with free samples, I was delivering my "all natural" speech. At the word *"natural,"* he interrupted to say that he would give this stuff to a lady at work who, in his words, "Thought everything should be natural." These words, coming from a farmer, were amazing. Here was a producer of natural products who did not perceive them as such. He clearly did not understand that we were engaged in marketing the same product; mine perhaps was a "finished product," of course, but what is more natural than Oats, Straw, Hay, Soybeans, and Corn?

My soap does not contain any of these plants, but does contain natural agricultural products from small agricultural holdings around the world that are traded globally on the commodities market daily, right beside his products. I began to think of the ways my products could affect the global scheme of things—for farmers were indeed producing my raw materials. It was important to me that these small farms, producing these fine essential oils and Coconut and Olive oils, would remain viable, not just so that I could profit from the sale of my soaps but because these raw materials are so well-made and beautiful.

I, too, am aware of the skill needed to produce essential oils and fine vegetable oils. These skills may not be widely available outside the families who have practiced them, with much trial and error, throughout many generations of growing and distilling. Small farms are the backbone of any civilization. The ability to grow food and other raw materials is crucial to economic stability. It is not a radical statement that when a group of people are not agriculturally self-sufficient and can no longer feed themselves, they become "political orphans," dependent upon other groups who can. These orphans then become "disposables"—they have moved off of the small holdings of land, and into the overcrowded cities where their skills are not utilized. What once was a self-sufficient, highly skilled, independent business man/woman/family now has to start over in a city already teeming with others in similar dire straits.

Perhaps this simplistic view would not stand with those who make a life work studying population trends and displaced peoples. But I do know that small agriculture is efficient, and produces superior results to large scale agribusiness, as it is now called.

Upon realizing this, I became acutely aware of the importance of incorporating "agricultural products" into as many consumer expendable goods as possible. The image "natural" has in our world is somewhat negative to certain portions of the populace. These are the people I wanted to reach; they are the key in the lock that would open the door to "Gaia" living. We need to convince them that living "naturally" is not simply trendy—it means survival. Recently, I saw a large roadside sign at an agricultural experiment station in northern Ohio that in three-foot letters declared, "Agriculture Grows Your Food," tempting me to add a mental graffiti note: "Agriculture could grow your clothing fabrics, body care, fuel, medicines, and more!" Farming saves lives, globally!

Delivering the Goods

I also realized several years ago that people sometimes buy a product because they have been educated about it, and sometimes they just like it and really don't know why. Both are valid reasons. Educating takes a lot of time. I love educating, but I understand simply "liking" too. Science tells us there is a primitive being inside us. They have sometimes used the term "limbic system," which is an easily remembered term, but does not carry the intrinsic shock value of their other name for this system, "reptilian brain." I rather like the latter term because it means something. If you do not have an abnormal repulsion for reptiles, you can understand that the function of the "reptilian brain" is to control basic functions just to keep us alive. That knowledge, paired with the anatomical exclamation point of the olfactory nerve being the shortest nerve in the body, going from the exposed mucosa of the nose directly into the deepest reaches of the brain, is a scientific explosion!

Scratch and Sniff

What does this say about humans, and all other animals as well? Smelling is important—*important*. Maybe even life saving. The studies on human pheromones bear out the likelihood that problems with infertility have links to our American pastime of scrubbing and anointing ourselves with every known synthetic ever concocted so that we won't *smell!* "I *smell*, therefore I *am*" should be our mantra! Actually, I do not like the smell of old human sweat, but our more subtle smells, the ones we aren't aware of, are probably most important.

I am always surrounded by smells, good and not-so-good. Because of my soap business, my house leaves a trail of scent up and down our road. The local hardware staff can smell my family members before they spot us in the crowded aisle of their burgeoning shop! My franchisee, Nickki Clark in London, was betrayed by scent when she sent an anonymous Valentine's card to a new beau! She was shocked, but I reminded her of how strong the scent of our little factory seemed when she first came to work with us, and how her little workroom in England drew people in off the street with the power of its scent. Even the little Skye Terrier "Jasper" trotted in to check us out when we first started pouring the essential oils around. Was he expecting to find an amazing garden?

Scent

Scent moves us all in the most fundamental ways. We cannot for one moment understand it. Yet we also cannot help but be mesmerized by its power. No one will deny the emotional tide that washes over us when we smell our newborn children, or get a whiff of our grandmother's bedroom. It is more fleeting perhaps than the sound of a favorite oldies tune, but it is more powerful.

Writers have written about it. Marcel Proust is probably the most famous one. But we all experience scent every day. Scent is so much a part of our safety mechanism that we frantically search the house, attic to cellar, when we smell hot plastic or "electrical" scent! We may avoid the perfume-spritzer girl at the mall, but we never avoid the smell of a home-cooked meal, or even the neighbor's barbecue. 'Fess up, all you vegetarians, it smells good to you too! That damn lizard brain!

I wanted people to use plants for medicine, because it works, and because it is a wonderful way to live. It also supports some wonderful people. Just as there is a reptile inside of everyone's brain, there is also a farmer. A cartoon rendition: Barney with a pitchfork! Everyone I have known in my life has liked to grow something once in a while. My maternal grandparents were successful farmers. My mother's house is filled with amazing house plants, some of which she grows from garbage (Avocado and Orange trees). All of my brothers and my sister garden. They also husband a few animals. My father, husband, brother, and brother-in-law are all tree planters. I don't know anyone who doesn't have at least a snakeplant in his or her home. We are all farmers.

We are all artists too. We all appreciate the colors and sounds and natural movements in our environment. Scent, that provocative telephone call from Barney with his pitchfork, calls us to garden, to farm, to cultivate. Scent, I believe, is the ultimate survival tool we humans have to preserve our continuance on the Earth. I do believe, as others do, that the Earth is mighty, and we will never bring her lazy heavenly roll to a halt; but we may indeed bring ourselves to an unnecessary end. Believe in what you do. Do something simple. Work hard, be kind, be honest with yourself and others. Be strong.

Epilogue

I do hope, dear reader, that you have not expected lists of essential oils and recipes, for you know, greater minds than mine have written all you need to know and are still writing! Please use every book located in the bibliography and you will expand your knowledge of aromatherapy and soap-making beyond even my own.

Acknowledgments

There is a bibliography in everyone's life that plots a map of one's personal, physical, and spiritual development. A bibliography of books, human encounters, and events. But, as far as my life in aromatherapy (or more correctly, herbalism) goes, certain names and books are easy to cite. Some of my favorite authors have passed from the Earth, but others live among us and have become cherished friends and acquaintances. I would like to acknowledge all of the people who have worked with my soap company in all of its aspects. And a special thanks to Jeanne Rose for saying to me, "You know, Barbara, you should sell this soap; it is really very good!" She has been my mentor, advisor, and formulator of some of our most popular soaps, but most of all a steadfast friend.

10

Your Medicine Tin of Five Essential Oils

Candace Welsh

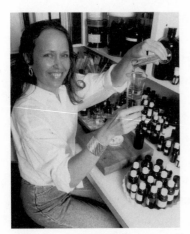

Candace Welsh holds a Master of Arts in Teaching and is a licensed massage therapist in the state of Florida, as well as nationally. She attended the Sarasota School of Natural Healing Arts. Her aromatherapy diplomas are from Joy Johnston of Canada, Dr. Dietrich Gumbel of Germany, Dr. Kurt Schnaubelt of California, Micheline Arcier of London, and Eve Taylor of London, England.

Manual lymph-drainage training from Hildegard Wittlinger of Dr. Vodder's School in Austria has also enhanced this work, as well as healing-touch training through the American Holistic Nurses' Association. Candace is currently on staff at the Florida Academy of Massage in Fort Meyers and Naples, Florida, as the aromatherapy instructor.

As "Oil Lady Aromatherapy," Candace gives aromatherapy treatments, does consultations and custom blending by appointment, lectures, and holds selective workshops on the "Medicine of Essential Oils" and "Touch with Oils."

"Your servant has nothing there at all," she said, "except a little oil."
—2 Kings 4:2

*T*he scope of aromatherapy is a vast field of study, reaching in many directions, and can be quite mind-boggling. There are well over four hundred essential oils. Understanding their qualities and practical uses can be a bit overwhelming at times for the beginner.

Essential oils are "essential" to the overall state of physical, mental, emotional, and spiritual health. It is crucial to the whole sense of well-being to have a few essential oils, and the understanding of their usage in the daily routines of life. One does not need to become an aromatherapist and work with dozens of oils to benefit from these precious liquids that nature so reverently provides for us. There are five major essential oils that serve as valuable medicine tools to enhance daily living.

Nature's essential oils are extracted from some part of a plant or tree through skillful and delicate processes of growing, picking, and extracting. They are like wine in the sense that wine is the juice from a grape. Although they are not plant juices, essential oils are fluids from some part of a plant. There are varying grades of essential oil quality based on environment, care, and processing.

Essential oils contain properties that make them good medicine. Many oils are antibacterial, antiviral, and antifungal. Because they also happen to smell so intensely, and because the olfactory tract connects directly to the brain, essential oils take the user's health to another dimension by affecting thoughts, memories, and emotions. Chemistry and aroma are what make essential oils profoundly valuable in enhancing health and vitality. They offer physical healing of the bodily tissue, and tremendous emotional comfort.

Through many years of practice, I have realized that with the use of a few essential oils, life is enriched and challenges can be met more effectively. The following five essential oils, a base oil, a mister, and a cotton compress cloth are the components of the medicine tin of essential oils. These items provide the tools needed to work out of the palm of the hand at home, as well as in our travels. Since essential oils are highly volatile, it is beneficial to keep them in dark bottles by themselves or in a clear bottle in a dark container. This way you make up what you need in the palm of your hand with some base oil as needed.

This chapter is devoted to the explanation of these five oils, their therapeutic properties, and what they can do for us. The best way to learn anything is to experience it first hand, so use these oils and note how you think and feel. You will come to know their value.

The Medicine Tin of Five Essential Oils

Lavender
(Lavandula angustifolia): the balancing oil

- the most versatile and useful essential oil
- the classical oil for a mental state of well-being

Properties
- antibacterial, antiinflammatory, analgesic, antirheumatic, sedative
- helps regulate nervous system, high blood pressure, blood sugar level
- tonic, astringent, restorative
- helps relieve stress, fatigue, and depression

Most Common Uses
1. *Burns, cuts, bites, bruises.* Apply 1 drop neat every ten to fifteen minutes as pain demands. After discomfort is gone or area is dried up, apply Lavender in base oil, or open a vitamin E capsule in your palm and add 1 drop Lavender. Use this as a healing salve.
2. *Wounds.* Wash with compress cloth to clean and disinfect, can also add 1 drop of straight Lavender to the skin around the outside of the wound. Do not use base oil with Lavender when the area is still wet. This keeps oxygen from getting to the area for healing. Add Lavender to base oil when area has dried up to help eliminate scarring.
3. *Headaches, stress, anxiety, depression, fatigue, insomnia.* Inhale from bottle; compress; use in bath; massage with base oil. Put one drop on pillow at night.
4. *Aches and pains.* Compress; bath; massage with base oil.
5. *Motion sickness.* Inhale from bottle; apply diluted to nose with base oil; can also add Peppermint.
6. *Metabolism, blood sugar or blood pressure imbalances.* Inhale from bottle; make palm blend with base oil and apply to nose.
7. *Purify air.* Inhale from bottle; use a mister or a diffusor. I keep a bottle of Lavender in my purse and another bottle in my kitchen cabinet. It continually amazes me how beautifully helpful this oil is for just about everything.

Tea Tree
(Melaleuca alternifolia): the oil of first aid

- the most versatile oil for all infections

Properties
- antibacterial, antiviral, antifungal
- tonic, astringent, stimulant

Most Common Uses
1. *Cuts, stings, bites.* 1 drop straight, every ten to fifteen minutes until discomfort is gone.
2. *Infections of all kinds.* 1 drop straight; compresses; make palm blend with base oil and rub on infected area (if area is not wet from infection).
3. *Acne.* 1 drop neat; use sparingly and cautiously.
4. *Athlete's foot, nail-bed fungus.* 1 drop neat; add to foot bath; massage by adding 1 drop to base oil in palm (if area infected is not wet from infection).
5. *Colds, flu, sore throat.* Inhale from bottle; use in bath or steam tent; massage by adding 1 drop to base oil in palm (if area infected is not wet from infection).
6. *Scalp infections.* Add 1 drop to shampoo in palm; also good with pet shampoos to enrich hair and skin.
7. *Mouth, gum, toothache, infections.* 1 drop straight on gum or lip; make palm blend with base oil and rub on gums; periodically add 1 drop to a little water and use as mouthwash; periodically add a couple drops to water in water-pik. Living in Florida has given me the wisdom that Tea Tree is the best choice for mosquito and red-ant bites. Put 1 drop on the bite right away, and add another as itching and discomfort demands.

Peppermint
(Mentha x piperita): the oil of digestion

- general tonic, refreshing and invigorating
- normalizing effect on stomach and head conditions
- promotes calm vitality due to a cooling and warming effect from its high menthol content

Properties
- antibacterial, antispasmodic, antiviral
- can be stimulating or calming (correct dosage is essential), can put us to sleep at night or wake us up during the day
- stimulates blood circulation and lymph flow, and helps detoxify connective tissue
- may irritate skin if applied directly; always blend with base oil

Most Common Uses
1. *Stomachache, sluggish digestion, flatulence.* Blend 1 drop with base oil in palm, apply to nose and massage abdomen in clockwise, circular, slow motion.
2. *Headache.* Inhale from bottle; blend with base oil and massage neck, head, shoulders, and abdomen; steam tent.
3. *Sinus, cold, flu.* Inhale from bottle; steam tent; bath; blend with base oil and massage nose, neck, and chest. Eucalyptus and Tea Tree can be combined with the Peppermint.
4. *Motion sickness.* Inhale from bottle; make palm blend and apply to nose, temples, ears, and abdomen. Lavender can also be used.
5. *General fatigue or sluggish mind.* Inhale from bottle; bath; massage.
6. *Aching body from sports or fever.* Combine with base oil and massage area. Eucalyptus can be added.
7. *In Ayurvedic medicine.* A Pitta-balancing oil, due to its cooling effect and sweet essence.

Peppermint is the oil I keep at my writing table. Periodically I pick up the bottle of pure Peppermint and simply inhale. It instantly clears my head, fights off mental sluggishness, and stimulates my creativity. This precious oil keeps me alert, clear, and focused. I am thankful for what it has added to my life.

Eucalyptus
(Eucalyptus radiata): the oil of respiration

There are many varieties of Eucalyptus. The most versatile are *Eucalyptus globulus* and *Eucalyptus radiata*. Either is quite acceptable. I use *E. radiata* in my medicine tin, because it is a little gentler, has a softer smell, and children prefer it.

Properties
- antibacterial, antiviral
- stimulates fluid circulation
- aids breathing

Most Common Uses
1. *Colds, flu, bronchitis, asthma.* Inhale from bottle; steam tent; baths; combine 1 drop with base oil in palm and apply to nose and use as chest rub. Before bed put 2 drops neat Eucalyptus on soles of each foot, and wear socks.
2. *Sinus infection.* Inhale from bottle; steam tent; combine with base oil and apply on and in nose; massage sinus areas above and below eyebrows, below cheekbones, and temples. Peppermint can be added.
3. *Joint aches and pains.* Combine with base oil and rub affected areas. Lavender or Peppermint can be added.
4. *Sore throat.* Steam tent, breathing through mouth. Make palm blend with base oil and massage ears, neck, and chest. Peppermint and Tea Tree can be added.
5. *Purify air.* Add to diffusor.
6. *Good morning oil.* Use after shower in the morning to breathe in the new day, to stimulate body functions, and protect your health. Breath brings in oxygen; oxygen gives life.
7. *In Ayurvedic medicine.* A Kapha-balancing oil due to its warm, spicy, stimulating effect.

"Eucalyptus" your way through the winter to keep yourself healthy. Apply a palm blend of base oil and 1 drop Eucalyptus to your nose and do a chest rub as well. Breathe and rest.

Orange Peel
(Citrus aurantium): the oil of tranquility

- cold pressed from the rind of the fruit (1,000 oranges make 2.5 cups of essential oil).
- sweet, warming oil promotes a feeling of well-being
- calms the nerves, soothes the heart rhythms

Properties
- antiseptic, antidepressant, anti-anxiety
- harmonizing to the body and mind
- may irritate skin if applied directly. Always blend with base oil. Do not use prior to sun exposure.
- good oil for children and older people, and all people who like the smell!

Most Common Uses
1. *Anxiety, depression, nervous condition.* Inhale from the bottle; combine 1 drop in base oil in palm and apply to nose; massage neck, abdomen, and lower back. Lavender can be added.
2. *Children.* Pour base oil into palm of hand, and 1 drop Orange (or 1 drop Orange and 1 drop Lavender) and apply a little to nose for a wonderfully calming effect at bedtime. Experiment to find out if rubbing hands, feet abdomen, or back is most relaxing, as this varies with the individual.
3. *Sleeplessness.* Combine with base oil for bath or abdomen massage; can also put in a diffusor with Lavender.
4. *Sluggish stomach.* Make palm blend with base oil and rub in a clockwise, circular motion on abdomen. Can add Peppermint or Lavender. This three-oil blend is delicious!
5. *Dry, aging skin.* Add 1 drop to body lotion in palm, or in a massage with base oil.
6. *Good night oil.* Use in bath or after shower to slow down and nurture self. Add Lavender, too.
7. *In Ayurvedic medicine.* A Vata-balancing oil due to its sweet, warming effect. A lady who owns a Montessori school makes a blend of Lavender and Orange at nap time, and has each child apply a little to his or her nose. Nap time finally became a real nap time.

Guide for Using Essential Oil in Your Daily Living

1. *Inhalation.* Breathe straight from the bottle, in a diffusor, or make a steam tent.

   To make a steam tent, boil water and pour it in a bowl, with 4 to 6 drops of straight essential oil. Close your eyes and inhale through the nose to treat sinuses or headache, or mouth to treat a sore throat or bronchitis. Inhale for

15 to 20 minutes. Put a towel over your head and bowl, forming a "tent" after the first few breaths. Massage back of neck during inhalation of oils.

2. *Compresses.* Apply to cuts, wounds, and skin problems. This disinfects and promotes cell regeneration.

   To make a compress, add 4 to 6 drops of essential oils to a half-cup of water, and mix well. Place a cotton handkerchief or cloth in the water to absorb the solution. Wash the cuts, or place the cloth on the skin and cover with plastic and a towel for approximately twenty minutes, or as long as is appropriate.

3. *Bath.* Consider baths as an ancient and therapeutic healing art. Nurture yourself with a soak for approximately fifteen to twenty minutes, three to four times a week.

   There are several methods for using essential oils in the bath.

   a. *Pure essential oil bath.* Make bath and get in, add 8 to 12 drops in water around you, swish and relax. Some oils, such as Orange and Peppermint, are too strong to be used in this way and may irritate the skin. Lavender is best for this.

   b. *Custom blend or palm blend bath.* After making your bath, make a small amount of essential oil blend, or palm blend diluted in vegetable oil. Massage the blend on/in nose, temples, back of neck, chest, solar plexus (abdominal area), and lower back, then get in the bath. Reapply the blend to chest and cover with warm washcloth. Close your eyes, breathe, and rest!

   c. *Hand or foot bath.* Use 6 to 8 drops of pure essential oils in a hand or foot bath. Tea Tree and Lavender are excellent. Make a foot massage blend in palm with a base oil, 1 drop Tea Tree and 1 drop Lavender.

4. *Shower.* Use custom blend or palm blend. Turn the water off, apply the oil blend while you are still wet, then towel off excess oil and water. A little oil can go a long way and should be massaged in thoroughly. Always apply a little to the nose first. Stimulating oils such as Eucalyptus and Peppermint are good in the morning; calming ones such as Lavender and Orange are good for the evening. Avoid applying oil to the soles of the feet, to prevent slip-sliding around on the tiles.

5. *Massage.* This reminds us of the tremendous healing powers of touch that have been practiced for centuries. Use a palm blend or a custom blend in the following ways:

   a. *Self massage.* With the blend in your palm, rub palms together and first apply some oil on and just inside the nose. Then work the temples, around the ears, and on the neck. The purpose is to make the nose-brain connection first. As the mind shifts, the body will follow. Additional significant areas for applying oils to your own body are chest, abdomen, low back, hands, and feet.

   b. *Massaging others.* With the blend in your palm, have them dip their finger in the oil and apply some on and just inside their nose. Then rub your palms together and apply oil around their ears and neck. Essential areas are hands, feet, head, back, or abdomen.

6. *Lavender mist.* Spray your face at any time throughout the day to cleanse, refresh, vitalize, and hydrate. The antibacterial properties of Lavender help clear the air and keep one healthy. A Lavender spritz is excellent to use while traveling in airplanes, cars, and in any confined spaces like offices, and is also good for sunburn relief, mouth spray, and hand spray. It is a useful application before or after make-up. The finer the mist, the better the effect.

   To make the Lavender spritz, add 2 drops of essential oil for every one ounce of pure water. Distilled water is preferable. Shake well before each misting, because essential oils alone do not mix with water. The Lavender mist is available in the medicine tin listed at the end of this chapter and contains distilled water, aloe juice, vegetable glycerin, and pure Lavender essential oil.

Measuring Oils

Combining these precious liquids means knowing that stronger is not better. Dosage is crucial. Too much of anything can be detrimental to our system and our environment and essential oils are potent. Overload gives us the opposite effect of what we set out to do.

The following measurements are very general guidelines to help you use your oils. Some essential oils are stronger than others. There is no set amount that fits all situations. For example, since Peppermint is very intense, and Orange is very sweet, 1 drop of Peppermint or Orange would suffice where 2 drops of Lavender might be used.

1. *Palm Blend.* Pour a good base oil in the well of your palm, add 1 or 2 drops total of essential oil.
2. *One Teaspoon.* Fill with base oil, add 2 to 3 drops total of essential oil.
3. *One Tablespoon.* Fill with base oil, add 4 or 5 drops total of essential oil.
4. *Shot Glass (one-half ounce).* Fill with base oil, add 6 to 8 drops total of essential oil.
5. *One ounce bottle.* Fill with base oil, add 10 to 15 drops total of essential oil.
6. *Two ounce bottle (or make in glass measuring cup).* Fill with base oil, add 15 to 20 drops total of essential oil.
7. *Palm healing salve.* Break open a capsule of vitamin E in palm, add 1 drop Lavender or Tea Tree. Good for healing skin abrasions after the wetness of infection is gone.

Additional Notes

- Use one-half dosage of essential oil drops for children (one drop in palm blend).
- Use palm blend for self-massage or when massaging another's hands, feet, head, back, or abdomen. The amount of oil that fits in your palm is enough to do that body part. There should be no extra oil on the skin when you are done. Rub it all in.
- Use the purest grade vegetable or nut oil you can find as your base oil. I use Jojoba oil because it is actually a liquid wax, wonderful for the skin (face too!), and does not go rancid.
- Remember essential oils are fat-soluble, not water-soluble.

Care of Products

Essential oils should be kept out of direct sunlight and excessive heat. Replace cap securely to avoid oxidation, and do not transfer to plastic bottles. Use the blends with base oils within a few months, although many will last longer. Pure essential oils, not blended in base oils, will keep for years if not exposed to heat, light, and air.

Some essential oils improve with age, others deteriorate. Change of color and putrid aroma are indicators. They are highly concentrated, should be used sparingly, and not used undiluted on skin. The exception is one drop of Lavender or

Tea Tree on burns, cuts, and bites. None of the products should be taken internally. Rinse out amber bottles with rubbing alcohol, then wash with hot water and soap, allow them to dry thoroughly, and reuse!

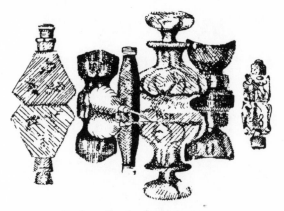

Perfume Bottles, by M.S. Moore

"Comforting" is one of the best words to describe the effects of essential oils. They are a liquid that provides a soothing mental and physical effect throughout life. They have helped me through two operations, menopause, and extreme fatigue. I've seen them help people through grief, loss, depression, and stress. They are a great comfort in times of change in life, birth, death, relationships, jobs, and in the aging process. Life is one change after another, and as long as we are alive, we will be changing. Essential oils are the liquids that help us flow through these changes with compassion and grace. Use essential oils, experiment with them, allow them to purify the air, cleanse your skin, clear your mind, and protect your health.

The Greek physician, Hippocrates, claimed the way to good health is to have an aromatic bath and scented massage every day. How could we go wrong with the tremendous healing powers of water, scent, and touch? Maybe these are worthwhile additions to your regime of good health care.

Today, the fast pace of life and excessive pollution create stressful environments that gradually break down one's physical, emotional, and mental state of health. The body is a storehouse of beautiful wisdom. It is our responsibility to look, feel, listen, and treat it with respect for the temple that it is. Using essential oils and touch to nurture the many aspects of our whole being with compassion is a beautiful way to do this.

11

Nurturing During Pregnancy with Aromatherapy

Ixchel Susan Leigh

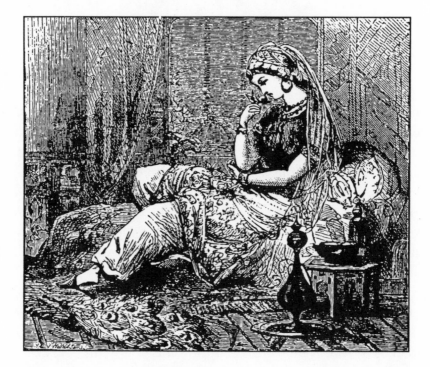

Ixchel Susan Leigh is an aromatherapist who has brought her expertise to help pioneer aromatherapy in the United States. Ms. Leigh is an educator, writer, spokesperson, consultant, and creator of aromatherapy products and treatments.

Ms. Leigh is the owner of *Essence AromaTherapy,* and the creator of *Crystal CandlEssence*™, a candle combining aromatherapy with color and gemstones to create scents-ability of well-being. *Essence AromaTherapy*'s collections can be found in specialty stores and spas throughout the U.S.

She consults for stores and spas around the country including The Golden Door in Southern California. She has also written articles that have been published in the United States and the United Kingdom. She has spoken at international conventions and taught seminars on aromatherapy.

Ms. Leigh is a member of NAHA, International Partnership in Aromatherapy (IPA), and American Alliance of Aromatherapy. She was nominated in 1992 by *Who's Who Among Rising Young Americans,* and cited for her accomplishments in American Society and Business.

*A*romatherapy is both an ancient art and a modern science. For thousands of years, people have been using oils infused with aromatic herbs, flowers, and other forms of plant life to enhance and restore beauty and well-being. Ayurvedic medicine in India was founded on the use of such infused oils.

Herbal therapy and Aromatherapy are closely related. Many of the perfumers and priests who used essential oils to prepare health and beauty treatments during the Middle Ages reportedly developed immunities to the plague epidemics of their times. Cleopatra enticed Mark Antony by wearing Rose-infused oil. And in more recent years, medical science began proving the remedial benefits of essential oils, helping the aromatic plants regain their age-old popularity. Today, in France and Germany, the health benefits of essential oils are so widely accepted that health-insurance programs pay for aromatherapy treatments.

Aromatherapy is especially vital in the months surrounding childbirth—when a woman is inspired to live in balance with the environment and to reduce her reliance on chemicals. Botanical essential oils are powerful healing agents, both physically and emotionally. And with proper care they produce no harmful effects. When used as recommended, many essential oils are nontoxic. However, pregnant or lactating women with serious health conditions are advised to consult with a health professional before using the oils.

Purchase *only pure essential oils,* which are available through reputable supply companies. Some oils are costly, as their production is limited. Two thousand pounds of Rose petals are needed to produce one pound of Rose oil. But rest assured, each healing drop goes a long way.

Applications for Pregnancy

Baths. During pregnancy, nothing is more pleasurable and comforting than a long, languorous bath. To prepare a bath, run very warm water. When the tub is as full as desired, turn off the water and add 5 to 10 drops of essential oil. The oils are volatile and will evaporate quickly if added while the water is still running. Disperse well, mixing vigorously by hand.

Choose the essential oils that best meet your needs and moods. The following blends are especially pleasing, and the oils may be used either singly or in combination.

Relaxing	Lavender *(Lavandula angustifolia)*, Rose Geranium *(Pelargonium graveolens)*, Roman Chamomile *(Chamamælum nobile)*, Neroli *(Citrus vulgaris flores)*
Uplifting	Lemongrass *(Cymbopogon citratus)*, Melissa *(Melissa officinalis)*, Palmarosa *(Cymbopogon martinii)*, Patchouli *(Pogostemon patchouli)*
Euphoric	Ylang-Ylang *(Cananga odorata)*, Sandalwood *(Santalum album)*, Rose *(Rosa centifolia)*
Tranquilizing	Lavender *(Lavandula angustifolia)*, Moroccan Chamomile *(Chamamælum mixta)*, Neroli *(Citrus aurantium)*

Inhalations. The sense of smell is one of our most powerful senses and is heightened during pregnancy. Olfactory messages travel immediately to the brain, where they stimulate feelings of pleasure or displeasure. Scents can also trigger memories and residual impressions of one's own infancy such as the sense of feeling loved, or the jolt of an unpleasant event.

When used to scent a room, inhalations create an uplifting atmosphere and generate a boost of energy. To prepare inhalations, try one or more of the following methods:

- Place 2 or 3 drops of essential oil on a cloth, and sniff as desired.
- Put essential oils in a diffusor, and diffuse the fine mist into the air.
- Fill a bowl with 1 pint of hot water, add 5 drops of essential oil, and set bowl in desired spot.
- Burn a candle scented with pure essential oils. The heat from the flame will melt the wax and in the process release the delicate oils within. Aromatherapy candles subtly scent the environment while adding a warm glow, refreshing the body, mind, and spirit.

Match the scent to the need, mood, or occasion. Inhalations can be made from the blends suggested above. In addition, consider the following applications, using the oils either singly or in combination:

For baby showers: Orange *(Citrus aurantium)*, Tangerine *(Citrus reticulata)*, Lemongrass *(Cymbopogon citratus)*

For summer gatherings: Bergamot *(Citrus bergamia)*, Rose Geranium *(Pelargonium graveolens)*, Bitter Orange leaves *(Petitgrain bigarade)*

For winter holidays: Frankincense *(Boswellia carterii)*, Fir *(Abies balsamea)*, Cedarwood *(Cedrus atlantica)*, Spruce *(Picea mariana)*

Special touches. As a mother-to-be becomes acutely aware of nurturing the new life within her, she realizes how important it is to nurture herself. Aromatherapy is a wonderful means of self-nurturing during these months of transition. To combine the emerging sense of motherhood with the deepening sense of womanhood, try daily baths with essential oils, or the special treat of aromatherapy massages by a health professional trained in prenatal care.

You can also tuck aromatherapy sachets in your lingerie drawer, or add a few drops of essential oil to the rinse water while washing your lingerie. Geranium *(Pelargonium graveolens)*, Ylang-Ylang *(Cananga odorata)* and Patchouli *(Pogostemon patchouli)* are ideal for this purpose. Be sure to apply oils to the water only, and never directly to the clothing, as they may leave permanent stains.

For freshening the air. To purify the air for labor, Frankincense *(Boswellia carterii)*, Lavender *(Lavandula angustifolia)*, Geranium *(Pelargonium graveolens)*, and Jasmine *(Jasminum officinale)* can be used in any of the "Inhalations" methods listed above.

Postpartum Care

For raising your spirits. Emotional ups and downs are common after giving birth. Frequent night feedings and postpartum blues can easily upset the balance required to care for a newborn 'round the clock. To stabilize your emotions and uplift your spirits, choose the bath or inhalation that best suits your needs. Especially helpful is Lavender *(Lavandula angustifolia)*, Rose *(Rosa centifolia)* or Neroli *(Citrus vulgaris flores)* for this time after the birth, as it can help ease mild depression.

For massaging your baby. A gentle massage can help ease the newborn's transition, and is a delightful way to initiate bonding with your baby. To make a soothing baby-massage oil, mix 1 ounce Sweet Almond oil with 2 drops Rose oil *(Rosa centifolia)*. A light, all-over massage with this simple oil is relaxing and soothing. This blend will also help relieve nipple soreness. Apply gently to the nipples. Although Rose is not harmful to the baby, remove any excess oils before breast-feeding.

For lactation. To help stimulate milk production, massage the following blend onto the breasts. Be sure to remove the oils before nursing.

   2 ounces pure vegetable oil
10 drops Clary Sage *(Salvia sclarea)*
10 drops Fennel seed *(Foeniculum vulgare)*

Essential Oils to Avoid during Pregnancy

Essential oils are highly concentrated forms of the medicinal properties inherent in plants. Many essential oils are naturally antibiotic, antiseptic, and safe for use with a minimum amount of education. The healing actions of these oils have been well-researched, and new reports detailing their positive effects are published regularly. A few essential oils, however, have been known to be toxic or allergenic, especially when used in large quantities. Other oils are considered to be abortives or neuro-toxins, and should not be used by pregnant women, as they may have harmful effects on the mother or baby.

Without the guidance of a professionally trained aromatherapist, it is recommended to avoid all essential oils that may be toxic during this time. Due to a woman's heightened sensitivity during pregnancy, skin irritation may develop. Stop treatments immediately if this occurs. Apply vegetable oil to dilute the effects, then wash with soap and water, and drink extra water to help flush the system.

Always use essential oils with respect for their powerful capabilities, and, always dilute essential oils before use when pregnant. Check several texts to determine the toxicity of an essential oil before use.

The following essential oils are *not* recommended for use during pregnancy due to their neurotoxic or abortive effects:

Aniseed *(Pimpinella anisum)*
Basil *(Ocimum basilicum)*
camphor (is always synthetic)
Caraway *(Carum carvi)*
Cinnamon bark or leaf *(Cinnamomum zeylanicum)*

Clove *(Eugenia caryophyllata)*
Fennel *(Foeniculum vulgare)*
Hyssop *(Hyssopus officinalis)*
Marjoram *(Origanum majorana)*
Mugwort *(Artemisia vulgaris)*
Myrrh *(Commiphora myrrha)*
Nutmeg *(Myristica fragrans)*
Oregano *(Origanum vulgare)*
Pennyroyal *(Mentha pulegium)*
Sage *(Salvia officinalis)*
Savory *(Satureia montana)*
Thyme *(Thymus vulgaris)*
Wintergreen *(Gaultheria procumbens)*

Many women are leading society in a reemergence of the commitment to a wholistic approach to living, balancing the sensitivities of humankind and nature. It is only fitting, then, that we make a commitment to raise our children with this sensitivity. For centuries, plant extracts have been used to improve the quality of life. Now, as increasing numbers of people are seeking comfort and peace of mind, spending more intimate time at home, luxuriating in baths, creating wonderfully scented rooms, aromatherapy is gaining renewed interest. Why? Because it is simple to incorporate into everyday living; because it is a powerful and nonintrusive means of healing; because it is an inviting and nurturing way to usher our children into the world.

12

Aromatherapy for Pregnancy and Birth

Susan Earle

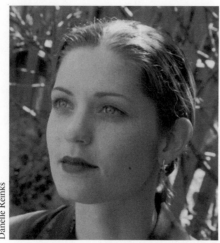

Danelle Reinks

Opening a book by Jeanne Rose uncovered the wonderful, aromatic, colorful world of herbs and aromatherapy to *Susan Earle*.

She was given the gift of creative writing and merciless editing by her parents, one a fifth-grade school teacher, the other a graduate degree professor. When offered opportunities by Jeanne Rose and the National Association for Holistic Aromatherapy, Susan began her career as an aromatherapy journalist, editor, student, and enthusiast. Her works have been published in magazines, aromatherapy courses, and in NAHA's *Scentsitivity Quarterly* newsletter.

Susan is currently a student of *The Herbal Studies Course*™ by Jeanne Rose, and is working toward Aromatherapy Certification, while obtaining a bachelor's degree in Health Sciences from San Francisco State University, working in her garden, participating in the administrative workings of NAHA, and, as always, typing away at the latest manuscript.

The following article was written from the perspective of a young woman who has not previously experienced the cycles of pregnancy and childbirth and has four marvelous resources to create an aromatherapy treatment plan for pregnancy: *Aromatherapy for Women & Children: Pregnancy & Childbirth* by Jane Dye, *Aromatherapy for Pregnancy & Childbirth* by Margaret Fawcett, *The Modern Herbal* by Jeanne Rose; and *Aromatherapy for Women* by Maggie Tisserand.

"With Child," "Bun in the Oven," and "Eating for Two" are all playful terms we use to describe the gentle, sacred, tender, powerful state of pregnancy. The emotions, realizations, and sensations a woman lives through during pregnancy and the birthing process are both unique and unifying. Each woman comes to different conclusions, learns different lessons, thinks different thoughts, and copes with different physical sensations, aches, pains, joys, and fears. Yet the experience is a unifying one. It is an opportunity to sense the connection of all women, to feel the honest power of creation, to unify with both spirit and Earth.

Living in such a joyful, frightening and exhilarating state is not easy. The demands of the growing being inside are added to those of your body, your partner, your friends, your employer, and your other children. Normally, you might respond by reaching for a sleeping pill, a potent herb, or a glass of wine. Maybe you would run a marathon or paddle a kayak. At varying points in your pregnancy, these things may no longer be possible, and some are considered dangerous at any time during pregnancy.

While pregnancy is a spiritual and meditative condition, it is also a physical one. The body, which is your friend and partner in creating a healthy, happy child may sometimes seem to turn against you. Your favorite breakfast may now turn your stomach inside out. Tables that were once easily pushed around the room may present a challenge and a strain. Standing up from a seated position is not the thoughtless activity it once was. Your skin is stretching, your breasts are swelling, and your feet are aching.

This constant focus on the physical state serves to strengthen the sacred nature of pregnancy. While she ponders the mystery of life that allows another living being to form and grow inside her, the pregnant woman is a reflection of Nature. Her body is the Earth, air, sun, and water that nurtures the seed. The realization of her body as a source of life, combined with the humble sense that we will never truly know the mystery of life, is an understanding that is sought by yogis, monks, and meditators of all religions.

Essential oils have sometimes been called the "spirit" of the plant. For some they symbolize the same union of the spirit of life in physical form that is found in the pregnant mother. Whether you use essential oils during pregnancy to emphasize this etheric state, or simply because you want to wear a bikini next year without rivers of stretch marks on your belly and breasts, experience shows that they work.

Jane Dye, Margaret Fawcett, and Maggie Tisserand have written wonderful manuals for aromatherapy during pregnancy. With these three books, an expectant mother, no matter what her past experience with aromatherapy, is in good hands.

There are numerous physical and emotional conditions that affect the pregnant woman. You may be familiar with the use of essential oils for stress relief, to cure colds, for beauty and body care. Such remedies are even more useful during pregnancy, as you will want to stay away from any toxins, harsh chemicals or medications. Be sure to spend some time researching the essential oils you have been using to ensure that they are safe for use during pregnancy. Some essential oils are neurotoxins and abortives, and are not safe for use by pregnant women.

The following essential oils are generally considered safe during pregnancy. (Fawcett, 1993) Please see the listing of Latin binomials at the end of the book. As you may be sensitive to smells, find your favorite aromas, use them in formulas, and surround yourself with them. Use a reliable and reputable source known for carrying only unadulterated, pure essential oils.

Dilute essential oils before use. Keep essential oils out of eyes.

Safe Throughout	Safe After Sixteen Weeks	Safe Late in Pregnancy and During Childbirth
Bergamot	Chamomile, Roman	Clary Sage
Frankincense	Jasmine	Cypress (small amounts)
Geranium	Peppermint	Rosemary
Lavender	Rose	
Lemon		
Mandarin		
Neroli		
Orange		
Patchouli		
Sandalwood		
Tea Tree		
Ylang-Ylang		

Some essential oils are *not* considered safe for pregnant women. According to Maggie Tisserand, Cinnamon bark, Basil, Pennyroyal, Hyssop, Myrrh, Savory, Sage, Thyme, and Origanum are not safe for use during pregnancy. Also considered unsafe are Anise seed, Camphor, Caraway, Cinnamon, Clove, Cedarwood, Fennel, Hyssop, Marjoram, Mugwort, Nutmeg, Tansy, Tarragon, Thuja, and Wintergreen.

As well as enhancing the emotional state and accenting the spiritual nature of pregnancy, there are numerous conditions throughout pregnancy, and during and after childbirth, that have been addressed safely and effectively with essential oils. Essential oils produce varying emotional responses depending on the memories and nuances of an individual. Choosing essential oils for emotional and meditative purposes during pregnancy is a very personal experience and can be a profound early experience for a mother and the developing child. Use your previous experience with essential oils, and the multitude of information available regarding the emotional and spiritual effects of essential oils, and experiment with those considered safe. Find the ones that work best for you.

As for the numerous physical challenges that arise in the varying stages of pregnancy and childbirth, essential oils are a good friend and a powerful ally.

Essential Oil Remedies During Pregnancy

Nausea

1 drop Peppermint in sugar or honey, taken every hour until nausea is relieved. One dose may suffice. (Tisserand, 1988)

Lavender compress to abdomen: Add 2 drops Lavender to a bowl of warm water. Soak small towel and apply to abdomen. Place larger towel over the top and rest thirty minutes. (Tisserand, 1988)

Maggie Tisserand also suggests surrounding yourself with pleasant aromas.

Stretch Marks

Prevention is recommended, though the following formula will also help with already formed marks.

20 drops Lavender
5 drops Neroli
in 2 ounces Wheat germ oil (Tisserand, 1988)

Back Pain

Massage with:

    8 drops Neroli

    8 drops Frankincense

    8 drops Sandalwood

    in 50 ml carrier oil (Dye, 1992)

Relaxation, Time-Out, Health, and Well-being

Use your favorite essential oils in a bath, foot bath, or massage throughout pregnancy. Clary Sage is a morale booster near the end of pregnancy. Lavender stimulates production of healthy white blood cells to ward off illnesses. Peppermint is cooling. Try Melissa, Bergamot, Lemon, or Orange for a citrus aroma, or Geranium, Rose, Jasmine, or Ylang-Ylang for a sweet scent. (Dye, 1992)

    Jane Dye recommends the following formulas:

Anti-stress	**Reviving**
3 drops Rose	3 drops Geranium
2 drops Frankincense	3 drops Rosemary
2 drops Lavender	2 drops Rosewood

Refresher

Hydrosols are a wonderful aromatherapy item for the expectant mother. They are mild in aroma, cooling to the skin, and wonderful refreshers. They can be added to the bath, used in a spray bottle to spritz the face, the feet, or any part of the body that needs refreshing. These are a must for any mother who is late in pregnancy during the hot summer months.

Pre-Labor Perineal Massage

According to Jane Dye, perineal massage can be helpful to prevent tearing or the need for episiotomy. Begin with a bath of 4 drops each of Geranium and Lavender essential oils. Empty the bladder. Use a massage oil of two drops of Lavender and one drop Geranium in a 2.5% dilution of base oil such as Almond oil. (Dye, 1992) Lubricate your two index fingers or thumbs and the perineal area. Insert fingers 3–4 cm inside the vagina and press the perineal floor toward the rectum and to the sides in a U shape. Dye describes the clitoris at 12 o'clock and the massage work taking place between four and eight o'clock. Massage with gentle pressure for approximately one minute, or until a slight burning or tingling occurs. (Dye, 1992)

This massage should be practiced for the last few weeks of pregnancy and, as the birthing time draws near, the area will become more supple. (Tisserand, 1988)

Cystitis

A massage for the whole body, or for abdomen, hips, and lower back, should be at 2.5% dilution of equal parts of either Chamomile, Lavender, and Cedarwood; or Chamomile, Bergamot, Fennel, and Eucalyptus. A compress over the lower back and stomach could contain Chamomile and Sandalwood, or Chamomile and Eucalyptus (2 drops of each oil). (Dye, 1992)

Hæmorrhoids

For the hæmorrhoids that often come during pregnancy, Jane Dye recommends two drops of Geranium and one drop of Cypress to one inch of KY Jelly applied twice a day after cleansing.

Labor

Whether you are a nervous and excited first-timer, or whether you are an old pro, essential oils can ease the stress and physical pain of childbirth. Essential oil massages during labor can also calm any nervous partners, and give them an activity other than pacing and fussing nervously over the laboring mother.

Labor Massage

Maggie Tisserand recommends the following blend for a firm massage to the lower back with the heel of the hand, between contractions, when needed.

> 14 drops Clary Sage
> 5 drops Rose
> 6 drops Ylang-Ylang
> 2 ounces vegetable oil

Pain Relief

Maggie Tisserand recommends a Clary Sage compress to the lower abdomen, just above the pubic hair. This should be performed only when the woman is lying down, and is to be applied warm and replaced when it cools.

When labor begins, all sources encourage the mother to remain relaxed. More easily said than done! Essential oils in a diffusor are helpful, and a warm, aromatic bath can be taken when contractions become stronger. The mother should rest in a comfortable position and use essential oil massage over shoulders, back, hips, and legs, with firmer pressure on painful areas. An alternative to the massage is a warm essential oil compress. (Tisserand, 1988)

The mother should occasionally stand and stretch her legs, to prevent cramping. A brisk essential oil massage, working up the legs and massaging towards the heart, will help circulation. (Fawcett, 1993)

Again, the essential oils to use are at the discretion of the mother. Lavender aids relaxation; Chamomile releases inner tensions; Bergamot and Mandarin renew energy; Rose or Jasmine will both serve to relax and boost confidence.

The Modern Herbal, by Jeanne Rose, has a wonderful description of natural childbirth from pregnancy through caring for a sick child. She has this to say about the care of the perineal tissue during the birth:

> Once the baby is actually coming out, the best way to prevent tearing is to birth the head quite slowly so the perineum has time to stretch. The perineal tissue is very elastic, but will tear if you stretch too fast. As the baby's head becomes visible, oil the head and the labia with Olive oil. It's best not to actually touch the perineum—just drip the oil on it at the point of maximum stretch, which will keep the tissue moist and elastic. Often it will tear *just* where you touch it. (Rose, 1987)

Ms. Rose also suggests placing the baby on the mother's belly or between her breasts as soon as the baby comes out, which is important for bonding between mother and child.

After Labor

Healing the Perineum

After an episiotomy or torn perineum, a Comfrey root herbal sitz bath aids in the healing process. Simmer 1 oz. Comfrey root in 20 oz. water for 20 minutes. Cool, and pour into a basin just big enough to sit in. Sit for at least 20 minutes. Maggie Tisserand recommends adding 2 drops Cypress and 3 drops Lavender. Cypress is astringent, and Lavender encourages growth of new skin. (Tisserand, 1988) Margaret Fawcett recommends Tea Tree, which is antibacterial, and Lavender.

Breasts

Your breasts may become very sore and inflamed, or you may suffer from cracked nipples. Yet experts agree that breastfeeding is vitally important to the health of the child and, as an early lesson in sacrifice, the new mother will find that hungry babies have no patience for the mother's discomfort. Once again, essential oils can be a saving grace. Be certain to remove all traces of essential oil before the next feeding.

To increase or balance milk production and flow. (Dye, 1992)
> 1 drop Fennel
> 1 drop Geranium
> 1 drop Clary Sage
> in a compress to cover the breasts

To tone the breasts (exercise is also recommended). (Dye, 1992)
> 10 drops Lemongrass
> 5 drops Geranium
> 5 drops Clary Sage
> in carrier oil

Cracked nipples. (Dye, 1992)
> 90% sweet almond oil
> 10% Wheat germ or Jojoba
> Add Lavender, Neroli, or Melissa to 3% and roll nipple gently between finger and thumb immediately after feeding.

For sore breasts. (Dye, 1992)
> 2 drops Roman Chamomile
> 2 drops Geranium
> 1 drop Lavender
> Apply in a compress

Mastitis

Mastitis is inflammation of the mammaries if the breast is not completely emptied of milk, or when milk ducts in nipple get clogged

Massage with Essential Oil to Prevent Mastitis

After each breastfeeding, perform a massage with essential oils added if desired. Massage any swollen areas until they are softened. Use essential oil of Peppermint if skin feels hot, Rosemary if it feels swollen. Massage toward the nipple and finish by massaging the whole breast. Remove all traces of essential oil before the next feeding. (Fawcett, 1993)

If Mastitis is Present

To reduce heat:

Compress of 1 drop Geranium; 1 drop Lavender; 2 drops Rose in a bowl of warm water. This should be applied every hour or so, and the nipple should be washed before feeding.

If fever occurs, try the breast compress while soaking the feet in Eucalyptus. A Lavender bath may also be useful. (Tisserand, 1988) It's nice to have a partner or a friend prepare the bath or compress and footsoak for you, as it may not be feasible for you to do it yourself in a fevered and swollen state.

Many essential oils are safe for use in relieving childhood ailments, and many aromatherapists recommend regular massage of your child with essential oils to aid health and vitality, and to provide a bonding experience between child and parent(s).

As always, the new mother should take proper care of herself, using essential oils to aid stress relief, sleep, and relaxation, and to ease depression. If your experience with essential oils began with your pregnancy, now is not the time to stop using them! Continue to learn about and explore the myriad uses of essential oils for health and well-being, for you and your growing family.

Essential Oils Considered Safe for Use by Pregnant Women
Bergamot, Chamomile (Roman), Clary Sage, Cypress, Frankincense, Geranium, Jasmine, Lavender, Lemon, Melissa, Mandarin, Neroli, Orange, Patchouli, Peppermint, Rose, Rosemary, Sandalwood, Tea Tree, Ylang-Ylang

*Essential Oils Considered **Unsafe** for Use by Pregnant Women*
Anise seed, Basil, Camphor, Caraway, Cedarwood, Cinnamon, Clove, Fennel, Hyssop, Marjoram, Mugwort, Myrrh, Nutmeg, Origanum or Oregano, Pennyroyal, Savory, Sage, Tansy, Tarragon, Thyme, Thuja, Wintergreen

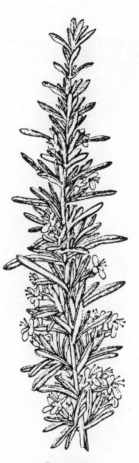

Rosemary
(*Rosmarinus officinalis*
verbenon)

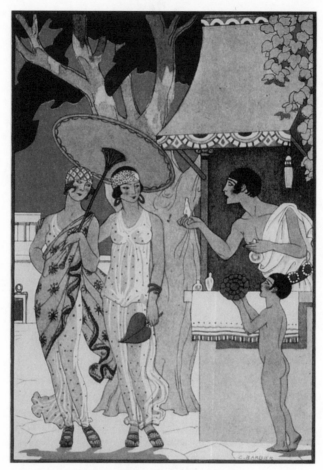

Ancient Greece, by Georges Barbier

III

A Scentual Mix

13

Magic at Our Fingertips

Emilee Stewart

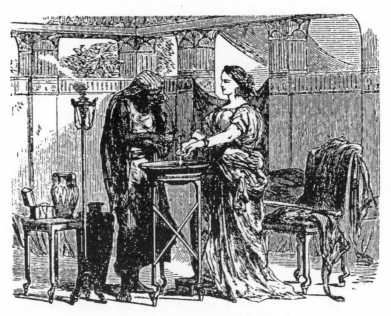

Judith preparing to meet Holofernes

Emilee Stewart is an international health and beauty therapist, and founder of one of the first aromatherapy centers in the United States located in North Carolina.

Ms. Stewart has been actively involved with massage, herbs, and aromatherapy for over twenty years. She has studied and worked with international leaders of aromatherapy. She is a fellow of the Society of Health and Beauty Therapists, and most recently was inducted as a member of *Who's Who* worldwide. Emilee has maintained a private practice in the central Florida area for the past ten years. She conducts seminars and speaking engagements on the healing qualities of aromatherapy. Her business, Private Universe, features custom blends of essential oils.

*I*magine a time more than three thousand years ago, when the oldest of the seven wonders of the world was being built, stone by stone. On the fertile land along the Nile, fragrant stands of Orange, Lemon, and Juniper, brilliant clusters of Geranium, and cascades of intoxicating Jasmine scented the air.

It's no wonder the Egyptians were among the first to explore the therapeutic and aromatic properties inherent in Earth's flora and fauna. As their knowledge passed from one generation to the next, from one culture to another, aromatic medicine, perfumery, and pharmacology took root as an integral part of our civilization.

Is it coincidence? Of all the seven wonders, the great pyramids of Egypt still stand today. And in our busy, high-tech world, the art of aromatherapy has once again come of age. Aromatherapy is now on the leading edge of natural healing.

Nature has given us a bountiful gift. At the heart and soul of plants and trees are unique and powerful qualities. Essential oils capture this life-force, and aromatherapy transfers this essence to us in a way as natural and simple as the taking of a breath.

Researchers at Columbia University have made a ground-breaking discovery: A family of genes in nose cells are responsible for detecting odor and transmitting it to the brain. Our sense of smell is unique in that the olfactory nerve receptors are the only receptors in direct contact with the outside world. Located just beneath the brain, level with the bridge of the nose, these sensitive hairs pick up the fragrant molecules and transport their message directly to the limbic system, passing the blood-brain barrier. The limbic system is the cerebral core of emotions and memory. It controls the entire endocrine system. As we become more health conscious and strive to live a more natural way of life, aromatherapy gives us the opportunity not only to live closer to nature but to let her "magic" soothe our weary needs.

My aromatherapy center located in Raleigh, North Carolina was designed as a holistic center to encompass the healing principles involved in achieving a balanced state among mind, body, and spirit. These principles include the belief that the environment in which aromatherapy is performed is as important as the therapy itself. In the center, I created a harmonious combination of sight, sound, and surroundings including pleasing architecture and decor as well as an abundance of plants. This environment, together with the fragrant aromas of the essential oils and their properties, creates a truly healing atmosphere.

Although the authenticity of the essential oils and their properties is of paramount importance, there is a deeper, spiritual side to aromatherapy that is lost in today's commercialization of the art. Everywhere you look in the marketplace, you see aromatherapy products. There is even a line of aromatherapy lipsticks!

It is time that we who are aware of the deep value of aromatherapy begin to question where all this is leading. We need to ask ourselves, "Are we, as a group, productively moving to enhance and build an awareness and understanding of the authenticity and true properties of the art of aromatherapy, or are we giving in to commercialism, and simply riding the wave of a popular fad?" If it is merely a fad, we will watch aromatherapy crest and fade, as all fads do, and eventually be replaced by another popular fancy. While many enterprising marketers exploit the ancient art of aromatherapy, there are many practitioners, teachers, writers, and aromatherapy enthusiasts dedicated to the preservation and conservation of the art and science of aromatics used for generations for worship, health, and beauty.

Essential oils are part of nature's handiwork. Like any art or beautiful symphony, the oils need a master hand to bring out their noblest qualities. The masterpiece created by the special oil and the aromatherapist working together is like a symphony played upon one's finest feelings. At the magical touch of the beautiful essences, the secret chord of our being is awakened. We vibrate in harmony, and our minds speak while we listen with an inner silence. Memories long forgotten are remembered with new significance. It is through communion and harmony with these special essences and essential oils that we can understand their properties and use them respectfully, giving thanks for the rich resource nature has offered us.

As individuals, we can't expect to change the world, but we can change the environment that immediately surrounds us. What we do as individuals affects our world and reaches out to touch many lives. It is our responsibility to maintain the integrity of the art of aromatherapy in all of its uses.

14

Scent, Soul, and Psyche

Julia Lawless

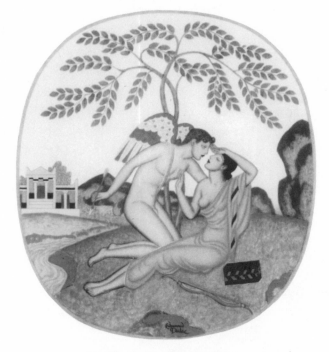

from *The Marriage of Cupid and Psyche*,
illustrated by Edmund Dulac, from the collection of Albert Seligman

Julia Lawless is a qualified aromatherapist and member of The International Federation of Aromatherapists. Her family business supplies essential oils and other natural products.

Julia is the well-respected author of *The Encyclopaedia of Essential Oils*. In her latest book, *Aromatherapy and the Mind*, she explores the historic evidence of psycho-aromatic traditions.

When burned, herbs were seen to release their inner virtues. The scent of
Bay thus evoked the presence of Apollo, as well as the qualities of prophecy
and clairvoyance.

*O*ur present culture pays little attention to the needs of the heart—our emotional, feeling nature has been subjugated to the constraints of reason for so long that we now find ourselves in a spiritual wasteland. Compared to the great civilizations of the past, we do not honour enough the inner or unseen realm of the mind, the subtle expressions of the psyche.

At one time, incense was burned upon temple altars and at household shrines on a daily basis, fragrant flowers were strewn on the floors of churches and dwelling-places, and the evocative power of perfume was understood as the silent language of divinity and human emotion. Now, having banished the ancient gods and goddesses, how are we to show our respect?

The Symbolic Imagination

I do not feel like writing verses;
but as I light my perfume-burner
with Myrrh, Jasmine, and incense,
they suddenly burgeon from my heart
like flowers in a garden.

Scent inspires the imagination and frees the spirit. In poetry, flowers are often used directly as a symbol of the soul, for their fragrance has an intangible quality that reaches to our most intimate depths. To the primitive mind, the child's eye or the poet's pen, everything in the physical world can be seen as an expression of the more subtle, immaterial realm.

To the ancients, there was far more to a plant than simply its tangible form, for each herb carried a whole series of associations with mythology, astrology, and folklore. To the mind's eye, the scent, shape, and colour of a plant, its habitat and manner of growth all helped to convey its innate quality. This essential, underlying property was known as the "virtue."

The Bay tree, for example, with its radiant shining leaves, evergreen growth, and heady, narcotic scent was associated with the sun, the sign of Leo, the god Apollo, and the "virtues" of strength, protection, courage, inspiration, prophecy, and insight. The leaves were made into wreathes to crown victors and great artists or poets; it was planted by the door of houses to keep evil "at bay"; and was used as incense by the pythia, the high priestess at the temple of Apollo in Delphi. When burned, herbs were seen to release their inner virtues. The scent of Bay thus evoked the presence of Apollo, as well as the qualities of prophecy and clairvoyance needed by the pythia to transmit the message of the oracle.

In Western fairy tales, trees and plants are often involved as life tokens, the life force of a person being involved with a tree planted at birth. In Grimm's story *The Juniper Tree*, a murdered boy is buried beneath a Juniper tree with his mother, only to be reborn like a phœnix from its depths:

Then the Juniper tree began to stir itself, and the branches parted asunder, and moved together again . . . At the same time a mist seemed to arise from the tree, and in the centre of this mist it burned like a fire, and a beautiful bird flew out of the fire, singing magnificently, and he flew high up in the air, and when he was gone, the Juniper tree was just as it had been before.

In this story, the Juniper tree is the source of new life and hope from which the released soul arises. In the original myth of the phœnix, the fire-bird dies and is reborn from the aromatic ashes of fragrant wood. The "spiritual bird" arises from the depths of the pyre like incense from a fragrant fire.

Indeed, the ancient Egyptians believed that the phœnix first brought incense to the Land of Punt in his claws, and that the scent of incense was his own scent. The Hebrews thought the phœnix was a god reincarnated, and the Egyptians saw him as the soul of Osiris, the god whose breath smelt of Myrrh and incense. According to the Egyptian legend, at the end of his long life, the phœnix builds himself a nest of Frankincense and Cassia on which he dies, and from his corpse arises the new phœnix. Thus the phœnix, like scent, depicts the vital essence or spark of life, the immortal soul; in this sense, it can be equated with the "fire-water" of the shamans and with the "quintessence" of the alchemists. As Gaston Bachelard says in *Fragments d'une poetique du feu*, "*Odours in and of themselves make myths possible . . .*"

Slowly, however, with the growth of rationalism in the West, the symbolic imagination was repressed—only poets and children were allowed to speak in the language of the heart:

Rational thought, in its pursuit of objective knowledge, denies the validity of subjective visualization. Its diabolic methodology has supplanted the symbolic perspective, and the material world is perceived as existing in its own right quite dissociated from the person observing it.

Yet the symbolism that has accumulated about particular plants or flowers in the course of time, together with the significance of their fragrance, is still very much a part of our collective cultural conditioning today. This underlying mythic language still communicates itself, often via the unconscious, and conditions our response both to its form and to its scent. Symbolism and myth still speak to us in the language of the unseen, just as scent communicates itself to our soul directly, influencing our mood and emotions in a subtle manner.

The gods and goddesses are not dead—it is just that we no longer see them or believe in them! To reawaken their power is to reinvest matter with spirit, to perceive the virtues concealed within the external manifestation of form. The virtues of the deities reside within ourselves and in nature; the virtues of plants express themselves through scent and through their "essence." To honour the presence of the spirit within is to become attuned to a way of seeing using the "mind's eye" and the symbolic imagination.

The Doors of Perception

Using aromatics and herbal drugs to open the doors of perception was a domain of expertise specific to the traditional shaman. The shaman featured largely in primitive forms of medicine because he or she was able to travel back and forth across the invisible barrier that divides matter from spirit, and act as a mediating influence:

The shaman himself must be a master of psychological control . . . He rejoins that which was once a totality—man and the animals, the living and the dead, man and the gods . . . and in providing this integration, the shaman provides his magical cure.

Within a contemporary context, the shaman's magical flight could be seen as a form of psychotherapeutic practice. Indeed, the key to health from the shamanic perspective was seen to lie predominantly in the domain of the psyche—and one of the principal ways of gaining access to this realm was by the use of herbs and aromatics.

An important part of the shaman's rigorous and challenging training was acquiring knowledge about medicinal plants, including those with hallucinogenic powers. Those plants that had curious psychic effects included aromatics such as Hemlock *(Conium maculatum)*, Mugwort *(Artemisia vulgaris)*, Bay *(Laurus nobilis)*, Nutmeg *(Myristica fragrans)*, and Cannabis *(Cannabis sativa)*.

Such knowledge has survived to the present day. In 1985, the Chumash medicine woman Chequeesh told researcher Will Noffke that she had learned of her native heritage by utilizing the "dream herb" Mugwort—a plant that is used to produce a narcotic (and toxic) essential oil. Hemlock, a poisonous aromatic plant with a foetid smell, was a vital part of the European witch's arsenal, and enabled her to fly away on her broomstick—the equivalent of the shaman's magical flight. In the Hindu Kush, the sibyl inhales fragrant smoke from the sacred Cedar in order to induce a trance-like state before pronouncing the oracle, much like the pythia of Delphi. On the island of Madura, off the north coast of Java, the spirit medium, generally a woman, sits with her head over a censer of incense until she is overcome and eventually collapses. Upon recovery, her voice is purportedly that of the spirit which has taken over her soul. In Uganda, the mediums light up an herbal pipe and repeatedly inhale deeply until they have worked themselves up to a frenzy, at which point the gods speak through them.

In eastern Asia, shamanism and animism predate the more familiar mainstream religions like Buddhism, Confucianism, and Hinduism. Cannabis was used in India and China as early as 1500 B.C. for sacred ceremonial purposes, and the ancient Scythians used it in the form of a narcotic vapour bath. The main active constituents in Cannabis are a resin and a volatile oil; the Indian name for this part of the herb is *charas*. It is the resinous exudation from the aerial parts that contains a large percentage of a red essential oil. In India today it is still smoked by the sadhus, or wandering holy men, as part of their religious life. Since Cannabis or Marijuana is also commonly used in the West as a mind-altering drug, there can be no doubt that certain aromatics can have a profound effect on the psyche or consciousness of an individual.

However, many of the so-called "magical" herbs or oils are dangerous if they are not handled correctly and in the right proportion. Such substances can easily be misused and abused if their power is not respected. As the Native American medicine man Chief Maza Blaska of the Ogalala tribe says:

From Wakan-Tanka, the Great Mystery, comes all power. It is from Wakan-Tanka that the Holy Man has wisdom and the power to heal and to make holy charms. Man knows that all healing plants are given by Wakan-Tanka; therefore are they holy.

Implicit in the ancient use of herbs and aromatics for healing purposes was an awareness of the sacred dimension within the ritual, and the need for a correct attitude toward the process for it to be effective. The fragrant plants that were used to make holy oils or incense for fumigation were often seen as having an identity in their own right, a personality that had to be respected if they were to work. Healing rituals were often accompanied by chants or incantations that honoured the soul or spirit of the plant. In ancient Egypt, hymns were sung to Nefertum, "god of the sacred Lotus," a plant renowned for its narcotic properties:

I invoke Nefertum, in the following of Ptah. Thou art guardian and protector of the perfume and oil makers, protector and god of the sacred Lotus. Osiris is the body of the plants, Nefertum is the soul of the plants, the plants purified. The divine perfume belongs to Nefertum living forever.

The scent of the Lotus was identified with the soul, its immortal aspect. It is also known that the ancient Egyptians pressed Lotus blossoms to acquire their juice. Added to wine, this "perfumed extract" would produce a powerful psychoactive drug which could produce visionary experiences or dreams. The fragrance scholar Morris noted that this is the "first instance of the association of inhalation of perfumes with inhalation of hallucinogens." Medicinal plants and aromatics were thus used to open the doors of perception or gain access to the realm of the unseen so as to restore unity. The importance of the spiritual dimension on such a journey was vital for the success of the healing operation, as well as for the personal safety of the shaman-priest acting on behalf of the troubled soul.

The Subtle Essence

The essence is like the personality or spirit of the plant. It is the most ethereal and subtle part of the plant, and its therapeutic action takes place on a higher and more subtle level, having in general a much more pronounced effect on the mind and emotions.

Shamanic practices are still in evidence in various parts of the world. In South America, for example, certain shamans called *perfumeros* actually perform their cure specifically through fragrances. They are especially sensitive to the nuances of body odour, and seek to transform the "aura" of their patient by manipulating their diet and prescribing plant aromas.

Both the rain-forest Indians and the Mestizos, the mixed Spanish-Indian population, use perfumes, floral waters, and aromatic plants in their healing rituals. The basic idea is that good-smelling fragrances protect against bad spirits by strengthening the aura, whereas bad-smelling fragrances, like rotting meat, damage the aura. The aura is considered to be the energetic-emotional envelope around the body. Each tribe has a classification of good and bad smells.

As part of the ritual, the shaman often takes Ayahuasca, a hallucinogenic jungle vine, which enables him or her to discern or smell the cause of the illness, which is usually attributed to evil spirits or sorcery. Tobacco is also revered as a magical plant throughout the Amazon and used to communicate with and nourish the spirit world. Some tribes use the scent of the Amazonian Basil *(Ocimum mircanthum)* to relieve anxiety and banish fearful visions. The Kuripakos of the Amazon collect the solidified resin from the *Protium crassipetalium* and burn it to "purify the house" following an illness.

The Mestizos say that shamans cannot do a proper healing without perfume. They have an altar of Christian and native power objects that must be purified and activated before a curing ceremony can take place. They say that fragrance is the link that holds all of these power objects together for healing, so it is essential.

Often while in a trance state, the shaman hears and sings magical healing songs while using a bunch of herbs to beat out a rhythm. The healing is also carried out in various other ways—sometimes the patient is given an aromatic bath and then rubbed with fragrant oils; sometimes the shaman puts some perfume into his or her own mouth, and after inhaling Tobacco smoke, blows it onto the patient. This is called *florecer,* which means "to blossom" or to make whole. The shaman's breath is also thought to have a healing power, and the breath itself is considered a vehicle for the revitalization of the soul.

Just as the soul, or essence, of mankind had to be persuaded to depart temporarily through fumigation in order for a spirit to enter the oracle, so it was commonly thought among many peoples that the soul would leave the body with the last breath at death . . . The common themes running through these observations are the notions that the breath, the soul, and odour are in some way interconnected, and that a being can be protected from evil outside influences in much the same way as the gods can be assuaged.

In *Perfume: The Story of a Murderer,* Süskind too identifies essence with breath, and breath as the medium that carries scent, unlike words, pictures, or sounds, into the very soul of the person:

For scent was a brother to breath. Together with breath it entered human beings, who could not defend themselves against it, not if they wanted to live. And scent entered into their very core, went directly to their hearts, and decided for good and all between affection and contempt, disgust and lust, love and hate. He who ruled scent ruled the hearts of men.

In this context, it is interesting to note that the olfactory cells are also the only place in the human body where the central nervous system is directly in contact with the external environment. When we smell something, there is a direct contact between the molecules of the scent and our own receptors—it is an intimate, essential type of encounter. While neurons of the visual or auditory system lead to the brain's cortex, the seat of abstract reasoning and analysis, the neurons of the olfactory system lead to the hypothalamus, which controls the subjective experience or "inner" response—memories, feelings, moods, and the body's hormones.

Vibrational Healing

A contemporary healer who, like the traditional shaman, has access to the spirit or supernatural world has been told that he was given a dimensional doorway that made him open to a vast store of energy. During his healing sessions, he manifests aromatic oils and ash, which literally pour from his hands, filling the room with scent.

. . . the interesting thing is that the aromatic oil will often start as one aroma and when a person has received it, their energy takes over and it might change several times. It's personalized to them . . .

The idea that aromas can be "personalized" to an individual corresponds with Marguerite Maury's method of revitalizing her patients using a "strictly personal aromatic complex" or "individual prescription" that was perfectly adapted to that person's temperament and state of health. Present-day writing on astral magic also emphasizes the value of specific personalized perfumes as a medium for healing. According to one theory, odours created by the volatilization of particles of matter emit vibrations that have a profound effect on the behaviour of all living creatures and especially on their "astral double" or "aura":

A perfume adapted to a person's astral sign will therefore tend to maintain his native humoral balance and auto-immune reactions through the unconscious reactions it provokes in the organism. It thereby acts as a charm that will enable the individual to improve his natural abilities and avoid imbalances. Each sign of the zodiac and each day of the month correspond to specific propitious aromas.

Some ancient writers even allotted a perfume to each day of the week: Saffron on Sunday; Mastic on Monday; Cassia on Tuesday; Cinnamon on Wednesday;

Aloes on Thursday; Ambergris on Friday; Musk on Saturday. By association, the fragrances are used to evoke or to form a link with the archetypal forces they represent. The choice of scent should therefore be attuned to the needs and personality of the individual if it is to be effective. In *Magical Aromatherapy*, Scott Cunningham explores the "merging of human and plant energy" and the way essential oils or ethereal oils (as they are called in Germany) can be utilized together with visualization to manifest specific changes.

Like traditional shamans, contemporary spiritual healers see essential oils as having a particular affinity with the subtle energy or "aura" of an individual, and having a revitalizing and harmonizing effect. In *Subtle Aromatherapy*, Patricia Davis further investigates the connection of essential oils with the chakras of the body, and the way in which they can be used to activate and balance energy within the subtle body. The base chakra, for example, is associated with Patchouli, Myrrh, Vetiver, Frankincense, and Elemi; the heart with Rose, Inula, Bergamot, Melissa, and Jasmine. In the practice of subtle aromatherapy it is "the vibration or subtle energy of the plant that is the healing factor." This is, however, harder to explain or examine than the physical properties of medicinal plants. Davis continues:

. . . *so how can we set about discovering these subtle healing properties? We can take a look at how plants have been used in the past, in shamanic traditions, in the ceremonies of many different religions, their symbolism in art, their meaning in myth and folklore . . . Finally we can study the plants themselves, for they can tell us much about their hidden abilities.*

Examining the traditions of the past with an open yet discriminating eye is a key to the future understanding of plant medicine, including the psychological effects of aromatic oils.

© 1994, *The Aromatherapy Quarterly*, Autumn, 1994, No. 42. As edited by Séza Eccles of the *Aromatherapy Quarterly*. Reprinted by kind permission of the editor. *The Aromatherapy Quarterly* can be contacted at 415-663-9519 in the USA and (011 181) 44 392-1691 in the UK.

15

Goddess Traditions
and Aromatherapy

Leila Castle

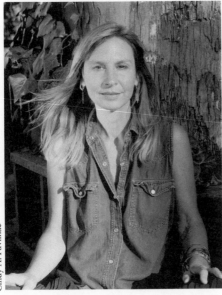

Cindy A. Pavlinac

Leila Castle is a native Californian born of French ancestry. Her interest in fragrance began as a child living beside the Berkeley Rose Garden, where she was caught by gardeners stealing armloads of roses to make perfume. Her study and teaching of goddess traditions spans over twenty-five years, and includes many years of travel to sacred places and research into the magical and transformational use of fragrance.

She was introduced to aromatherapy and essential oils in 1987 by aromatic consultant John Steele, with whom she has worked closely. Her forthcoming book, *Earthwalking SkyDancers: Women's Pilgrimages to Sacred Places,* (North Atlantic Books, 1996) is a collection of women's stories of the sacred feminine at sacred places worldwide. She lives in Point Reyes, California with her two children, making luscious aromatic blends for the well-being and happiness of as many people as possible.

hile recently attending a conference on ethnobotanicals at the Mayan temple ruins of Palenque in southern Mexico, I learned indigenous Lacondon Mayan stories about this enchanted sacred place from German anthropologist Christian Rätsch, who had once lived with the Lacondon. The Tuberose is the sacred creation flower of the Lacondon. They believe it grew from Palenque and gave birth to the first goddess and god, who in turn gave birth to all other beings. It is a beautiful story of the union of female and male deities emanating from this intoxicating flower.

At midnight on the full moon we entered the temple ruins and took part in a ritual honoring Ixchel, the Mayan goddess of the moon and rainbow. I will always associate the warm, luminous quality of the moonlight and the scent of burning Copal and Tuberose with her.

During a meditational journey, I entered one of the newly excavated temple ruins deeper in the rainforest, still beautifully decorated with brightly painted frescoes of floral design. Several goddess-like Mayan women greeted me. Their long, shiny black hair hung loosely as they gently laid me down on a healing altar covered with Tuberose flowers. As they anointed and massaged my hair and body with a fragrant Tuberose-infused oil, they told me that the spirit of this plant was a healing blessing to me and that it would always be a part of me that I could bring back to the world through my aromatic work. I melted into a buttery-sweet Tuberose bliss, experiencing a deep, sacred, feminine healing energy.

When I returned home from that pilgrimage, I made a botanical perfume blend with essential oils and absolutes for Ixchel to honor this experience and to share the healing energy of it with other women and men. The blend consisted of Tuberose, Jasmine, Vanilla, and Ambrette absolutes with Citruses.

Originally perfumery was a means of experiencing union with the goddesses and gods through the offering of fragrance while reconnecting with the living Earth, with Gaia. According to *The Magical and Ritual Use of Perfumes* by Richard and Iona Miller the original meaning of the word *therapeuein*—"to heal" in Greek— was to serve the gods.* With its roots embedded in the rich soil of the most ancient cultures that revered the Great Goddess, aromatherapy does this marvelously.

According to the research of the late archaeologist Dr. Marija Gimbutas, in the peaceful, egalitarian, Neolithic goddess cultures of Old Europe the sacred feminine

---

*Editor's Note: According to the Shorter Oxford English Dictionary, therapeuein means 'to minister to, treat medically.'

was regarded as the source and unity of all life in nature. The Great Mother who births all creation from the darkness of her womb was a metaphor for nature. As the cosmic giver and taker of life, she was also Mistress of the Plants, and of the death and renewal of plant life. She was Mother Earth, a pregnant goddess ripe with the fertility of the Earth and all creatures, mother to wild plants and domesticated grains. This was a world where the pregnancy of the Earth and women were revered as the same, where images of the vulva sprout buds and branches of trees. This is the mother culture of the Western civilization that stretched from Scandinavia to the Mediterranean, from Ireland to the Middle East.

Our present aromatic craft of healing with the essences of plants shares much with the knowledge of the priestesses and women in these Neolithic goddess cultures who preserved an ancient tradition of botanical wisdom from Paleolithic times based on deep attunement and direct experience using plants for the well-being of their communities. In the several-thousand-year period that followed the destruction of these cultures by the violent invasion first of Kurgan warriors, then of Christianity, the ancestors and inheritors of this ancient tradition of botanical wisdom were the witches, or wicca, the wise women.

The witch-Goddess that survived in European folklore was skilled in the use of medicinal herbs and balanced the interwoven web of human, animal, and plant vitality. Midwives, herbalists, counselors, and general practitioners were all educated in the language of herbs and healing. Healing was the domain of women—the art of healing linked to the activities of motherhood—combining wisdom, nurturing, tenderness, and skill. In her book on natural healing methods, *Liber Simplicis Medicinal,* St. Hildegarde of Bingen (1098–1178) recorded that women healers in the early Middle Ages knew the healing properties of 213 varieties of plants, fifty-five trees, and dozens of mineral and animal derivatives.

Unfortunately, most of these women were murdered for this knowledge during the Burning Times that swept Europe during the fifteenth- and sixteenth-century Inquisition. An estimated nine million "witches" were executed for the crime of healing, as well as those who consulted healers, because they had gone to witches instead of to God. It is from the ashes of these women that the technology of modern medicine emerged.

In its use of the most concentrated form of herbalism—essential oils, the distilled essences of botanicals—aromatherapy can be understood as a rebirth of this ancient knowledge, a very suitable one for our present time and need because of its incredible accessibility to masses of the population, especially in urban areas where toxins and pollution are strong. We are literally bringing the spirits of the botanical realm of nature, of Gaia, into our homes, workplaces, and daily lives as never before. What a wonderful way to return us to the forest and garden, and to a more healthy, nurturing, and pleasurable way of life.

In *Sacred Pleasure,* Riane Eisler writes about the relationship of pleasure and pain to the evolutionary trends of partnership and domination. She associates our original evolutionary orientation toward pleasure, empathy, and nurturing with partnership cultures that regarded the feminine as divine. The trend toward domination, enforced by the threat of pain, control, and warfare, is characterized by warrior cultures that later emerged and evolved about five thousand years ago, in which the feminine is devalued as well as the body, sexuality, and nature.

Our practice of aromatherapy today is an aspect of our original evolutionary trend toward partnership values, along with the ascension in current awareness of the environment, ecology, holistic and alternative healing methods, feminism, women's spirituality, and Gaian consciousness. All these trends are working to heal the destruction caused by the devaluation of the feminine, the body, sexuality, and nature. As a direct descendant of ancient botanical wisdom, intertwined with and dependent upon the health of the Earth for the therapeutic value of essential oils, aromatherapy reflects the nurturing, caring, and pleasure-oriented values of partnership by its deeply sensual methods of application such as massage, bathing, and perfumes, and by its pleasurable effects.

Our sense of smell is a primordial, erotic human experience. Our first scent perception is of the female essences from our mother's body, her blood and milk. Women's sense of smell is strongest during pregnancy. Sperm finds the egg by its scent. This erotic and life-enhancing nature of fragrance is beautifully expressed in the goddess art and myths of many cultures worldwide.

Aphrodite, the Greek goddess of love and beauty, was called the Golden One, associated with the goldenness of Honey, the sweet nectar of women's aroused sexual fluid, and the radiance of sexual pleasure. She is a goddess of perfume, represented by fruit, flowers, and nectar as sexual organs. In the Homeric Hymn to Aphrodite, from *Goddesses of the Sun and Moon* by Karl Kerenyi, she prepares herself to meet her lover:

> *She went away to Cyprus, and entered her fragrant temple at Paphos, where she has a precinct and a fragrant altar. After going inside she closed the bright doors, and the Graces gave her a bath, they oiled her with sacred Olive oil, the*

kind that gods always have on, that pleasant ambrosia that she was perfumed with. Having put on all her beautiful clothing, having ornamented herself in gold, Aphrodite, lover of laughter, hurried away to Troy, leaving sweet-smelling Cyprus, quickly cutting a path through the clouds high up.

In tantric traditions in ancient matrilineal India, menstrual blood was called "the flower," and vulva/yoni-shaped flowers were used in rituals. The Lotus is the symbol of both enlightenment and the yoni. Sandalwood paste was used to anoint the vulva in rituals. One of the offerings in tantric rituals is scent—perfume, incense, and flowers. All the senses are offerings of enjoyment to the deity that is an image and embodiment of our own true nature.

Xochiquetzal is the Central American Aztec goddess of love, sexuality, and pleasure. Her name means Precious Flower. Hummingbirds, butterflies, and flowers are her symbols. She seduces Quetzalcoatl, who then becomes Xochipili, Prince of Flowers. We often speak of the notes, chords, and harmony of fragrances in an attempt to describe their qualities. It is not surprising that Xochiquetzal is also associated with song, as are the celestial deities of fragrance and music, the Ghandarvas and Apsaras of India.

In ancient Sumeria, the Queen of Heaven and Earth—Inanna—was represented by a priestess in the sacred marriage ritual that bestowed the king with power to rule through his ritual sexual union with the goddess. The poetry that describes this union in the myth of Inanna, translated by Samuel Noah Kramer, is some of the earliest known writing, and expresses a deeply erotic awareness that is still integrated with nature and the sacred feminine. In preparation for the rite, Inanna perfumes her sides with scented oil after she baths her "holy loins" and sprinkles sweet-smelling Cedar oil on the ground. Rushes are also cleansed with Cedar oil, which are then arranged for the bed . . . "A bridal sheet to rejoice the heart, a bridal sheet to sweeten the loins, a bridal sheet for Inanna and Dumuzi."

Sharing the Nectars

I make aromatic goddess blends to help us remember these primordial feminine scents as contemporary women, and to return to an awareness of the sacredness of women and life. The perfume blends are made to invoke aromatic experience of different aspects of the Great Goddess in her various manifestations through many times and places in the world. I research herbal, aromatic, archeological, mythic, archetypal, textural, poetic, astrological, and magical sources to find references and correspondences to fragrances, incenses, plants, or flowers associated with and attributed to different goddesses. I marry this information with my knowledge of the effect and fragrance of the oils and how they blend, to actually create a change of consciousness for the user that matches and elicits the quality of the sacred feminine.

Magic is defined as *the art of changing consciousness at will,* and scent has the power to evoke and access deeper and altered states of consciousness. Perfume then becomes magical, transformational, not only aesthetic or cosmetic. Having worked with many of these goddesses through study, ritual, and practice for a long time, they have a familiarity that I can enter into to find the fragrances. We could call this archetypal or sacred perfumery.

The first goddess blend I made was "Aphrodite." Falling in love, and very much under her enchantment at the time, I wanted to create a fragrance that expressed the passion I felt as well as the beauty of my femaleness. I used Geranium, Sandalwood, and Rose absolute, each attributed to Venus, because this is the planet associated with Aphrodite. I chose oils that are among the most deliciously aphrodisiac to evoke her nature: Jasmine absolute, Clary Sage, Neroli, and Ylang-Ylang. The blend was and continues to be very successful, not only for me, but for the many women who have also experienced its luxurious sensuality.

It gives me great pleasure to do this—not only to be able to work with the oils themselves, but to share them, knowing that I am providing the women and men who use and enjoy them with the finest quality blends made with pure essential oils and precious flower absolutes that will nurture their bodies and souls. I call it sharing the nectars. Another form of flower power!

And as I work with the oils myself, I experience my own profound levels of physical, emotional, spiritual healing. We are healing thousands of years of destruction of feminine values and wisdom, the dissociation of sexuality and spirituality, the separation of mind, body, and spirit, the disconnection between people and nature, and the war between men and women. The plant spirits that we call essential oils are some of our great and generous allies in this present unprecedented moment in the history of the planet, as we face a global healing crisis of staggering proportions. I hope we can succeed, and that aromatherapy will be a means of that success. Healing us through the beauty, gentleness, and pleasure of the flowers, trees, and wild, green, growing things is a way that Gaia is working to rebalance and heal herself.

16

A Healing Partnership:
Oils and Crystals

Tricia Davis

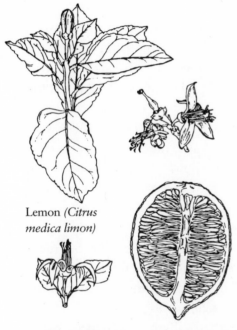

Lemon *(Citrus medica limon)*

Patricia Davis was born in London, educated "all over the place" because of wartime evacuation, and returned to Parliament School after the war. Her early ambitions were to be either a dancer or a painter from 1952-1955. While working as a bi-lingual secretary and studying dance and painting part-time in the early fifties, Ms. Davis first encountered aromatherapy.

After eighteen years of motherhood, Ms. Davis trained at Esalen in massage and aromatherapy, and opened a practice in North London.

In 1982, she founded the London School of Aromatherapy, from which she retired in September, 1994. The school is now run by her daughter. Ms. Davis also launched *The Aromatherapy Quarterly* in 1983, and served as its editor until 1990.

Deeply involved in the foundation of the International Federation of Aromatherapists (IFA), Ms. Davis served on the working party that brought the International Federation of Aromatherapists into being, and later on the Council and Education Committee, which she chaired in its early years.

The author of *Aromatherapy, an A-Z* (1988), *Subtle Aromatherapy* (1991), and *A Change for the Better* (1993), Ms. Davis now lives in Devon, where she paints, writes, and cultivates her garden.

I was given my first crystal about eight years ago by the French aromatherapist Yves de Maneville. It was a small, clear Quartz point, and although I have acquired many larger, more brilliant and impressive crystals since then, it has a special place in my affections—much in the way one remembers a first love. Yves also showed me some simple ways of using essential oils and crystals together, and for several years I was quite content to limit my use of crystals to clear Quartz and these simple techniques.

Gradually, though, I began to acquire more and different crystals and gemstones, although I did little with them beyond placing them in a sunny spot and enjoying looking at them. As my collection grew, so did my curiosity, and I knew I needed to study them in depth to understand their healing energies. It was not until I moved to Devon that I found the right teachers.

I was shopping in Totnes' famous Friday market on a brilliant April morning when a shaft of sunlight struck rainbows off a transparent turquoise crystal on the other side of the marketplace. Weaving my way through the junk stalls and organic vegetables, I hurried across to where this wonderful colour had attracted my attention, and asked the stall holders what it was. By the time they had explained what the crystal was (an Aqua Aura), and its special properties, I knew these were the people from whom I wanted to learn. Luckily for me, they had a new course starting a few weeks later, and I embarked on a miraculous voyage of discovery. If you can cast your mind back to the moment when you first came across essential oils, you will know what I mean: the excitement of discovering each stone in turn, its special properties and uses in healing, its very personality.

As I learnt more about the healing action of crystals, it became clear that there were many analogies with essential oils, and I even ventured to take a few oils to some of the classes. Caroline and Simon, our teachers, had a genuine interest in the oils too, and were already using them in burners in their healing room.

As my knowledge of crystals expanded, I quite naturally began to incorporate them into aromatherapy treatments, especially as at that time I was being drawn more and more toward the practice of aromatherapy at a subtle or spiritual level. Crystals lend themselves ideally to this kind of work, although they have plenty of applications in straightforward physical treatments too.

If you would like to use crystals as part of your aromatherapy practice, it is probably best to start simply, and decide how far you want to develop this aspect of your work as you gain personal experience of them. A lovely starting point might be to buy a piece of Amethyst matrix to place in your healing room. It has an ability to absorb and transmute negative energy, and so is very good to have in any place where healing work is done. It will benefit both you and your clients.

Progressing to ways of using crystals more directly with your aromatherapy clients, a simple beginning could be to place three or four clear Quartz points on the massage couch while you are working. If you have three Quartz crystals, you can place one above your client's head and one below each foot. With four, place one at each corner of the table, angled toward your client. If the person you are working on is depleted and in need of an influx of healing energy, you should place the crystals with their points toward the client's body; but if the person is overactive, stressed, or holding in too much energy, you should place them with points outward to channel off excessive energy. Do remember, though, that whenever energy is taken away, something must replace it, so turn the crystals around during the closing stage of your massage to channel in healing.

As the previous paragraph implies, crystals are able to direct energy to where it is needed, and this is no "airy fairy" idea but scientific fact. The fact that crystals can receive, store, amplify, and transmit energy has been understood and utilized by scientists in applications ranging from the early "cat's whisker" radios to the most complex and sophisticated computers, and we can apply the same principles to healing with crystals, whether alone or in partnership with essential oils. If you accept the fact that there is an inexhaustible fund of healing energy available in the Universe, you will see that there is a clear analogy between crystal healing and those early radios: Healing energy surrounds us at all times, just as radio waves do, and crystals enable us to focus that energy where and when it is needed, just as a listener could make the radio waves audible when wanted. Of course, crystals are not the only way of "tuning in" to the power of healing—meditation, visualization, and prayer are some of the other ways of doing so, and in aromatherapy we can think of the plants and their precious essences as another means of touching that Source.

To what extent you want to develop the use of essential oils and crystals conjointly in your practice will depend partly on your personal feelings and partly on your clientele. If your practice is very much geared to treating physical problems such as back pain, skin problems, etc., your clients may not be very receptive to methods other than straightforward physical massage. However, if you work with people who understand the potential of aromatherapy on the emotional, psychological, and spiritual levels, they are likely to be sensitive to the added dimension that crystals can bring to such work. Most of us work with a cross-section of clients, and you will have a sense of who would, or would not, appreciate the introduction of crystals into their treatments.

About eighteen months after I completed that first course (I have since completed the intermediate and advanced training), my teachers and I embarked on some joint work. Working through each chakra in turn, we explored intuitively the relationship between oils and chakras, stones and chakras, and oils and stones. Simon and Caroline already had a deep knowledge of crystals and how they relate to chakra energies, and I had done a considerable amount of work with oils and chakras, so the main emphasis of our work was on how the oils and the stones resonate with and enhance each other. It was a very enriching process for all three of us, and the greatest delight and excitement lay in the discovery of just how precisely the character and action of certain stones and oils mirrored each other.

A Colourful Correspondence: Chakras & Stones

In healing and balancing the chakras, coloured crystals or gemstones are very significant, though clear Quartz has a part to play, too. Whereas clear quartz, being transparent, resonates with every colour of the spectrum and can channel all vibrations of healing energy, the coloured stones are more specific in their application and resonate with the energies corresponding to the stone's own colour. As the energy of each chakra is associated with a specific colour, it is not difficult to select stones that harmonize with those energies. Starting with red at the base chakra and working through the spectrum, it is possible to find stones in colours that correspond to every chakra, though to limit the choice of stones only to such direct "matching" would be rather simplistic. All the same, it can be a good starting point.

Stones that are a true red in colour are not common, but there are a number of reddish stones that can be used to stimulate and strengthen the base chakra. Garnets and Rubies represent a true red, but are costly. However, you do not need big pieces, and they do not need to be of the gem quality that jewelers use. Even small pieces embody the specific healing energy associated with red, and would be valuable assets in a collection of healing crystals. Also associated with the base chakra are stones that are earthing and grounding in their action, many of which are black, dark brown, dark green, or sometimes combine more than one of these colours. If you are planning to use them in partnership with essential oils, you might start by considering the oils that have a grounding effect, and making comparisons. Many of the oils that benefit the base chakra are found among those classified as "base notes." Have a good look, as well as a sniff, and you will see that several of them are dark reddish or brown in colour (try Myrrh and Patchouli).

Moving upward to the second, or sacral, chakra and its associated colour, orange, many of the same remarks hold true: There are not many bright orange stones but many of the "red" ones can equally well be considered orange, being red-orange-rust in tone, and some of these harmonize with the sacral chakra as well as the base. We should also consider here the fact that each chakra influences, and is influenced by, those above and below it, so there will always be a degree of overlap in the stones and essential oils that you might use to balance each one. Several of the oils that have a particular affinity for the sacral chakra are also base notes, and some are valuable in working with the base chakra too.

For the solar plexus, yellow stones such as Citrine, Sulphur, and Yellow Jasper are easily identified, but a number of green stones can also be very valuable when working here. Green is generally thought of as the heart chakra colour, so here again you can see the principle of overlap at work. The flow of energy is quite often blocked between the solar plexus and the heart, so using stones that resonate with both of these centres is very valuable. At the same time, you can think about oils that have an "opening" energy, and perhaps massage movements, either on or off the body, which might help to shift blocks and restore the natural flow of energy. Juniper, which is as much a detoxifier on the psychic plane as on the physical, is often an appropriate choice.

The heart chakra is of tremendous importance, forming the link between the three lower and the three upper chakras. If the heart chakra is closed, energy cannot flow freely between the upper and lower chakras, and our physical energies cannot nourish our mental, emotional, and spiritual aspects. At this centre, we use both pink and green stones: green corresponding with the heart centre's place in the spectrum as it relates to the seven major chakras, and pink because it resonates with the love associated with this chakra. Here we can find some of the clearest correlations between oils and stones. Rose Quartz is the heart chakra stone par excellence, and its energy parallels in every way that of Rose oil. Bergamot is another heart chakra oil, resonating with some of the green healing stones such as Peridot or Aventurine.

Continuing our journey through the chakras, we can find a very direct "match" between Blue Chamomile and several blue stones, such as Blue Lace Agate, that are beneficial to the throat chakra, but when we come to the brow chakra, or third eye, the correspondences are far more subtle and we need to look much more at the energies of the respective oils and stones rather than any obvious colour relationship.

The same is true to some extent of the crown chakra. There are quite a number of essential oils and an equally large selection of crystals that resonate with crown chakra energy, and it is not always very obvious why they relate to each other as perfectly as they do. To understand these relationships or resonances, it really is necessary to work with and experience the oils and stones, and feel the corresponding energies. I'll give just one example here: Neroli embodies, for me at least, the pure white-gold radiance of the crown chakra and of the eighth and higher chakras that are not located within the physical body. Consider for a moment the Orange blossom that yields this precious oil: the pure white flowers with their golden stamens radiating out from the centre, borne on branches high above the ground. More than any other oil, Neroli speaks of purity and of Spirit.

Developing Your Own Intuition

You will realize that I have given few actual examples of oils or stones in this article, and there are several reasons for this. One is that there are several oils and a number of stones appropriate to each chakra, and the choice will always depend on the needs and energy levels of a particular client at a specific time. There are also quite a few stones and oils that are applicable to more than one chakra. Be wary of writers-teachers who make didactic statements that this crystal corresponds to that oil, without any alternatives or correlations. There will always be exceptions to any rule, and a fluid and intuitive approach will lead you to the right choice far more often than following rigid rules. Using your own sensitivity and intuition to seek out oils and stones, handling these and sitting with them in meditation, and placing them at different points on your own body, will teach you more than any article or book, and when you begin to feel the character of each stone you will find that your existing knowledge of essential oils will often suggest interesting combinations.

Yet another reason for not tying in oils-to-stones-to-chakras too rigidly is that there are other factors to consider along with the underlying spectrum-colour idea. For example, an individual chakra may need either calming or stimulating, so you might choose oils or stones that have such effects, regardless of the fact that they are not of the colour or energy usually associated with that chakra. You might use a red stone and a tonic or stimulant oil on the throat chakra if the energy feels very depleted. Red stones are generally very energizing, wherever they are placed on the body. Conversely, blue stones and some of the green ones have a generally calming and soothing action, so you might place them over any chakra that feels too "full" or over-active. You can arrive at such choices in exactly the same way you decide when and how to use a tonic or stimulant oil, or a sedative or anti-inflammatory one.

You need not, of course, restrict your use of crystals and gemstones on the body to the energy centres alone. You might place energizing stones on or around an injured limb to encourage healing, or over the thymus to stimulate the immune system; or you could place cooling, soothing stones over an area of inflammation.

Grounding, earthing stones can be placed on or near a client's feet, or in their hands. I'm sure you will have noticed that a client can feel a bit "spacey" at the end of an aromatherapy treatment, especially if you have done a lot of energy work; in such instances it is very useful to give them a piece of Hæmatite to hold in each hand for a while. This is one of the most grounding stones (it is a form of iron ore), and will quickly restore the person to a more balanced state.

Practical Guidelines for Crystal Work

If you are not drawn to working with healing stones directly on your clients' bodies, or if your clientele would not welcome it, there are still ways to bring the healing energy of oils and crystals together in your practice. You can increase the potency of your essential oils by placing clear Quartz crystals in a grid pattern around the bottle, or simply by putting a small crystal in the dish in which you have mixed your oils for a treatment.

If you want to work with crystals, be as careful about selecting and buying them as you are when buying essential oils. Get to know your suppliers; and ask them where the crystals come from. Some are mined destructively by blasting with explosives, and some operations are carried on until a site is totally depleted of its crystals. If you wish to use stones for healing, try to avoid such exploitation and ravaging of Gaia. Instead, look for crystals that have been hand-cut by craftsmen who respect the Earth and will not strip a source bare. Such mining is usually small scale and often carried out by the same family for generations. You can see similarities with some of the traditional producers of essential oils, many of whom have been growing the herbs organically and distilling on-site for many years within one family.

When you buy, or are given, a new crystal, welcome it and get to know it before you use it in healing. Firstly, wash the crystal in a solution of sea salt and spring water. Hold it in your right hand, then in your left. Bring it close to your heart and welcome it as you feel its energy. Particularly if you are new to crystal work, it is a good idea to use a new crystal on yourself for a while before trying it with anyone else.

Crystals should also be washed each time they are used in healing. Pour non-carbonated water into a bowl and add sea salt until no more will dissolve, then place your crystals in the solution. Quartz crystals should be left in salt water overnight, but coloured stones need only be dipped in and then dried carefully. Crystals also like to be placed in sunlight, so on a bright day, you can place the bowl of salt water out of doors, or indoors in a sunny spot; or put your crystals out in the sun even if they are not in need of cleansing at that moment. You'll see how much more they sparkle when you bring them in, after absorbing the powerful solar energy.

Please do not be tempted to rush out and buy a few crystals and start using them (with the exception, perhaps, of an Amethyst to place in your healing room). Crystals and gemstones are extremely powerful therapeutic agents, just as essential oils are, and should be studied in just as much depth, and used with equal care and responsibility. This article has been, of necessity, only a brief introduction to the subject. If you want to know more about working with oils and crystals together, my book *Subtle Aromatherapy* contains a section based on the research that Caroline, Simon, and I carried out, which I mentioned above. For the best guide to crystals and gemstones, I strongly recommend the *Crystal Trilogy* by Katrina Raphaell, who is one of the world's inspired and dedicated teachers of crystal healing. There is as much rubbish written about crystals as there is about essential oils, and it is important to find sources you can trust.

Once you start studying crystals, you will realize the learning is never finished! As with essential oils, there is always something new to discover, a new aspect of some oil or stone you thought you knew well, an unexpected experience, an insight shared by a colleague. Many of us are working with essential oils that were virtually unknown, or not generally available, a decade ago. In the same way, crystal work is being extended as new ones come to light. Sometimes there are stones long been known to geologists, whose healing energies are only now being discovered; but there are also stones only found in recent years. These are often of particular relevance to the needs of the present time.

Crystals enable us to bring the energy of the mineral kingdom into our healing work, just as essential oils enable us to draw on the healing energies of the plant kingdom. In nature, plants and minerals live in the most intimate harmony; plants drawing upon the minerals for their very nourishment, and it feels good and seemly to bring them together again for the healing of ourselves and our fellow humans. Both plants and minerals are the gifts of Gaia to humankind, and we owe her our continuing thanks whenever we use them.

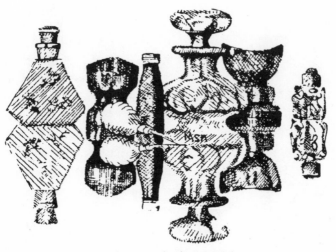

Perfume Bottles, by M.S. Moore

17

Perfumery with Rare Essences

Christine Malcolm

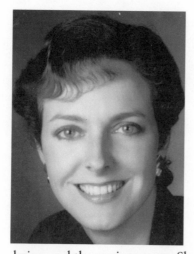

Christine Malcolm is owner of Santa Fe Botanical Fragrances Inc., a natural-perfume company that develops fragrances gathered globally from botanical aromatics and a member of the American Society of Perfumers, Society of Cosmetic Chemists, and Women in Flavor & Fragrance Commerce since 1970. Christine has worked in the fragrance supply industry in research and development for several major companies in quality control, sensory evaluation, and creative perfumery.

At Ohio State University in 1984, she received an honors in Experimental Psychology for conducting research in olfactory perception related to human well being and the environment. She studied Preventive Medicine at the Ohio State School of Medicine, and is certified in natural therapeutics from Dr. Scherer's Academy of Natural Healing in 1986. She is director of ARIA, Aroma Research Institute in America, which she founded in 1987. She lectures and writes for magazines worldwide, and is currently documenting the botanical-fragrance industry in several countries.

*T*he smell of one's persona is very individual, like a fingerprint. Fears, hopes, and wishes emanate in the effluvia of the emotions that a person generates. This effluvia is a combination of thoughts, food intake, and environment.

Modern fashion encourages us to hide from each other. We live close to each other, but mask our odors in order to be acceptable, so that none of our ethnic and emotional differences are predominant.

Anyone who is very odor perceptive will understand that we are a pre-packaged persona. Natural perfumery recognizes that these individualities can work with aromas to create a pleasing scent. The difference between natural perfumes and synthetic perfumes is that the synthetic ones smell the same on everyone, while natural perfumes have organic bases and greater mutability, causing them to interact with the oils of the body. While the scent may be recognizable as Jasmine or Rose, this interaction produces an individualized print as the aroma changes.

Technology for obtaining botanical aromatics has improved since the 1940s and, because most fragrances on the market over the past fifty years have been predominantly synthetic, original creations by a new generation of perfumers are possible.

Under-utilized production facilities are being put back into service and new ones are being built, taking advantage of recent technological innovations and providing better and more consistent extraction methods to obtain a wider variety of aromas for the natural perfumery palette. Over three thousand essential oils have been identified from the large number of plant species, and only several hundred have been commercialized. Of the 300,000 to 500,000 flowering plant species in the world, only ten percent have been examined even in a cursory fashion. Only one percent (3,000 to 5,000) of those have ever been cultivated. A tremendous reserve of potentially useful plant aromas or essential oils have never even been discovered.

I was trained in commercial perfumery, which emphasizes the use of synthetic ingredients sprinkled with naturals, and it has been an interesting transition to reorient myself to only natural essential oils, absolutes, gums and resins.

The commercial perfumer usually trains as an apprentice for a minimum of six years, and must have the ability to "visualize" a scent, and construct it using the olfactory memory, just as an artist draws upon memory of color and form. When I create a fragrance, I try to materialize the moods and imagery of a scent, and capture what I already have a mental picture of, on paper. This can be accomplished by anyone who has a good relationship with essential oils who knows the oils from both the olfactive realty and memory impression, so that utilizing them as a paint palette is easily done. This knowledge is gained by using the oils on a daily basis. When using aromatic chemicals, there are thousands to commit to memory, while only the knowledge of twenty to forty essential oils is necessary to create aromatherapy blends. The novice perfumer begins learning the craft by making simple blends of two, three, four, and five essences in varying combinations.

Essential oil blending does not have to be complicated, because the majority of the work is already accomplished by nature herself! There is a depth and dimension in essential oils that cannot be compared to aroma chemicals, no matter how similar the molecular structures. Essential oils themselves have long evolutionary and cultural histories that contribute to their multidimensionality.

Over the years, I have delved into the mystery of perfumes and the intimate histories behind each natural aromatic. I have been passionately in pursuit of familiarity with aromatics, which I accomplish partially by creating blends. My compositions utilize earth-borne ingredients, and result in simple but mysterious fragrances that are harmonious and aesthetically satisfying. Creating perfumes from a natural palette is challenging, and opens possibilities far beyond the treasured fragrances of the past.

It is only necessary to know five essences to begin. Put a drop of essential oil on blotter paper, and smell the oil from the paper. Putting the essential oil or resin in a vehicle such as Jojoba, vegetable oil, or alcohol to dilute it will enable you to have a better opportunity to decipher the nuances of the aroma. Ten percent dilution is a good starting point. Try Lavender, Clary Sage, Patchouli, Geranium, or Lemon. Write your first impressions of the aroma in a notebook. Everyone will have a different perception of the same aroma. Vocabulary that describes colors, textures, shapes, and emotions is very useful in order to describe your perceptions.

Let the aromatic dry down a bit and smell it again, continuing to add information to your written description. Is it very diffusive, or heavy? How long does the aroma last? Terms like woody, fruity, citrus, green, mossy, or herbal can help you to describe and remember the aromatic. Does it have a minty, nutty, tea, hay, tobacco, or other characteristic note? Is there a burnt note? This is usually indicative of an oil that was distilled at too high a temperature.

Evaluate the forms and shapes that come to mind. Is it sharp, round, smooth, voluminous? What type of personality does it allude to? Is it sultry, aggressive, shy, angry? Is it scattered or tight? The more you can describe it, the better you will remember it. Any word that you can ascribe to it will be helpful.

Where does it go in your body? Is it highly volatile? Does it go directly to your brain? Does it delicately come into your chest? Note the difference between the initial impression and the middle and final stages, referred to as the dry-down or base notes.

I would describe Violet leaf absolute as cool, cucumber-like, earthy, high pitched, green, and narrow. It is a note that stays with you for a while. Petitgrain, on the other hand, has a more voluminous presence. It is citrusy but floral. It seems to me to be a more complicated aroma. It is a good mixing oil, whereas Violet leaf absolute is a good highlighter, even though it will last through all three stages of evaporation. Geranium always has an intriguing top note. It reminds me of a metallic Rose. It is cool and sometimes crisp. It is a great top note, but stays until the middle. Sandalwood is very subtle, yet it is a wonderful cohesive choice to pull the other aromatics together, and lasts till the end. It creates a musky aroma. It is a precious woody note that keeps a blend together.

Taking a bath in which you have put a single oil or combination is also a helpful means of getting to know the aromas. There are books available on the market that can give you ideas of descriptive words. If you are truly interested in becoming a blender yourself, try not to use the formulations of others until you have worked with the oils yourself.

Creating perfumes can open up a whole new dimension to your being and I encourage you to try it. Techniques come with your preferences for different aromatics. If you are crazy about Cinnamon, chances are most of your blends will include Cinnamon. As you start to work with your own palette, a signature of your creativity is forming. The most important difference between artists is their specific choice for their color palette. The same principle applies to a perfumer's palette.

Make a clean and peaceful space for yourself, one where you can sit and smell and ponder the aroma. After you have familiarized yourself with each aroma, start to visualize, in an olfactory way, the combination of two or three of the oils. Try Basil, Lemon and Vetivert. Close your eyes and imagine Lemon, fresh and clean, tart and diffusive, in combination with Vetivert or Patchouli. These two essential oils are woody and earthy. Imagine most of the blend to be Lemon, with the added weight of the woody notes. Visualize in your smell-memory what the two in combination are. Try different combinations, 50/50 and 25/75. Now actually put them together, to smell for yourself what they actually are like. Keep notes.

After you have the proportions that smell the way you desire, imagine a third oil such as Basil or Cinnamon bursting off the top of the fragrance. Now you have a good start to add other nuances such as Ylang-Ylang, Jasmine, or Geranium. Add more spices like Cardamom, Coriander, Pepper, or Clove. If you want to warm it up use heavy balsamic notes such as Benzoin, Labdanum, Cedar, and Sandalwood. Be careful not to overpower the blend with one note. Rosemary or Peppermint will wipe out a carefully balanced blend although there may be times when you are deliberately looking to enhance one major note in a fragrance composition. Do not limit yourself, but do proceed very slowly by adding one new note at a time, developing a vocabulary and aromatic memory for each aroma before working with it.

Using this method, you will teach yourself about perfumery and how aromatics react with each other. Some essential oils are synergizers, that is, they enhance the oils they are added to. Some help to mellow and round out a blend. There is no absolutely correct way to blend. To create a blend for yourself or another person, you first need to consider how sensitive you are to aromas. You may be the type of person who only likes to have a semblance of aroma in your space. Always ask your prospective patron how much scent they can tolerate. Many people claim to have allergies or sensitivities to aromas. In many cases, a person's acceptance of essential oils is stronger than their tolerance for synthetic aromas, and many people who consider themselves sensitive to aromas are able to enjoy essential oils without any side effects.

Always let the client smell several oils to see what they are drawn to. If they like to cook, they may enjoy the aroma of spices and herbs. Do they enjoy the scents of flowers? Or do they enjoy hiking through the woods? Ask questions that give clues to their activities and associated scents that go with them. Always ask which aromas, if any, they do not like. By process of elimination and clue-seeking, you will come up with the appropriate blends. If you want the blend to be specifically aromatherapeutic, you can ask questions about their present state of emotional and physical health.

As a perfumer who specializes in creating natural perfumes and synergy blends, it is my hope that those of you interested in essential oils will consider the broader definitions of what aromatherapy means. A drop of essential oil is simply added to a chemical formulation does not make the product aromatherapeutic. Let us not limit aromatherapy to an allopathic design whereby the oils are used only as remedies. Aromatics can be worn for aesthetics, because they bring pleasure to the wearer and purpose to the environment. Blends of aromas can exist just as they are—precious aromatics brought forth from the Earth. Using a natural perfume reflects the way in which we honor ourselves by honoring the Earth. The legitimacy of past wisdom must be appreciated and applied along with present technologies. By taking into account the old and the new, the inner and the outer, we see that they can be artfully blended to provide the sustenance needed to afford us encouraging alternatives.

Botanical Perfume Formulations

A relaxing blend based on Lavender *(Lavandula angustifolia)*:

In a one or two ounce glass bottle (depending on intensity of fragrance desired), combine:

35 drops Lavender *(Lavandula angustifolia)* flower
24 drops Bergamot *(Citrus bergamia)* peel
20 drops Sandalwood *(Santalum album)* wood
12 drops Geranium *(Pelargonium graveolens)* leaves
 2 drops Frankincense *(Boswellia carterii)* resin essential oil
 2 drops Carrot *(Daucus carota)* seed
 2 drops Parsley *(Petroselinum sativum)* seed
 2 dops *Cistus labdanum* resin essential oil

Fill with Jojoba oil or grain alcohol.
This is approximately 5-10%.
To make a bath oil, use a 1/2-oz. bottle.

Lavender *(Lavandula angustifolia)*
also combines well with Cedarwood
(Cedrus libani), Clove *(Eugenia*
caryophyllata), Clary Sage *(Salvia*
sclarea), Jasmine *(Jasminum officinale)*
Oakmoss *(Evernia prunastri)*,
Patchouli *(Pogostemon patchouli)*,
Pine *(Pinus spp.)*, Citrus oils,
Evergreens and Ylang-Ylang
(Cananga odorata).

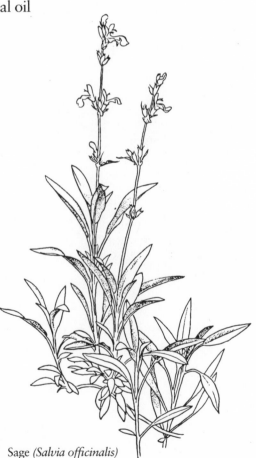

Sage *(Salvia officinalis)*

For an exotic, uplifting blend, try the following. It is a delightful Lily-of-the-Valley fragrance with a precious woody undertone and sweet Oriental nuance.

    30 drops Geranium *(Pelargonium graveolens)* leaves
    20 drops Sandalwood *(Santalum album)* wood
     7 drops Rose absolute *(Rosa spp.)* flower
    15 drops Bergamot *(Citrus bergamia)* peel
    15 drops Lavender *(Lavandula angustifolia)* flower
     3 drops Benzoin resin absolute
     2 drops Frankincense *(Boswellia carterii)* resin essential oil
     2 drops Coriander *(Coriandrum sativum)* seed
     2 drops Basil *(Ocimum basilicum)* leaves
     1 drop Cardamom *(Elettaria cardamomum)* seed

Neroli is an emotionally uplifting scent that can impart an ethereal nuance to a floral fragrance. This blend is not only uplifting but also very grounding. To make a 7.5% blend, add 1 ounce Jojoba oil to the following essential oils:

     2 drops Jasmine *(Jasminum spp.)* flower
    10 drops Neroli *(Citrus aurantium)* flower
    12 drops Sandalwood *(Santalum album)* wood
     6 drops Petitgrain *(Citrus aurantium amara)* leaves
     4 drops Frankincense *(Boswellia carterii)* resin essential oil
     6 drops Ylang-Ylang *(Cananga odorata)* flower
     3 drops Orange flower absolute *(Citrus aurantium)* flower
     2 drops Vetivert *(Andropogon zizanioides)* resin essential oil
     5 drops Bergamot *(Citrus bergamia)* peel or Tangerine *(Citrus reticulata)* peel
     5 drops Patchouli *(Pogostemon patchouli)* resin essential oil
     5 drops Clary Sage *(Salvia sclarea)* leaf

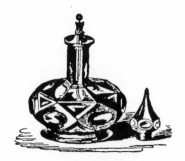

Perfume lamp

18

Essential Oil Blends to Perfume Your Body

Jeanne Rose

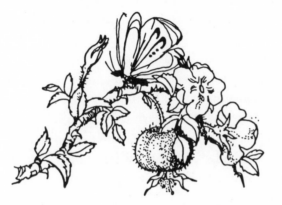

*Y*ou are the alchemist's apprentice now. Mixing and blending natural botanical-based scents is just part of your day's work. You bathe and cleanse in yummy fragrant soap, and use left over essential oil drops to scent your laundry. You make particular blends to inhale for health and apply nature's pure lotions—made of vegetable oils, beeswax and essential oils, and preserved with Grapefruit seed extract—for the health of your skin. Now you need only make your scented blends to use as perfume to fragrance your body.

The formulas that follow are simple to make. Just make the essential oil blend, pouring the essential oils directly into a two-dram vial (1/4 oz. bottle). Shake the mixture at least fifty times to let every molecule of each scent thoroughly incorporate. Age at least two weeks. This is your blend. Then add the carrier oil or alcohol.

147

Adding vegetable oil makes an oily perfume or massage oil, and adding alcohol makes a perfume or cologne.

Perfume Oil • Make your blend in a two dram vial, shake it thoroughly, let it age and meld two weeks, then fill the bottle with Jojoba oil. If the scent is too strong, pour into a 1/2 oz. bottle and add more Jojoba oil. Use sparingly, directly after the bath, applying the oil blend to the body before toweling off.

Massage Oil • Make your blend, shake the bottle thoroughly, let it age and meld two weeks. To every ounce of vegetable oil, add 2-10 drops of your perfume blend, depending upon the strength of the scent that you prefer. Shake thoroughly before using.

Bath Oil • Make your blend in a two-dram vial, shake it thoroughly, let it age two weeks, then top it off with unscented Turkey red oil (water-soluble oil). You can use it in the bath, or pour it into a 1 oz. bottle and add a sudsing agent such as liquid soap. Use only 1/4 oz. per bath.

Perfume • Make your blend in a two-dram vial, shake it thoroughly, let it age two weeks, then top the bottle with alcohol, shake thoroughly, and age it again two weeks. Use this in a spritzer over the body, particularly the pulse points.

Cologne • Make your blend in a 2 oz. bottle, shake it thoroughly, let it age two weeks, then add 1/2 oz. perfume alcohol, shake thoroughly, and age it again for two weeks. Now add distilled water to fill the bottle. Shake thoroughly. Can be applied directly and spritzed on the body via a mister or spray bottle. Shake before each use.

Blends for the Body

Floral or Sensual Types

1. **Oriental**

Pogostemon cablin (lvs)	5 drops
Boswellia sacra (eo)	5 drops
Rosa centifolia (flw)	5 drops
Coriandrum sativum (sd)	3 drops

2. **Sensuality**

Nardostachys jatamansi (rt)	200 drops
Rosa centifolia (flw)	100 drops
Lavandula angustifolia (flw)	50 drops
Matricaria recutita (flw)	1 drop

3. **Mexico Beach**

Vanilla planifolia (pods) CO_2	5 drops
Cryptocarya massoïa (bk)	1 drop
Jasminum officinale (flw) abs.	3 drops

4. **Mexico Beach #2**

Cryptocarya massoïa (bark)	3 drops
Citrus sinensis (pl)	20 drops
Jasminum officinale (flw) abs	3 drops

5. **Floral Floral**
   5 drops of each:
   Citrus aurantium bigarade (flw)
   Rosa centifolia (flw)
   Jasminum officinale (flw) abs.
   Cananga odorata (flw) extra
   Lavandula angustifolia (flw) SPA wild
   Vanilla planifolia (pods) abs.

6. **Floral Spring**

Cedrus atlantica (wd)	6 drops
Cananga odorata (flw) #3	6 drops
Rosa centifolia (flw)	2 drops
Citrus paradisi var pink (pl)	5 drops

Herbs & Spice or Men's Types

7. **Fields of Grass**

Cymbopogon martinii (lvs & flw)	5 drops
Citrus limonum (pl)	2 drops
Pelargonium graveolens Bour. (lvs)	3 drops
Piper nigrum (berr)	1 drop

8. **Candy Store**

Ravensara anisata (bk)	5 drops
Cinnamomum zeylanicum (bk)	1 drop
Citrus sinensis (pl)	10 drops
Vanilla planifolia (pod) abs.	1 drop

9. **Spice Islands**

Piper nigrum (berr)	2 drops
Coriandrum sativum (sd)	2 drops
Myristica fragrans (sd)	1 drop
Cinnamomum zeylanicum (bk)	2 drops
Syzygium aromaticum (bud)	2 drops
Citrus limonum (pl)	20 drops
Citrus reticulata, red (pl)	20 drops
Citrus paradisi (pl)	10 drops

10. **Desert Spice**

Citrus aurantium var *bergamia* (pl)	20 drops
Citrus sinensis (pl)	20 drops
Boswellia sacra (eo)	10 drops
Citrus aurantium var. *amara* (lvs)	10 drops
Citrus aurantifolia var. *limetta* (pl)	5 drops
Lavandula angustifolia (flw)	10 drops
Coriandrum sativum (sd)	10 drops

11. **Lady Killer**

Citrus sinensis (pl)	8 drops
Nardostachys jatamansi (rt)	2 drops
Cinnamomum zeylanicum (bk)	1 drop

Woods & Forest

12. **Floral Night**

Pogostemon cablin (lvs)	6 drops
Cedrus atlantica (wd)	3 drops
Citrus aurantium bigarade (flw)	3 drops
Pelargonium graveolens var. *Bour* (flw)	3 drops
Salvia sclarea (lvs)	3 drops

13. Dark Green Woods & Moss

Pogostemon cablin (lvs)	5 drops
Salvia sclarea (lvs & flw)	4 drops
Santalum album (wd)	8 drops
Rosa centifolia (otto)	2 drops
Tree moss abs.	1 drop

14. Yerba Buena

Picea mariana (ndl)	15 drops
Pseudotsuga douglasii (ndl)	15 drops
Pinus pinaster (ndl)	9 drops
Abies grandis (ndl)	6 drops
Mentha spicata (lvs)	2 drop

15. Dark Green Woods Santal

Pogostemon cablin (lvs)	5 drops
Salvia sclarea (lvs)	5 drops
Boswellia sacra (eo)	2 drops
Santalum album (wd)	3 drops

16. Dark Green Woods & Leaves

Pogostemon cablin (lvs)	6 drops
Salvia sclarea (lvs)	4 drops
Cupressus sempervirens (ndl)	3 drops
Citrus paradisi var white (pl)	3 drops
Citrus aurantium var. *amara* (lvs)	2 drops

17. Green Harmony—Greece

Pseudotsuga douglasii (ndl)	5 drops
Lavandula angustifolia (flw)	4 drops
Citrus aurantium bigarade (flw)	2 drops
Citrus limon (pl)	3 drops
Galbanum/Olibanum 1:3	1-2 drops

18. Grounding

Nardostachys jatamansi (rt)	5 drops
Pogostemon cablin (lvs)	2 drops
Citrus paradisi var pink (pl)	2 drops
Cananga odorada #1 (flw)	2 drops

Refreshing Citrus Types

19. Floral Summer

Cananga odorata extra (flw)	3 drops
Pelargonium graveolens (lvs)	5 drops
Lavandula angustifolia (flw)	3 drops
Salvia sclarea (lvs)	3 drops
Citrus aurantium spp bergamia (pl)	4 drops

20. Cool Harmony

Juniperus communis (berr)	6 drops
Salvia sclarea (lvs)	4 drops
Rosmarinus officinalis var verb (lvs)	1 drop
Mentha x piperita (lvs)	1 drop
Citrus aurantifolia var. *limetta* (pl)	3 drops

21. Tropical Beach

Cryptocarya massoïa (bk)	5 drops
Salvia sclarea (lvs)	10 drops
Nardostachys jatamansi (rt)	10 drops
Citrus paradisi, pink (pl)	10 drops

22. Green Harmony—Herbs

Cedrus atlantica (wd)	3 drops
Salvia sclarea (lvs)	5 drops
Citrus aurantium spp. bergamia (pl)	6 drops
Juniperus communis (berr)	3 drops
Ocimum basilicum (lvs)	1 drop

23. Floral Citrus

Citrus aurantium bigarade (flw)	6 drops
Citrus paradisi var white (pl)	2 drops
Citrus reticulata var red (pl)	2 drops
Citrus sinensis var CA (pl)	2 drops
Commiphora myrrha (eo)	1 drop

The essential oil blends have all been given by their Latin binomials so that you will know exactly which oils to use to duplicate these body perfumes. Since there are so many incorrect names in many books for the various Citrus types and parts, here is a listing of the Citrus types separately, with their common names:

Citrus aurantifolia var. *limetta* is Lime peel oil

Citrus aurantium var. *amara* (lvs) is Orange petitgrain or leaf oil

Citrus aurantium var. *bergamia* is Bergamot peel oil

Citrus aurantium bigarade is Orange flower oil or Neroli

Citrum limonum is Lime peel oil

Citrus paradisi is Grapefruit peel oil and comes in pink or white

Citrus reticulata, green is Tangerine peel oil

Citrus reticulata, red is Mandarin peel oil

Citrus sinensis is Sweet Orange peel oil

The initials: abs = absolute

flw = flower   ndl = needles

rt   = root   pl   = peel

bk   = bark   berr = berries

wd   = wood   sd   = seed

lvs   = leaves

Resource

Christine Wildwood has written a wonderful blending book called *Creative Aromatherapy*. The subtitle perfectly explains what is contained within its pages: *Blending and Mixing Essential Oils and Flower Remedies for Health and Beauty*, published by Thorsons, an imprint of HarperCollins, London & San Francisco, 1993. Some of the inspiration for the formulations come from this book.

19

Culinary Aromatherapy

Mindy Green

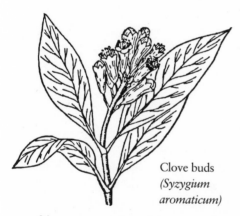

Clove buds
*(Syzygium
aromaticum)*

Mindy Green has a background in herbalism spanning twenty-three years. Her fascination with the healing power of plants led to the study of aromatherapy in 1978. With over a decade of experience in the natural-foods industry in the U.S. and Canada, she is also a licensed æsthetician and massage practitioner, and holds a degree in Wholistic Health Sciences. An herbalist, aromatherapist, and cosmetics consultant, Mindy is a co-director and faculty member of the California School of Herbal Studies, where she draws on fifteen years of teaching experience to share her skills in cosmetic and herbal preparations, laboratory procedure, aromatherapy, plant identification, natural skin care, and wild-foods cooking.

She is a co-founder and consultant for Simplers Botanical Company, a founding member of the American Herbalists Guild, and associate editor of the American Herb Association Newsletter. She has lectured in the U.S. and Canada, and is a contributing writer to several aromatherapy and herb publications. Mindy is proud to contribute to the herbal renaissance in America, and has just co-authored a book on the use of essential oils and herbs called *Aromatherapy: The Fragrant Art of Healing*.

*C*ulinary herbs themselves have always been a mainstay of creative cooking, and will continue to be so. Herbs add flavor, color, and nutritional value to all recipes. But have you ever considered topping a Geranium sponge pudding with a dollop of Neroli whipped cream, dreamed of a trio of scented sorbets, or imagined real Rose ice cream?

Iced herbal tea with a splash of aromatic hydrosol is heavenly on a hot summer day! Or how about flavoring your favorite jar of Black Tea, or your sugar bowl, with a few drops of essential oil?

It is a snap to make your own Lemon or Peppermint extract. Try oil of Dill in potato salad, or Caraway oil in cream cheese. There is no reason to confine essential oil and hydrosol use to cosmetic or therapeutic applications. Aromatics are wonderful in the kitchen, and with a bit of experience, a few guidelines, and a creative mind, the culinary possibilities are endless. I hope that reading this chapter and trying a few of the recipes will elevate your cooking creations to new heights of inspiration.

Safety is an important consideration in the kitchen, just as it is with any aspect of aromatherapy. Be sure you use pure oils from reliable sources, not synthetic scents or flavorings. Essential oils extracted with carbon dioxide are ideal for culinary use because their flavor is often stronger and more true to the plant. Absolutes are never used in the kitchen because solvent residues may be left as a by-product of their extraction process.

In general, it is wise to use only those oils that you would normally think of as foods, such as Citrus oils or seed oils such as Anise, Dill, Celery, Cumin, or Coriander. There are also a few suitable essential oils from flowers and medicinal herbs, including Rose, Neroli, Geranium, Lemon Verbena, Mint, and Melissa. All of these taste great in bubbly water, too. And of course, there are the essential oils from common spices, such as Ginger, Cinnamon, Clove, Nutmeg, Cardamom, and Black Pepper. Oils from commonly used culinary herbs such as Thyme, Rosemary, Oregano, Savory, Marjoram, and Sage are great for savory dishes, but are a bit tricky to work with as their flavors can be somewhat bitter or overpowering.

Essential oils evaporate as food is heated, so yield their best flavor and aroma when uncooked. It is best to use the oils in fresh-food dishes such as salad dressings, cold soups, blender drinks, or uncooked desserts. In cooked dishes like soups and sauces, add the oils at the last minute. Only one to three drops are necessary. With dishes that need to be baked, such as casseroles or cakes, you may need to add a bit more essential oil to compensate for what will evaporate during cooking.

What makes the difference between a delectable success and a culinary failure is the same basic principle that makes a success or failure of any aromatherapy blend: *dosage*. (The quality of your essential oils should also be good.) Experiment, but be conservative until you get the feel of how essential oils react with food. Start with one drop, and go from there. A little bit really does go a long way, especially when you consider how much of a plant is needed to make one drop of essential oil. It takes more than thirty Roses to make one precious drop of Rose oil.

Aromatic hydrosols can add some flair in the kitchen as well. Many gourmet or traditional ethnic cookbooks call for Rose water or Orange blossom water in exotic dishes, but imagine using Lemon Verbena or Rosemary water in some of your own recipes. Hydrosols are much milder in flavor than essential oils, and are safe to use (as long as the plant they are derived from is nontoxic), so are less of a concern. There is little information on the medicinal uses of hydrosols, but it is known that the Romans drank Rose water for a hangover. Hydrosols are best kept refrigerated.

The following recipes should help get you started, and spark your own imaginative ideas for creating the most exotic culinary delights. With a little inspiration, you can dramatically dress up and add excitement to almost any recipe. Share your favorite creations with us!

Extracts

Making your own flavoring extracts from essential oils is easy and economical. Extracts provide a good way to minimize dosage when one drop of an essential oil is too much. Any culinary essential oil can be made into an extract, but the technique is especially appropriate for oils that are harsh, strongly flavored, or very expensive. These include Peppermint, Rose, Lemon, Basil, and Ylang-Ylang.

The usual carrier for commercially made extracts is alcohol, but vegetable glycerin and vegetable oil are perfectly suitable and mix well with the essential oils. Glycerin is sweet and soluble in most media. I have been making my own Rose extract for years, and have learned that glycerin is the best carrier for this particular essential oil. I have tried alcohol and found that, when cold, the Rose essence forms a waxy film on top of the alcohol. However, alcohol works well with the Citrus oils and Peppermint. Shake all extracts before using. Start with five drops of essential oil per ounce of carrier, and adjust to suit your taste.

Basic Aromatic Extract Formula

> 5 drops essential oil
> 1 ounce carrier
>> Use 1/2 to 1 teaspoon in a recipe.

Sweet Recipes

Aromatic Honeys

Aromatic honeys are a delightful way to introduce even the staunchest skeptic to the pleasures of essential oils. Essential oils from herbs, spices, seeds, and flowers make excellent honeys. Some favorites are Angelica, Ginger, Cardamom, Rose, Peppermint, and Bergamot. You can use the oils individually or in combination. A few ideas for compatible flavors are Peppermint and Ginger, Rosemary and Lemon, or Cinnamon and Orange. These honeys are perfect for flavoring coffee or tea, and are effective digestive aids when taken after a meal. They are also very handy for making instant tea when traveling; just add one teaspoon to a cup of hot water and enjoy. I prefer to use a light honey, but dark honeys work as well.

These honeys will keep forever, but some may crystallize. To reliquefy, loosen the lid and place the jar in hot water until the honey melts. Never heat these honeys in the microwave.

Basic Aromatic Honey Formula

> 1/4 cup honey
> 1-2 drops essential oil
> Begin with one drop; it is usually enough. Stir well.

Aromatic Whipped Cream

If you really want to impress and delight your dinner guests, you'll try this. The idea came from fellow herbalist and aromatherapy enthusiast Diana DeLuca. She served a Neroli whipped cream that was out of this world! I was so taken with the topping I can't remember what it was served on. Since then I've discovered it is delicious with chocolate desserts. I have also experimented with other essential oils and had many pleasant results. Cardamom whipped cream on gingerbread is fabulous, and these creams make exotic toppings for cappuccino or hot chocolate.

Next I'm trying Black Currant whipped cream atop Apple cobbler! How about Mandarin cream on angel food cake? Don't the possibilities excite you? Exotic simplicity is thrilling and scrumptious!

For a low fat topping, add essential oils to yogurt.

Basic Aromatic Whipped Cream Formula

> 1/2 pint whipping cream
> 1–2 drops essential oil

Whip the cream to desired consistency, add essential oil and mix well. Start with one drop only. Add sweetener if desired.

Peppermint Tapioca

Quick and easy, this pleases children of all ages. The digestive attributes of peppermint are so fine, you could call this a medicinal dessert.

> 3 tablespoons "quick cooking" tapioca
> 2 3/4 cups milk
> 1/3 cup honey
> 1 egg (optional)
> 1 square (1 ounce) semi-sweet chocolate (optional)
> 1–2 drops Peppermint oil

Mix together everything except the peppermint oil and let the tapioca soak for 10 minutes. Cook over medium heat, stirring until the chocolate is melted. Bring to a boil, lower heat, and cook five more minutes. Let cool 15 minutes. Add Peppermint oil to taste, and pour into dessert cups. Serve warm or cold.

Midnight-at-the-Oasis Balls

We've all heard the saying, "Open sesame" (often mistaken for "open, says me"), from Ali Baba and the Forty Thieves—but did you know it referred to the strengthening and virile powers that this vitamin-E-packed seed contains? Try these suggestive delights on your lover on a warm, sultry night!

> 1 cup hulled Sesame seeds
> 2 tablespoons tahini or Almond butter
> 2–3 tablespoons honey
> 1 tablespoon finely chopped Dates

1 teaspoon Cardamom powder
1 teaspoon bee pollen
1/2 teaspoon Ginseng powder (optional)
1/2 teaspoon Vanilla extract
1 drop Rose oil

Grind the seeds in an electric coffee grinder. Add the Rose oil to the Vanilla to help disperse it. Mix all ingredients together thoroughly, and form into balls. Roll in shredded Coconut, Cocoa powder or whole Sesame seeds. Refrigerate and serve at just the right moment!

Lemon Geranium Sponge Cake
The addition of Geranium oil in this low-fat dessert adds a delightful floral hint.

1/3 cup honey
3 tablespoons flour
1/4 cup fresh Lemon juice
1 teaspoon grated Lemon peel
2 eggs, separated
1 cup milk
5 drops Geranium oil

Preheat oven to 325°F. Beat together honey, Lemon juice, rind and flour. Add yolks, milk and Geranium oil and mix again. In a separate bowl, beat egg whites until stiff, and fold into the Lemon mixture. Pour into a buttered 8-inch-square baking pan or individual custard cups, and place in a hot water bath. If available, lay fresh Rose Geranium leaves on top of the pudding. Bake for 45 to 50 minutes, or until cake is set and knife comes out clean. Serve warm or cold.

French Toast with Flair

2 eggs
1/2 cup milk
1 tablespoon pure Maple syrup
1 drop Cinnamon bark essential oil

Mix all the wet ingredients well and soak the bread thoroughly before frying. Bergamot, Anise, or Cardamom are nice substitutes for the Cinnamon oil. Cinnamon is strong, so if you find one drop too much for your palate, try one teaspoon of homemade essential oil extract, or dilute with more milk.

Essential Oil Blender Drinks

Peach Blush

> 3 ripe Peaches
> 1 cup plain yogurt
> 2 tablespoons honey
> 4 ice cubes
> 1–2 drops Mandarin essential oil

Whiz everything together in a blender. Start with one drop of essential oil and taste before adding more.

Jitterbug Perfume Spritzer
(Variation on a theme)

> 1/2 cup Strawberries
> 2 tablespoons honey
> 1 tablespoon Beet juice
> 1 teaspoon bee pollen
> 4 fresh Melissa leaves
> 2 cups mineral water
> 1 drop Melissa essential oil

Blend all ingredients in blender and serve with a fresh Jasmine blossom in each glass. If you don't have the Beet juice, soak 1/4 cup grated beets in the mineral water for 10 minutes, and strain. If you've ever read *Jitterbug Perfume* by Tom Robbins, you'll know why this is in there!

Strawberry-Rose Ice Cream

> 1 cup fresh strawberries
> 3 tablespoons nonfat dry milk powder
> 1/4–1/3 cup honey
> 3/4-cup plain yogurt
> 1 cup heavy cream
> 2 drops Rose essential oil, diluted in a little glycerin

Blend all ingredients in the blender until smooth. Churn in an ice cream maker until frozen. When my children tasted this, they thought it was "too perfumey."

Since I absolutely love Rose, I thought it was to-die-for! You may wish to try just one drop of Rose oil the first time you make this.

Cooking with Aromatic Hydrosols

Hydrosols (also called hydrolats) are easily added to many recipes, and you are limited only by what is available. It is safe for an adult to ingest an ounce or two of an aromatic hydrosol at one sitting, but you will find that you do not need nearly that much for flavoring. Rose and Orange blossom are the most readily available hydrosols and can often be found in your supermarket or gourmet deli. (These are frequently called for in Middle Eastern recipes.) Be sure you are not using an artificially scented water, or a product loaded with preservatives or emulsifiers. Also beware of distilled water scented with essential oils, which are often sold as hydrosols. (See the source list for companies that sell pure quality hydrosols.)

Hydrosols, like essential oils, are best in recipes that require no cooking. Always smell and taste your hydrosol before adding it to a recipe. Poorly made hydrosols can taste burned or overcooked. A hydrosol suitable for flavoring should be fragrant and fresh. One tablespoon of hydrosol is plenty to flavor one cup of water, but you will notice the fragrance and flavor with just a sprinkle. Try them in bubbly water, champagne, or over ice cream!

Lavender Lemonade

> 2 cups prepared Lemonade
> 2 tablespoons sweet Lavender hydrosol

Simple, with a hint of Lavender fragrance. For a special touch, add ice made with fresh Lavender flowers frozen into the cubes.

Refreshing Mint Julep

> 2 cups water
> 1/2 cup fresh Spearmint leaves
> 2 tablespoons Lemon Verbena hydrosol

Rub the Mint leaves to release the essential oils, soak them in 2 cups cold water overnight, and strain. Add hydrosol, and serve with ice cubes frozen with fresh Borage flowers.

Orange Rosemary Sorbet

> 1/4 cup water
> 2 tablespoons honey
> 2 cups fresh-squeezed Orange juice
> 1/2 teaspoon finely chopped, fresh Rosemary leaves
> 2 tablespoons Rosemary hydrosol

Gently warm water and honey together until the honey melts. Add Orange juice, hydrosol, and Rosemary leaves. Churn in ice cream maker, and serve in chilled bowls for a refreshing, fat-free dessert.

Savory Recipes

Flavored Vegetable Oils

Flavored vegetable oils are the savory version of the extracts described above. This is a great way to tone down the strong flavor of essential oils such as Thyme, Oregano, Basil, Savory, Rosemary, and Sage. Just one drop of these oils can sometimes be too much, especially for light flavoring or when making small portions, so having a prepared dilution is handy. Flavored oils are nice for making croutons or as a base for salad dressings, and are also wonderful for basting grilling vegetables or fish. Essential oil of Lemon in Olive oil makes a terrific marinade or dip for French bread.

Oils make a better carrier in this instance than glycerin or alcohol, not only because these will be used in savory dishes rather than desserts, but because the vegetable oil tones down the harshness of these essential oils more effectively than any other carrier. Olive oil lends itself very nicely as a carrier for food flavoring, but you can use canola, sesame, safflower, or other vegetable oils instead. Use 1/2 teaspoon or more of the prepared oil in any recipe. For a lighter flavoring, use less essential oil, or make an infused oil from the herb itself. Whenever possible, add these flavorings just before serving.

Basic Flavored Vegetable Oil Recipe

> 4 drops essential oil
> 1 ounce vegetable oil
> Try a combination of essential oils.

Wild Miso Soup

The addition of wild garden greens and herbs makes this soup a real immune-booster.

> 1 cup leafy wild greens
> > (Dandelion, Dock, Mustard, Lamb's Quarters, Mustard, Mallow)
>
> 1 Onion
>
> 1 Carrot
>
> 3 Shiitake Mushrooms (if dried, soak for 30 minutes in water)
>
> 1 slice Astragalus root
>
> 1 tablespoon Ginseng rootlets
>
> 1 tablespoon fresh Ginger
>
> 1/4 cup Lovage leaves
>
> 1 quart water
>
> 3 tablespoons dark miso
>
> 1 drop Thyme essential oil, diluted in 1 teaspoon vegetable oil (or 1 teaspoon flavored oil)

If you are not familiar with the wild weeds in your area, use Chard or Kale. The Astragalus and Ginseng rootlets may be purchased by mail order or from an herb or natural food store.

Sauté chopped Onion, Mushrooms, Ginger, and Carrot in a bit of Olive oil for five minutes. Add chopped wild greens, Lovage, Astragalus, Ginseng, and water. Bring to a boil, cover and simmer for about 20 minutes. Remove from heat. In a cup, mix the miso with a little soup stock to thin, and add it to the pot. Add the diluted Thyme oil, stir well, and serve. If you reheat this soup, use low heat and watch it carefully; boiling destroys important enzymes in miso.

Essential Creamy Gazpacho

A cool treat on a hot summer day!

> 3 large fresh Tomatoes, peeled and seeded
>
> 1/2 Avocado
>
> 1 cup plain yogurt
>
> 1 Cucumber, peeled and seeded
>
> 2 tablespoons fresh Cilantro (Coriander leaf)
>
> 2 tablespoons white wine
>
> Juice of 1/2 Lemon

1 clove Garlic
1 green Onion
1 tablespoon fresh Mint leaves
1/2 teaspoon salt
freshly ground Pepper
1–2 drops Oregano *or* Dill essential oil

Start by whizzing the Tomatoes in the blender. Add the other vegetables, and pulse just until everything is chunky. Add 1 drop of the essential oil, mix well, and taste. Add another drop if needed. Chill for at least one hour before serving.

Savory Cheese Torta

Stunning creations suitable for centerpieces, tortas are as elegant as they are versatile.

8 ounces cream cheese, softened
8 ounces sharp cheddar, grated
3 tablespoons chopped Chives
1 teaspoon Paprika
2 garlic Cloves, pressed
1/3 cup sun-dried Tomatoes
2-3 drops Sweet Basil essential oil
10 whole Basil leaves
1/3 cup Pine nuts, lightly toasted

Soak the dried Tomatoes in hot water to soften, if needed; drain and chop. Line a two-cup bowl or other mold with two layers of cheesecloth. Arrange small Basil leaves in a circular pattern in the bottom of the bowl. Stir the cream cheese into a smooth consistency and add the Basil essential oil, Paprika, Garlic, and Chives. Press half the cream-cheese mixture into the mold, being careful not to disrupt the Basil leaves. Add the dried Tomatoes as the next layer, then the Pine nuts. Layer in the grated cheddar and press lightly. Finish with the rest of the cream cheese. Fold the cheesecloth over the mixture, cover and refrigerate overnight.

Before serving, unfold the cheesecloth from the top of the mold and invert the bowl onto a bed of Lettuce. Lift off the bowl and carefully unwrap the cheesecloth. Your creation is beautiful!

This is a very versatile recipe. You can create a variety of tortas by using different cheeses and layering with chopped Olives, pesto, marinated Mushrooms, Artichoke hearts, different nuts, other herbs, and various essential oils. Go wild!

Herbed Vinaigrette Dressing

This dressing is especially good on organic baby greens with gorgonzola cheese and lightly toasted hazelnuts .

  1/4 cup balsamic vinegar
  1/2 cup Olive oil
  2 tablespoons water
  1 teaspoon honey
  1 teaspoon prepared Dijon Mustard
  1 clove Garlic
  1/4 teaspoon salt
  2 drops Black Pepper oil
  4 drops Basil oil
  2 drops Thyme oil

Whiz everything together in the blender. Pour onto salad and toss well.

There are endless variations on the use of essential oils in the kitchen. I hope this sampling of ideas and recipes inspires your imagination. Just remember, start conservatively, be safe, and enjoy being creative!

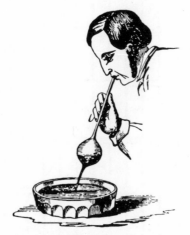

Pipette to draw off small portions
of otto from the water

Culinary Aromatherapy

Use only 1 drop of essential oil per 4 servings.

	Anise	Basil	Blk Pepper	Cardamom	Cinnamon	Clove	Coriander	Cumin	Dill	Fennel	Geranium	Ginger	Grapefruit	Jasmine	Lavender	Lemon	Lime	Mandarin/Tangerine	Marjoram	Massoïa	Nutmeg	Orange	Parsley	Pprmint.	Rose	Rosemary	Sage	Thyme	Vanilla	Ylang
MEAT	※	※	※		※	※		※				※	·		※	※	※	※	※	※	※	※	※			※	※	※		
CHICKEN	※	※	※		※		※	※		※		※	※		※	※	※	※	※	※	※	※	※			※	※	※		※
FISH	※	※	※	※	※		※	※	※	※	※	※	※		※	※	※	※	※			※	※			※	※			
EGGS		※			※		※		※						※		※	※		※	※	※	※			※	※	※		
CHEESE	※	※	※		※		※	※	※	※		※			※	※	※	※	※		※		※			※	※	※		
VEGGIES	※	※	※		※		※	※	※			※			※	※	※	※	※	※		※	※			※	※	※		
RICE	※	※	※	※	※	※	※			※		※		※	※	※	※	※	※	※	※	※	※		※	※	※	※	※	※
SALAD	※	※	※		※		※	※	※	※		※	※		※	※	※	※	※		※	※	※	※		※	※	※		
PASTA	※	※	※	※	※		※		※	※	※	※	※	※	※	※	※	※	※		※	※	※	※	※	※	※	※	※	※
DESSERT PASTRY	※			※	※	※	※			※	※	※	※	※	※	※	※	※		※	※	※		※	※				※	※
BREAD	※	※	※	※	※	※	※	※	※	※	※	※	※	※	※	※	※	※	※		※	※	※	※	※	※	※		※	※
CAKE	※	※		※	※	※	※			※	※	※	※	※	※	※	※	※		※	※	※		※	※	※			※	※
SORBET ICE-CREAM	※			※	※	※	※			※	※	※	※	※	※	※	※	※	※	※		※		※	※				※	※
FRUIT	※	※	※	※	※	※	※	※	※	※	※	※	※	※	※	※	※	※	※	※	※	※	※	※	※	※	※	※	※	※

A Fragrant Dinner From Around the World

Apertif	Orange Petal Wine Spritzer
Appetizer	Mushrooms stuffed with Almonds & Spinach scented with Orange EO & Mushroom EO
Fish Course	Ossetra & Sevruga Caviar set in flower servers
Beverage	Chilled Russian Imperial Vodka scented with Lemon EO
Meat Course	Baked Marrow Bones in a Coriander Broth
Soup Course	scented with Coriander EO
Wine	Round Hill 1990 Napa Valley Zinfandel
Cleanse Palate	Spearmint Sorbet with Fall Flowers
Fowl Course	Garlic Thai Chicken with Lemon Grass scented with Ginger EO
	Jasmine Rice with Jasmine EO
	Green Beans Julienne with Dill Weed
Wine	Sausal 1990 Alexander Valley Chardonnay
Salad Course	Selected Lettuce simple Olive Oil & Lemon Juice dressing scented with Black Pepper EO
Beverage	Glacier Water from Canadian glaciers
Cheese Course	Roquefort Aromatherapy Sweetmeats of Bergamot, Bitter Orange and Mastic on Lavender Honey Thins
Wine	Muscat de Beaumes de Venise
Dessert	Figs in a Garlic Port Sauce
Wine	Schramsberg 1988 Napa Valley Cremante
Finale	Madelines scented with Grapefruit EO
	Germain-Robin Special Reserve Christmas Brandy
	Cuban Cigars
	Coffee with Cardamon

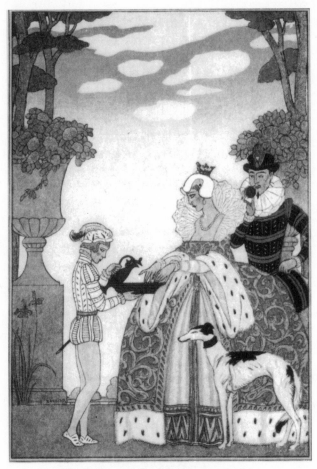

Elizabethan England, by Georges Barbier

IV

The Oils

20

Benzoin

Shirley Whitton

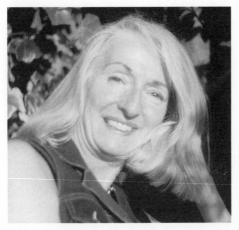

Shirley Whitton's love of herbs and flowers began as a child growing up on her father's market garden in Surrey, England. She has always been captivated by the natural perfumes and colours of the herbs and flowers that are still a part of her daily life. Over the last ten years she has studied classical and scientific aromatherapy, various forms of massage, reflexology, and colour therapy.

Shirley Whitton is an author, researcher, and aromatherapist and runs a flourishing holistic-therapy practice at her home in West London, and works with people with learning difficulties. She is the author of *The Fragrant Year*, published under the pseudonym of Jane Grayson.

Styrax benzoin (Dry). *Styrax parallenloneurus* (Perkins). Family: Styraceae.
Gum Benzoin. Gum Benjamin. Sumatra Benzoin. Palembang Benzoin and other
species of the N.O. Styraceae trees native to Thailand, Sumatra and Java, including Siam Benzoin *(Styrax tonkinenses)*.

*B*enzoin has been available as a gum in the West for many centuries, but its
natural home is the Far East. In native Malayan culture, it was used for
ceremonial purposes, and as an incense and fumigation to drive away evil
spirits. Its appeal in the West has been more functional and cosmetic, with a repu-
tation as a warming panacea for respiratory conditions. Many of us have used its
tincture, Friar's Balsam, as an inhalant, although these days this remedy is more
likely to have the active principal, Benzoic acid, taken from other gums, such as
Tolu or Peru Balsam, in which it is also present in large quantities.

Benzoin fascinates me as an aromatherapist because of its ability to cross with
ease the boundaries between perfume and medicine. I use it regularly, especially in
the wintertime, to provide a sweet and stable base for many blends, and as a valuable aid in appeasing, balancing, and gently releasing emotional tension. It is also
excellent in clearing pulmonary congestion and healing chapped, cracked skin. I
will talk about these properties in more detail later, but for now a look into the history of this gentle friend will help to give a better perspective on the growth of the
perfume trade in general, for Benzoin's history is inextricably linked to the development of perfumery in the Western world.

Early records show that Benzoin was imported by the Chinese, and later the
Egyptians via the Red Sea. In Egypt, it never attained such a high spiritual significance as did Frankincense and Myrrh, both of the latter resins coming from the
famed Land of Punt. Nevertheless, Benzoin was an essential part of the unguent-
maker's kitchen: Papyrus recipes tell us it was pounded, heated, and made into
balls and cones, along with other substances such as Pine, Juniper, Galbanum,
Storax[1], Cypress, and Labdanum. The enduring quality of Egyptian perfumes is
well known, and was proven at the opening of Tutankhamon's tomb in 1922. At
that time, the use of heavy animal extracts such as civet, musk, and ambergris
appears to have been unknown and Benzoin, a lingering base note, must have been

---

1. Storax is Liquid Amber *(Styrax officinalis)*, often confused with Benzoin

of great value to them.[2] Its gently tenacious quality remains largely unrivaled to this day, and it will always be a popular vegetable fixative for many perfumes.

The Greeks called it "Silphion," but used it less extensively, since their preference was for lighter, more herbal fragrances. The Romans knew it too, and it is quite possible it would have traveled with them. However, in England, it was probably at the height of its appeal between the fifteenth and seventeenth centuries, when all the major ports were bustling with trade in spices and other newly discovered treasures from the East.

Queen Elizabeth I loved her "Benjamin," which she had powdered into a dry perfume, together with another warm favourite, Sweet Marjoram. During the Elizabethan era, the use of perfume reached unprecedented heights. Everything, it seems, was impregnated with scent: notepaper, clothes, hangings and entire rooms; the latter art and fashion having reached these islands from France via Moorish Spain and Portugal.

The Spanish had been under Arab domination for more than five centuries, and the Arabian love for, and lavish use of, perfume was now part of the fabric of Spanish society. A well-regulated trade between Spain, Portugal, and the Middle and Far East was centred around Lisbon and Seville, working with "divers tall ships of London, with certain other ships of Southampton and Bristol." As we became a major sea-faring nation, the trade routes opened up and Benzoin, called "luban-jawi" by the Arabs, began to arrive, packed alongside silks, spices, and many other treasures in large quantities.

The Arabs controlled all the major routes through Persia to China, India and the Malay Archipelago and, even as far back as the sixth century, they were using Ceylon as a major trading centre: "The island being, as it is, in a central position, is much frequented by ships from all parts of India and from Persia and Ethiopia, and it likewise sends out many of its own. And from the remotest countries . . . it receives silk, Aloes, Cloves, Sandalwood, and other products."

To maintain their monopoly, the origin of many of the Arabian imports was a close and jealously guarded secret. The search for this mysterious Far Eastern source was thought to have been Columbus's original mission, and it is said that the Portuguese were well aware that he was going in the wrong direction, but did

---

2. Egyptian recipes frequently refer to "oil of ben," which has led to some confusion, but this is not in fact Benzoin; it is Horseradish, which was also used in cosmetics and cooking.

nothing to stop him. It was only a matter of time, however, before they were forced to relinquish part of their stranglehold, and court records for the East India Company in 1601 state clearly that the British priority was to go: "toward ye Islands of Sumat, Java and other ye parts thereabouts entendinge to trade those islands and places for Papper Spices Gould and other m'chandizes wch are likest to yeald ye most profitable return for ye Adventurers."

As expensive luxuries arrived from far and wide, in France and then in England, the fashion in perfumery spread amongst the wealthy classes, developing largely out of the manufacture of scented leather gloves, also inherited from Moorish Spain. The basic method of perfuming the leather was to steep it in a mixture of "ottos" mixed with gum, of which Benzoin was the most popular: "Take gloves of calf-leather, or better still, Spanish leather, and wash them first in Rose-water, then in Malmsey wine, dry them, shaking them well. When quite dry, rub them well inside and out with half and ounce of Labdanum and the same amount of liquid Styrax, which should be melted in a crucible over heat. *[Editor's note: Styrax is different from Storax.]* Then soak the gloves in the mixture which follows: take half an ounce of Florence Iris, Benzoin, Liquidamber, Clover, Cyperus, Sweet Rush, Sandalwood, dry Roses, of each half an ounce: mix well together into a fine and subtle powder, and strain through a fine bag. Soak the powder in Rose-water over heat, and then put in your gloves, leaving them for a whole day. Dry them, and give them another soak in the said solution, but in this last soak add to the liquid six grains of ambergris, the same again of musk and civet, and soak the whole with oil of Benzoin." From *The Ornamentation of Ladies* by Giovanni Marinello, published in 1562.

Elizabeth I wore scented gloves all the time, even in bed, since they were a valuable aid in whitening the skin. Perfumed necklaces and girdles were also common, and little balls or beads were often laid on hot coals to perfume rooms, always with the main ingredients being gums, of which Benzoin was an essential part: "Take 1 ounce of Benjamin, 1 ounce of Storax, and 1 ounce of Labdamin. Heat in a mortar, very hot, and beat all these gums to a perfect paste; in beating of it put in 6 grains of musk, 4 grains of civet. When you have beaten all this to a fine paste, wet your hands with Rose-water, rool it round betwixt your hands, and make holes in the beads, and so string them while they are hot."

The use of perfumed ornaments as a vehicle for poisoning was widespread and then, as now, perfumes and cosmetics were open to adulteration. Common vendors traded at fairs, peddling highly dubious "mixtures" that often included white lead: this was a well-known, highly toxic skin lightener that invariably led to a slow death, a terrible price to pay for vanity. Instructions from Elizabeth to Lord Cecil insisted that: "No manner of perfume, either in apparel or sleeves, gloves or such like, or otherwise, that shall be appointed for her majesty's savor, be presented by any stranger or other person, but that the same be corrected by some other fume."

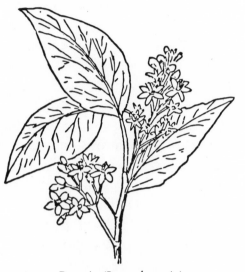

Benzoin *(Styrax benzoin)*

During the reigns of the Louis XIV, XV, and XVI, heavy perfumes gave way to the lighter "spirits of wine" such as the Eaux de Colognes, and Benzoin was still the main fixative and often a principal ingredient in these concoctions. It also had an important role to play in the perfuming and powdering of wigs, but now we find more recipes for it as a room fragrancer, such as the favourite "oislet de Chypre," which was a small "bird" made of gum-paste, filled with perfumed powder and placed in a cage. Often, it took the form of a censer which, when lit, released the sweet, vanilla-like fragrance into the room.

It had become the tradition for tradesmen and craftsmen to protect themselves by forming guilds; the largest of these, and by far the richest by the end of the sixteenth century, was that of the grocers. For a long time, they held the monopoly over all the spice and perfume substances, and had become very skilful at cutting out the middleman. However, with the rise of the medical profession, the growing, widespread use of distillation and the preparation of alcohol, fierce competition arose from the apothecaries.

This was the time when the boundaries between perfume and medicine were beginning to be defined, and from then on, the use of Benzoin was modified and began to move in a more therapeutic direction. The resin became much more familiar as a tincture sitting on the apothecary's shelf, or as the occasional addition to the cassolet on top of the physician's walking stick. Despite this development, however, Benzoin's popularity as a fixative in perfumes has never waned, and continues to this day. On the rare occasions when an enfleurage is produced, Benzoin is still used as a purifier and preservative for the mixture of suet and lard with which the glass plates are covered.

The two species most used in perfumery are Benzoin Siam resinoid, *Styrax tonkinensis,* and Benzoin Sumatra resinoid, *Styrax Benzoin.* The first has a sweet, balsamic, chocolate-like fragrance that is extremely tenacious. The second is warm, sweet, and powdery. Both are used as fixatives, although the first is also used quite frequently to provide a balsamic note to a perfume. Sumatra Benzoin contains Cinnaminic acid, which gives it its pleasant balsamic smell; Siam Benzoin does not.

In the Gamut of Odours, (a scale of odour classification similar to musical notation) arranged by Septimus Piesse, the famous French perfumer, Benzoin is placed among the deep bass notes, only four places up from the bottom on his musical scale. Its capacity to linger makes it of great value in creating a blend designed to soothe the senses, and remove deep-seated fears. Madame Maury said that it "creates a kind of euphoria; it interposes a padded zone between us and events."

My own experience with it is exactly this. On an emotional level, Benzoin's powers of penetration are very great. It has the ability to hold the senses in a kind of velvet glove, whilst it slices through inner resistance. Although gentle and inoffensive, it is also very incisive, and once we begin to work with it properly, it will soon reach a deep and personal level and help us to reveal hidden aspects of our nature. For those who have become too inward-looking and silent, its reassuring warmth creates a stable base from which to examine congealed doubts and fears and get them moving again.

Benzoin is an oleo-resin, or resinoid, which means that to obtain the best fragrance it must be subjected to a process involving the use of a solvent that is then removed with alcohol. Unlike Frankincense and Myrrh, Benzoin is not distilled after that, but remains as a resinoid; to do otherwise would destroy a lot of its aromatic constituents—hence its sticky consistency. New extraction processes, such as carbon-dioxide extraction, use less solvent and, as a result, are yielding better-quality fragrances. For therapeutic integrity, nevertheless, we are well-advised as aromatherapists to search out Benzoin that has been dissolved in wood alcohol, or even to buy it in solid form and melt it down as necessary.

Benzoin has no contraindication, although there is a very slight risk of sensitization, usually when it is found in blends or tinctures that include Peru or Tolu Balsam. It is thought that this is not from the Benzoin itself, but is a cross-sensitization that occurs in such mixtures. There might also be a small risk of sensitization due to residues from the solvent extraction process.

Generally speaking, though, Benzoin is gentle and benign if used carefully. The gentleness of its nature is mirrored by the care and consideration with which it is harvested in its native environment. The process is long and complicated, but the solar energy that it absorbs and conserves during this time has an important effect on the human body and psyche; it is indeed a hot, dry remedy, full of the sun.

It is a pathogenic product, which means it only exudes the resin when the plant has been wounded. This is not done until the trees are seven years old, when incisions are made in the trunk. After a time, the liquid, balsamic resin either collects beneath the bark or exudes from the incisions. When it is sufficiently hardened, it is collected in the form of "tears." The first three years' collection provides the finest resin, and after that the resin is known as the "belly." Finally, when the tree is felled and the remainder scraped out, this resin is called the "foot."

Its chief aromatic constituents are vanillin (an aldehyde), benzoic acid, and esters of benzoic and Cinnaminic acids.

On a physical level, it is invaluable as an expectorant and in the treatment of catarrh. It is a good pulmonary antiseptic, useful for most problems related to the lungs, as well as asthma, bronchitis, and laryngitis. It is a urinary antiseptic, and stimulates the flow of urine as well as the general circulation. It warms and tones the heart. It is also a cicatrisant, wonderful for chapped, sore or cracked skin, dermatosis, acne, eczema, psoriasis and, in certain cases, ulcerated wounds. It is effective for frostbite or bed sores, since it protects and disinfects the skin. It also is useful in cases of arthritis, gout, or rheumatism.

Benzoin blends well with other balsamic notes, such as Frankincense, Myrrh, or Cistus, and can be relied upon to provide a lovely base to many blends; it will also encourage the higher notes to stabilize and stay around far longer. Other good companions include Cypress, Juniper, Lemon, Coriander, and many of the spice oils; also the precious oils like Rose, Jasmine, and Sandalwood. I find it an extremely adaptable oil, and have mixed it successfully with Chamomile, both Roman and German, to provide a soothing, healing blend for the treatment of PMS and a whole range of menopausal symptoms.

It is well worth experimenting with this oil, provided that, as with most other oils, it is treated with due respect and used sparingly. Too much can be overpowering, but actually can do little harm, and it will always lend a beautiful baseline to a carefully selected blend. It is a shoulder to cry on and a warm blanket with which to collect the tears. To quote Tisserand in *The Art of Aromatherapy,* "To understand the action of Benzoin you only have to think of its planetary ruler, the Sun: heating, drying, energising, uplifting and eventually soporific. What is there more pleasant, more euphoric, than to bathe in the warm sun?"

The Women's Oils Introduction

Susan Earle

Spikenard and Rose—the blending of those—that's what girls are made of.

I remember breathing deeply of a powdery pink aroma while laying on the grass of my Nana's backyard when I was very young, and she and my grandfather were still alive. Last year, while sampling unknown essential oils from an un-marked blotter, I recognized the safe and summery aroma as that of the Roses border-ing my Nana's yard, combined with the light, intoxicating scent of the dewy grass. Whenever I am graced with the scent of Rose, images of my Nana's hair, white as clouds, her round Swedish-blue eyes, and silky layered slips arises, just out of reach, like a reflection in a pool of water.

As with a woman, the charm and beauty of the Rose lies in its paradoxes. The vibrance of even the lightest vanishing shades of pink and yellow call the observer to delve with body and soul into its velvety depth. Though they appear delicate, the petals have a flesh that declares a proud sense of self. They are at times grandiloquent, at times a whisper; at times flamboyant and complex, at times simple. In form and in fragrance the Rose is an image of soft Femininity and her sultry sister Sensuality.

Jasmine is the intoxicating fragrance of the memory of a lover's voice, so clear you may turn to answer, only to find yourself cradled in the melancholy of its lonely, tran-quil fog. It echoes with casual eloquence. It is the innocence of a girl. It is the desire, hate, love, joy, fury, lust of a woman.

It is late at night, and in the land of the half-asleep I feel the car turning the corner onto the street where I live. Snuggled warmly in my mother's soft lap, I am dancing a lazy dance with her breath, her low voice occasionally giving harmony to the rythmic pumping of her heart. Spikenard is the warmth of a mother's lap. It is the honest joy and relief of reuniting with a dear friend. It is the security of the womb. It is a protec-tive embrace from Mother Earth.

There is traditional symbolism accompanying many aromas, especially those which have been used for centuries. The aromas of essential oils hold different meanings for each individual. Study the history of essential oils, learn their chemistry, know their uses. But above all, be still, close your eyes, breathe deeply, and open to the personal sym-phony of images, emotions, and memories each oil conducts for your pleasure alone.

21

The Women's Oils
Essential Oil Profiles of Rose, Jasmine and Spikenard

Victoria Edwards

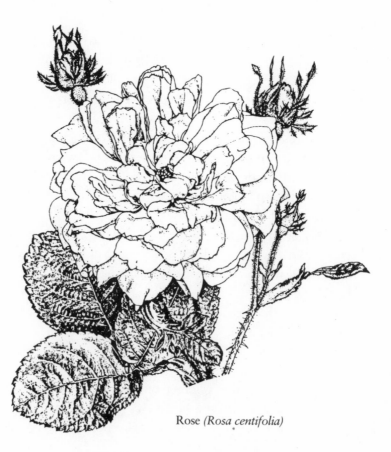

Rose *(Rosa centifolia)*

A Rose Is a Rose. . .

Rosa spp.

*T*he numerical expression of the Rosaceae can be seen in the floral envelope, which has five petals, five leaves, and twice five sepals. Slice an Apple (Rosaceae family) crosswise and you will see the five-pointed star pattern. The five aspects of the Rose to be explored here are the historic, the cultural, the symbolic, the physical (medicinal and cosmetic), and the spiritual.

Commonly considered the most beautiful member of the Rosaceae family, the Rose originated in Asia Minor and is one of the oldest flowers in cultivation. It was grown five thousand years ago in the ancient gardens of western Asia and North Africa. Roses have been mentioned in poetical work since the dawn of creation. Roses grew in the mythical gardens of Semiramis, Queen of Syria, and Midas, King of Phrygia.

According to Greek legend, Flora, the deity of flowers, walked through the woods one cloudy morning and found the body of a beautiful nymph. Saddened to see such a lovely creature dead, she decided to give her new life by transforming her into a beautiful flower surpassing all others in charm and beauty. She called on the other deities to help her: Aphrodite, to give beauty and to bestow the three graces, brilliance, joy, and charm; her husband, Zephyrus, the west wind, to blow away the clouds so that Apollo, the Sun, could send his blessing through his rays; and Dionysius, the deity of wine, to give nectar and fragrance. When the new flower was finished, the gods rejoiced over its charming beauty and delicate scent. Chloris collected a diadem of dewdrops and crowned the new flower the Rose, as queen of flowers. Aphrodite presented the Rose to her son Eros, the deity of love. The white Rose became the symbol of charm and innocence, and the red Rose the symbol of love and desire.

When Eros, in turn, presented a Rose to the deity of silence to induce him to conceal the weaknesses of the gods, the Rose became the emblem of silence and secrecy. In ancient Rome, things spoken "sub rosa" (under the Rose) were part of Venus's sexual mysteries, not to be revealed to the uninitiated.

The rosary was an instrument of worship of the Rose, which ancient Rome knew as the flower of Venus. Five was the Marian number because it was the number of petals in the Rose, and also in the Apple blossom. The mature Apple was the symbol of motherhood, fruition, regeneration, and eternal life. Five was considered proper to Marian devotion because Rose-Mary was the reincarnation of

Apple-Eve. The five-fold Rose and Apple were also related to numerous pre-Christian images of the goddess, the witches' pentacle, the five-pointed star of Ishtar, and the Egyptian symbol of the uterine underworld and rebirth cycle.

At Chartes Cathedral, the window called the Rose of France shows in its center the Virgin in her majesty. In the great age of cathedral building, Mary was worshiped as a goddess in her "Palace of the Queen of Heaven." At Notre Dame she was often addressed as the Rose, Rosebush, Rose garland, Rose garden, Mystic Rose, or Queen of the Most Holy Garden. There are many documented accounts of apparitions of Mary to various saints, either with Roses or the odour of Roses present. The church, the garden, and Mary's body were all mystically one; for she was Lady Ecclesia, the church, as well as "the pure womb of regeneration." Much like a pagan temple, the Gothic cathedral represented the body of the Goddess who was also the universe, containing the essence of the male godhead within herself. This interpretation was largely forgotten after the passing of the Gothic period. In later centuries, "Gothic" became an epithet of contempt, synonymous with "barbarous." The symbolism of the Palaces of the Queen of Heaven was no longer understood.

According to an old Persian legend, the caliph Sehangir, while walking with his beautiful bride in his palace gardens along the canals and fountains decked with Rose petals in celebration of their wedding, noticed an oily film on the surface of the waters, produced by the action of the sun on the Roses. Fascinated by the heavy scent of this oil, he ordered it bottled for later use. This attar (fragrance), in Persian also called *otto*, is still considered the most precious of all perfumes.

Fragrance is the rightful heritage of the Rose, and it is what we consciously expect of it. We cannot disassociate fragrance from the Rose.

> Of late there has been great uneasiness among flower lovers because of the numbers of scentless or nearly scentless Roses appearing on the market. It is hard to believe that a scentless Rose could have a great vogue, but there is that chill and soulless beauty Frau Druschki to the contrary. A trend toward mere beauty of person in Roses is greatly to be deplored! In Britain, to offset this trend, various awards for fragrance have been given, the most important of these being the Clay Cup. Offered annually for the Rose of good form and colour possessing in greatest degree the old Rose fragrance. The winner in 1929, 'Aroma.'   [Source unknown, c. 1930]

Fortunately this trend has been successfully reversed, and growers now are focusing on fragrance again. The most recent result of breeding for fragrance has reached fad status with the 'Pink Prelude.' Bred in sunny Antibes, on the Riviera, the scent of the bud is said to be 'the deepest mixed in.' Fast becoming the favored bloom of the jet set, 'Princess Caroline of Monaco had three hundred for her birthday,' the demand has created a scarcity, but a version is now being cultivated in California.

What is meant by the pure colour of Roses and sometimes designated as the "true old Rose scent" is the property of that great trinity that once constituted the chief Rose wealth of the gardening world: *Rosa centifolia,* the cabbage Rose, *Rosa damascena,* the damask Rose, and *Rosa gallica,* the French Rose. The hybrid perpetual and some hybrid tea Roses have the blood of one of these three coursing through their veins. The perfume of the Rose remains pure, uncloying, and sweet to the last whiff, nor does it lose its sweetness in death. Dried Rose petals hold a scent for years. In periods of extreme heat and drought, Roses grow appreciably less. Before a storm, the sweet odours will increase, and Roses are found to be more fragrant in autumn than summer.

Other Roses worth mention are the *Rosa rugosa,* Chinese Rose, and the *Rosa moschata,* which is making news for its Rosehip-seed oil. Hips are a fruit by definition. They contain seeds that are nourished by a pulpy flesh. Rosehip-seed oil contains a high amount of Gammalinolenic Acid (GLA), which is also found in Evening Primrose oil. So far, these oils are being found helpful for dissolving fatty deposits and healing scar tissue, as well as exhibiting a remarkable effectiveness in treating feminine problems associated with the menstrual cycle.

Medicinally, the Rose has historically held a place in traditional folk remedies. According to Chinese herbal texts, *Rosa rugosa* is prescribed in the form of an extract for all diseases of the liver, to scatter abscesses, and in blood diseases. Its fragrant, cooling nature, and its sweet taste, tinged with a slight bitterness, is believed to act especially on the spleen and liver, promoting blood circulation. According to Madame Maury, a pioneer of modern aromatherapy, the Rose is an antitubercular and antibacteriological agent, most active on the heart and eyes. She wrote that Rose oil exhibits a considerable influence on the female organs, by cleansing and regulating their functions.

The effect of Rose-Melissa oil (ratio of 1:2) on herpes roster and herpes simplex has been confirmed in studies in Germany. The oil is applied without dilution. An application of two or three times has resulted in the disappearance of the complaints in one or two days. According to Maggie Tisserand, a blend of Rose oil rubbed into the groin-area lymph nodes, combined with Lavender sitz baths, helped to ease outbreaks from the virus. In a holistic clinic in California, patients suffering from herpes have experienced recovery using Rose oil diluted in Rose water, in combination with Bach flower remedies taken internally, and utilizing positive affirmations.

Cosmetically, the oil of the Rose supports regeneration of the epidermis. Rose also has a beneficial effect upon the moisture content of the skin, and is useful in treating sensitive skin prone to inflammation or couperose conditions (small broken veins).

The Rose, above all, produces a feeling of well-being. The mental and emotional effects of Rose oil have proven very positive in treating various forms of depression. Postnatal depression, depression following the break-up of a relationship, feminine insecurity, and sexual dysfunctions are often responsive to therapy that includes Rose oil. It opens the heart, and soothes feelings such as anger, fear, jealousy, and anxiety.

Rose oil is a remedy for both skin and soul. Dietrich Wabner writes, "I cannot confirm the yin-yang or female-male classification. The harmonizing effect of Rose oil makes clear that no definite yin character is at work. Rose shows a balance of yin and yang." Relaxation and stimulation are both possible effects of Rose oil.

Combining an intoxicating scent with such tender and fragile beauty, it is no surprise that the Rose is renowned as an aphrodisiac. In India, Rose petals are traditionally scattered on the wedding bed. Used as a massage oil, sprinkled in the bath, or worn as a perfume, Rose oil evokes an erotic atmosphere. No wonder that lovers give each other Roses. The fragrance of the Rose has the power to unite physical and spiritual love. Rose oil is an aphrodisiac, yet it does not have the effect of arousing desire alone but instills this desire with a need for harmony. The fragrance of the Rose transforms love into the art of love. Superior to all scents in the floral realm, the Rose works simultaneously on the physical, emotional, and spiritual bodies, purifying and uplifting all three.

Spikenard . . . The Anointing Oil

Nardostachys jatamansi

It was some time ago that an acquaintance first spoke to me of his long search for Spikenard, or Indian Nard oil. My curiosity was aroused, for I knew little of this ancient oil. In 1988, I had my first opportunity to smell Spikenard, and the scent immediately evoked images of large stone tombs. I then began to search for more information regarding this ancient oil.

Dioscorides, a Greek physician, wrote of Spikenard two thousand years ago: "It smells like goats; the root is warming, drying, and diuretic, staying the fluxes and whites. It helps nausea, morbid hepatic, morbid renal, the superfluous lids of eyes and is anti-toxic."

> They [Spikenards] have a warming, drying & vertical faculties, & they stay ye fluxes of ye wome & ye whites. They help both the Nauseas, & the Stomachi rosiones & ye troubled with flatuosities & with the morbus hepaticus, & with the morbus regius, & with the dolor renum. They are good also for the superflous humors of the lids of the eyes, binding, & thickning they eye-lids. The inspersion of htem is profitable to take away the smell of ye sweat.
>
> From Dioscorides' Herbal, 1st century A.D.

The plant itself is a marvel in the botanical world. Identified as a "blooming rhizome," it presents a unique fusion of root, sprout, and flower. It develops two different kinds of subterranean sprouts simultaneously from one root—a purely vegetative one, and a flower sprout. This phenomenon is unique in plant life. The essential oil is mostly found in the subterranean sprout.

According to Dietrich Gumbel in his book, *Principles of Holistic Skin Therapy with Herbal Essences,* Spikenard is helpful in finding one's "inner balance" in the emotional, spiritual, and physical interplay of energies. Gümbel enthuses about Spikenard, saying that it has a harmonizing, relaxing effect on all organs and organ systems, and can successfully be used against all functional disturbances. This dramatic statement is supported by his theory that because the rhizome of the plant develops a "vegetative sprout" and a "flower sprout," it is seen to incorporate all three levels of the plant: root, leaf (or sprout), and flower. It therefore acts on all three levels of the skin and, correspondingly, has an "integrating," balancing effect on metabolism in general.

The plant, also known as *Nardostachys jatamansi,* grows in the mountains above the Ganges and Jumna Rivers. It is native to India, and abounds in the loftier regions of the entire

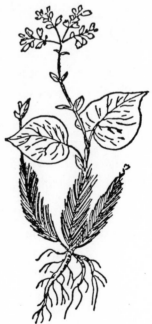

Spikenard
(*Nardostachys grandiflora*)

Central and Eastern Himalayas, extending from Kumaon to Bhutan, at elevations of 11,000 to 17,000 feet. It inhabits stony places, and varies in stature and amount of odour according to the elevation. The rhizomes are collected in abundance by the natives of the hills, and are used throughout the East in a dried state, in unguents and as a drug.

Jatamansee is the Hindu synonym for the "Sumbul," which in Arabian texts is the plant representative of the Greek *Nardos*. Sumbul is a common name for a variety of plants, not all of which are *Nardostachys*. Traditionally, *Spikenard* was harvested annually and brought down to the plains of India for trade. Alexander the Great wrote of the memorable aroma of the Spikenard wafting up as the elephants he and his troops rode upon trod these fragrant grasses. Spikenard is related to Valerian. Anyone familiar with the almost faecal fragrance of Valerian or its essential oil may be surprised to find that the odour of Spikenard oil is similar and yet more appealing. The peaty, mossy, humus-like odor of Spikenard is one of fresh earth.

With its androgen-parasympathetic and estrogen-sympathetic qualities, Spikenard has a harmonizing, relaxing and balancing effect on all organs including the skin. The oil redresses the skin's physiological balance and causes permanent regeneration. It should be used in particular for mature skin. The essential oil is also said to be cooling, antipyretic, and laxative. Traditional uses include the treatment of skin diseases, throat troubles, ulcers, leprosy, and diseases of the blood. Some very recent research at the University of Saugar in India has shown the essential oil to have useful antifungal and antibacterial properties.

Mughal Empress Nur Jehan, step-mother of the builder of the Taj Mahal, was an expert perfumer. She is said to have used a combination of Spikenard, Rose, Sandalwood, and Vetiver as a rejuvenating cosmetic preparation to make herself more attractive to the emperor.

There are many references to Mary of Bethany* anointing Jesus Christ with Spikenard oil, the very ritual of the Chrism. The future deliverer of Israel is called "The Messiah" or "The Anointed One." This appears in its Greek form as Christ (Zpiores). The ancient ritual of Chrism is referred to in the Nag Hammadi Library as more important than baptism. This ritual reaches even farther back, to King Mel-

---

* Mary of Bethany was not considered to be (Saint) Mary Magdalene until the time of Gregory the Great.

chisedek who first introduced the ritual of bread and wine and oil. Unction, the process of anointing with oils, is numbered among the seven sacraments. The Roman Catholic Church still administers the rite of Extreme Unction for the health of Soul and Body, Forgiveness, and Spiritual Strengthening.

The legends are many, and the romance and poetry of the descriptions irresistible. St. John recounts an anointing: "Then took Mary a pound of ointment of Spikenard, very costly, and anointed the feet of Jesus, and wiped his feet with her hair. And the house was filled with the odour of the ointment."

A more detailed description of such an event, identified as Magdalen's Last Anointing, comes from the revelations of St. Anne Catherine Emmerich as recorded by Clemens Brentano:

> To Mary, Jesus had announced his coming death, and she was inexpressibly sad. That morning, Jesus spoke of many things with his apostles... During his instructions Magdalen came back to Jerusalem with the ointment she had bought. Veronica saw to the purchases of the ointment, which was of three kinds, the most precious that could be procured. Magdalen had expended upon it all the money she had left. One was oil of Spikenard. The flasks were of a clear, whitish, though not transparent material, almost like mother-of-pearl (probably alabaster); they were in shape like little urns. Magdalen carried the vessels under her mantle, in a pouch which hung over her breast. While Jesus taught, Magdalen rose quietly from her seat, went up behind Jesus and cast herself at his feet, weeping bitterly. She bent her face low over the foot that was resting on the couch while Jesus himself raised to her the other that was hanging a little toward the floor. Magdalen loosened the sandals and anointed Jesus' feet on the soles and upon the upper part. Then, with both hands, drawing her flowing hair from beneath her veil, she wiped the Lord's anointed feet, and replaced the sandals. Magdalen's action caused some interruption in Jesus' discourse, and he said, 'Be not scandalized at this woman,' and then addressed some words softly to her. She now arose, stepped behind Him and poured over His head some costly water, and that so plentifully that it ran down upon His garments. As with her hand she spread some of the ointment from the crown down the hind part of his head, the hall was filled with the delicious odor.

From the Golden Legend of Jacob's de Voragine, St. Jacob, Archbishop of Genoa, 1230 A.D., we get an account of another such anointing. "As rich as Mary Magdalen was, she was no less beautiful; and so entirely had she abandoned her body to pleasure that she was no longer called by any other name than 'the sinner.' But when Jesus was journeying around the country preaching, she learned one day by divine inspiration that He sat at meat in the house of Simon the Leper. Thither she ran at once, but not daring to mingle with His disciples, she stayed apart. And she washed the Lord's feet with her tears and wiped them with the hair of her head, and anointed them with precious ointment. And henceforth there was no grace that He refused her, nor any mark of affection that He withheld from her. He drove seven devils out of her, admitted to her His friendship, condescended to dwell in her house, and was pleased to defend her whenever the occasion arose. And he could not see her in tears without Himself weeping for love of her." Magdalen also had the honor of being present at the death of Jesus, standing at the foot of the Cross; and it was she that anointed His body with sweet spices, Myrrh and Frankincense after His death."

Historical texts are full of descriptions such as these. Almost all accounts of Mary of Bethany (Magdalen) include her expression of devotion by anointing Christ with precious oils and ointments. Spikenard is consistently referred to when the precious substance is specified. An account of Mary Magdalen's death in France holds that the building held a beautiful scent of her being for weeks afterwards.

During a psychic reading I asked about Spikenard and was told that, in general use in this culture, the oil of Spikenard is for past pain, that people hold inside them. It is a cleanser, a resolver for that pain. It takes that judgment of the self and the pain, and lifts them simply from looping their energy into the chakra where judgment is. It draws the energy upward to the sixtth or seventh chakra. To use it, place a drop of oil on the chakra where there is pain, and another on the top of the head. The ancient ritual was to use it with high-pitched whistles or flutes, walking around the person anointed.

Also, Spikenard can be used with acupuncture to help release emotional aspects, or used in a deep massage on persons who feel that the pain in their lives is beyond their control. This oil ultimately gives control over that inside which is considered evil. I talked to a woman who drank Spikenard root tea throughout her pregnancy. She claimed to have used it religiously after reading about it, and attributes her wonderful and easy birthing experience to its use.

In general, Spikenard is considered to have anti-aging properties, useful for incurable skin problems and in spiritual work as an anointing oil for inhalation or application.

The Ultimate Jasmine for Aromatherapy Use

Jasminum sambac • *Jasminum odoratissimum* • *Jasminum officinale* • *Jasminum grandiflorum*

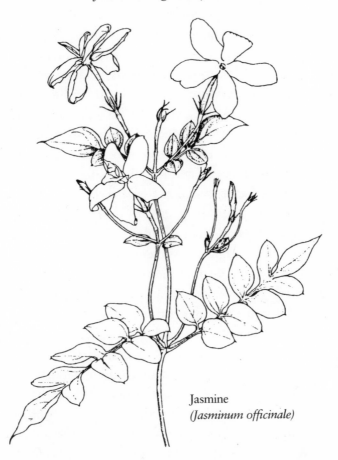

Jasmine
(*Jasminum officinale*)

Jasmine is often referred to as the King of Flowers and if the Rose is the Queen of fragrance, Jasmine is certainly the King. The name Jasmine is derived from the Arabic *yasmin*. Chinese Jasmine, *J. sambac,* is largely used for scenting tea and is known in China as *mo li*. The Hindus call it "Moonlight on the Grove" and "Mistress of the Night." Jasmine is one of the most expensive essences, along with Rose, and has long been a favorite of Eastern nations.

The Jasmine was associated with the rise of European perfumery in Italy during the Renaissance, and when Italian ways were transposed to France, the cultivation of this flower was included. Charles Gamier brought solvent extraction apparatus to northern Egypt in 1912, and from that beginning the Egyptian industry has burgeoned. Today, French Jasmine from around Grasse is fine but very little is produced. In 1984, Egypt was responsible for eighty percent of world production.

The Jasmine plant is a creeper of the Oleaceae family, with white or yellow flowers, and requires plenty of sun and warm summers. It is cultivated in Algeria, Morocco, France, China, Egypt, Italy and Turkey, the French oil being the most expensive. Jasmine exudes its most exquisite perfume at dawn, the hour Paracelsus called "the time of balsams" *(balsamiticum tempus),* and the time Jasmine flowers are cultivated. Each flower must be picked by hand, a reason the crop has diminished in France. In Egypt, where both the *officinale* and Arabian *Jasmine sambac* forms are grown, teenage children pick the blooms because the plants are low growing in height and it is more difficult for adults to pick. India and China are becoming rivals, as manual labor is still extremely cheap. In India, the Jasmine is grown organically, and Neem extract is used to protect the plants from insects.

Upon picking, Jasmine can be treated by the ancient means of enfleurage or by solvent extraction to yield a fragrant concrete and absolute. It has been calculated that no less than eight million Jasmine flowers go into each kilogram of Jasmine oil; it takes more than 700 flowers to make one gram of concentrate. Jasmine is an exquisitely expensive, exquisitely delightful aromatic. Together with Rose and Neroli, Jasmine has the honor of being one of the highest priced plant scents.

Perhaps ninety-nine percent of all "oil of Jasmine" sold today is synthetic. This can be determined by the sickly sweet, chemical odor of such products, as well as the cheap price. Cost and your nose will determine whether the product is true Jasmine. True Jasmine oil is a beautiful mahogany, deep reddish-brown color. It blends very well with Rose and Citrus oils. It has a sweet, exotic bouquet which never fails to please. One or two milliliters of true Jasmine absolute sells for $40.00 and up.

When I first began to sample the Jasmine oils from different countries, I compared the quality and scents. Before the cost of customs charges, international shipping and broker fees, I found these prices for the finest *Jasminum grandiflorum* absolutes: Egyptian $1300 per kilo, Indian $1350 per kilo, French $1394 per kilo. The *Jasminum sambac* was the costliest at $2400 per kilo.

The *J. sambac*, which is grown organically, seemed to have four times the power and odor intensity of the *J. grandiflorum* variety. I began to note the reactions of customers, friends and other people. Smelling the Jasmine sambac concrete and rubbing a tiny amount on the temples created a feeling of bliss and happiness in almost everyone—almost an intoxication. No one disliked it! On further research, I discovered the Jasmine sambac concrete has no trace of a solvent or hexane.

Jasmine is a recognized aphrodisiac, but refers magically to the spritualization of sexuality. Jasmine awakens the spirit within the inner Temple of the self, representing the sacred prostitute Hetaera who belongs to no one but herself, the spirit who channels the love of the Divine so that the recipient may know the perfect union of opposites. Jasmine has the power to transcend earthly love.

Some experts detect animal-like undertones, and classify Jasmine as a yang (masculine) plant. These experts refer to the action of Jasmine as predominantly yang—warming, opening, and relieving spasms. It is indicated where there is cold, listlessness, spasm, depression, catarrh or other discharge. It is, like all absolutes, a fairly powerful oil. There is no danger of toxicity, but if it is over-used it will cease to be of benefit and may result in an increase of catarrh. Too much yang eventually turns to yin. Jasmine is considered more yang in its pure state, becoming more yin as it is diluted.

On the first page of his book *Magical Aromatherapy*, Scott Cunningham states, "Jasmine uplifts me." He goes on to write that Jasmine is associated with the element water and the moon. The magical influences are Love, Peace, Spirituality, Sex, Sleep and Psychic dreams. "Therefore, in direct opposition to aromatherapy tradition, I've classified Jasmine as a feminine (yin) plant ruled by the moon and possessed of the qualities of the element water," writes Cunningham. The beautiful blossoms and delicious scent seem related to feminine energy in general. In China, the fragrant flowers are symbolic of women.

Like the Rose, Jasmine has a marked effect on the female reproductive system. Traditional aromatherapists utilize Jasmine to alleviate women's reproductive problems and to facilitate childbirth. It relieves uterine spasm and also menstrual pain, whether in the abdomen or the back. It helps to relieve the pain of childbirth, promotes birth and promotes the flow of breast milk, so it is of great value as an ante- and post-natal massage oil. *Aromatherapy for Pregnancy and Childbirth* states that Jasmine is safe after sixteen weeks, i.e., not for use during the first trimester of pregnancy.

Jasmine oil works on the emotional and physical level, and is of great value in psychological and psychosomatic problems. Although it does have psychological effects, its use is especially indicated when applied to an emotional problem. Jasmine is a nerve sedative, and at the same time greatly uplifting. It is an antidepressant, and produces a feeling of optimism, confidence, and euphoria. It is most useful in cases where there is apathy, indifference or listlessness. It grants a sense of wholeness, and boosts self-confidence in relating to others.

In her book *Aromantics,* Valerie Worwood mentions the study in Japan by Professor Shizuo Torii which confirms the influence of Jasmine as stimulating to the sympathetic nervous system, which in turn controls our sexuality. Worwood writes that Jasmine is powerful, that it provokes the ultimate image of woman in man. Seductive, it gently lifts your darkest moods.

The scent and potential uses of Jasmine absolute far outweigh the high cost of the substance. Lawless says the flowers of *Jasminum sambac* are used for conjunctivitis, dysentery, skin ulcers and tumors. The root is used to treat headaches, insomnia, and pain due to dislocated joints and rheumatism. Since ancient times, Jasmine has been diffused from Persia and Kashmir throughout all of Europe, Asia, and North Africa, to be used in cosmetics, hair dressings, religious garlands, and as a perfume for tea. In China, and all over the Far East, the blossoms are used as a flavor in black teas, and in China specifically, they are used in cosmetics, to decorate the hair of pretty girls; and an infused oil was used in former times to massage the body after bathing.

In India, according to Mary Greer in *The Essence of Magic,* in India, Jasmine is the flower of Lakshmi, the goddess of luck, happiness and fortune. The flowers are still used in marriage and all spiritual ceremonies in India and the Far East. In India, where marriages are arranged by the parents, the rich bride and groom spend their wedding night in a bed of Jasmine flowers—sometimes as much as fifty kilos of them.

Because of the intensity of the odor, its scarcity and high cost, one drop of Jasmine absolute on a cotton ball is sufficient for most uses. The flower essence increases capillary action and is a general stimulant for the entire system, including the nasal passages, and can therefore be used to improve the sense of smell. According to Guenther's *The Essential Oils,* Jasmine absolute is used for hard, contracted limbs and problems with the nervous and reproductive systems. It is useful for cough and difficulty breathing; it disperses crude humours, and is good for cold and catarrhous constitutions, but not for the hot. Used in moderation, Jasmine is beneficial for hot, dry sensitive skin types, and because it is such a delicious scent it forms a welcome ingredient in any facial oil. It is sometimes used in conditions such as dermatitis or erysipelas, especially if accompanied by depression. Jasmine is the most exquisite of scents, and is used in many of the costliest perfumes; not one of the *grands parfums* is without Jasmine. Its complex and wholly attractive scent is as popular today as it always has been. Synthetic Jasmine is easily manufactured, but even to that a little of the absolute is added to cut the harshness.

Jasmine's powerful scent directly affects our emotional centers, making it an excellent choice for love rituals. Inhale the aroma, with proper visualizations, to enhance an ongoing relationship or to find a new one. With proper visualization, the aroma of Jasmine creates the mental, emotional and physical responses necessary for sexual arousal. For this reason it is also used to treat emotional sexual dysfunction (in women, the ability to enjoy sexual contact or to achieve orgasm; in men, the same two conditions as well as difficulty achieving or maintaining an erection, and lack of ejaculation). Sniff and visualize.

Jasmine's calming, soothing fragrance is also of tremendous help in relaxing our physical bodies. Rubbed lightly into the temples, Jasmine is soothing, anti-depressant, and relieves stress and headaches. To encourage sleep and produce psychic dreams, sniff the absolute. This beautiful fragrance lifts the spirits, quiets the nerves, and stifles worries about tomorrow. You need not visualize to reap these changes simply breathe.

An essence that strongly touches the god-spark in people, Jasmine has a profound spiritual effect. This scent can lull us into states of heightened spiritual awareness with the proper visualization. Be aware of the divine energy manifested within the odor. Breathe it in, and connect with the energy behind all in existence. It helps access your own inner wisdom by awakening you to symbols and metaphors that can vitalize your imagination and intuition. The "Mistress of the Night" lifts your spirits, relieves depression, heightens spiritual awareness, brings psychic dreams and treats emotionally based sexual dysfunction.

Jasmine is the essence of mystery and magic.

22

Mints Are Not Just for After Dinner

Linda Hein

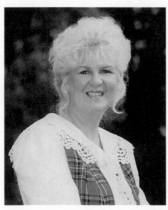

Linda Hein practiced as a licensed beautician in the sixties, beginning to listen to her clients' desires for health and well-being.

In the seventies, her family moved to a farm in Wadsworth, Ohio, where she took up the breeding and raising of Paints and Quarterhorses. She filled the farm with a diverse group of animals. Cows, chickens, pigs, goats, rabbits, raccoons, falcons, an eagle, foxes, a bear, a kinkajou, and also kids lived in harmony on their farm, along with the usual assortment of dogs and cats.

In 1992, Linda was asked to manage and assist in the opening of a local health-food store. In 1993, she moved on to the Mustard Seed Market, where she manages the health-and-beauty aids department. This position has afforded her the opportunity to further her education in aromatherapy and homeopathic treatments.

*I*n the first century A.D., the naturalist Pliny wrote that "The smell of mint stirs up the mind and appetite to a greedy desire of food." He recommended binding the head in a crown of Mint, which delights the soul and is good for the mind. Pliny, along with Hippocrates and Aristotle, judged it "contrary to procreation," while the Greeks were of the opposite opinion: they forbade their soldiers to eat Mint because it so incites a man to love, diminishing his courage. It was found that the Greeks, not Pliny, were correct.

In the Middle Ages, Charlemagne wrote in his *Capitularies* that Mint was to be specially cultivated for its therapeutic qualities.

In the seventeenth century, wild Mint or Spearmint took a foothold in what is now Great Britain. Found growing in the wild, it was first cultivated in 1750, spreading to the continent in 1770. The English herbalist Culpeper prescribed the herb as a "great strengthener of the stomach."

During the 1880s, English herbalists and doctors alike used Mint in special Family Dispensatory Chests, which contained "those drugs and herbs with which one person, at least, in every village ought to be provided."

Even in modern times, the Mints have been used in first-aid kits. During World War I, a resurgence of herbal healing began when other more traditional drugs were in short supply. The main herbs used were Garlic, Lily-of-the-valley, Sphagnum Moss, and Mint.

There are over 650 species found throughout the temperate regions of the planet.

Spearmint *(Mentha spicata)*—Brought to the New World by colonists, it has a light flavor, without the bite of menthol. It has sharply pointed, toothed, lance-shaped leaves, and is one of the most common garden Mints. It is also sometimes listed as *Mentha viridis*.

"The essential oil is composed of *l*-Carvone up to 56 percent, Terpenes, Limonenes, Phellandrenes and sometimes Linaloöl and Cineol. It is anti-inflammatory, calming, mucolytic, and tonic for the digestive system. It has a wonderful ability, when inhaled, to create a feeling of joy and happiness and therefore makes an excellent addition to stress relief blends. It is indicated for all sorts of respiratory problems and chronic bronchitis." (Rose, 1994)

Peppermint *(Mentha x piperita)*—Considered a hybrid of Spearmint and Watermint *(M. aquatica)*, it has a pronounced flavor and is the classic source of Mint essential oil. It has longer leaves than that of Spearmint, with purple stems. It has a rampant growth rate.

Its essential oil contains up to 48 percent Menthol, and up to 30 percent Menthone, with other constituents including Cineol and Pulegone. There are many chemotypes and strains of Peppermint, and classification and identification can be difficult. Its properties are cooling, viricidic, tonic, and stimulant, particularly to the heart, brain, and pancreas. It has hormone-like properties that regulate ovarian hormones. Use of the essential oil is indicated for insufficient liver or pancreas juices, flatulence and belching, headache and migraine, nerve pain, and prurulent eczema. It is a very good disinfectant for the air for seriously ill patients with AIDS, senility, or those with high fever. For gas in the stomach, whether human or pets, one drop in half a glass of water, sipped slowly will do the trick. Peppermint oil diffused will cool any room, even if it is very hot.

—*Guide to [325] Essential Oils,* by Jeanne Rose

Corsican Mint *(Mentha rotundifolia)*—Grown in the Mediterranean basin, this Mint has a pure, light flavor, and is used to produce the liqueur *Creme de Menthe.* Its leaves are only 3/8 inches long, and bright green. It is less hardy than the other Mints.

Field Mint *(Mentha arvensis)*—Also called Corn Mint. Known as the native North American Mint, it has a strong Peppermint-like flavor. Also known as *Mentha canadensis,* it has ovate, toothed leaves, and is a common weed in poorly drained soils. The variety *Piperescens,* or Japanese Mint, is the major source of commercial menthol.

The Menthol content of the essential oil can be up to 90 percent, and the Menthone content up to 20 percent, with other components. Menthol is considered an antibacterial and a soother for the motor nerves. It is stimulating to the brain but also associated with constriction of blood vessels. It has been used in sciatica, migraine, headache, or in blends to discourage all types of vermin. A teeny bit on a sugar cube or in honey can be used for indigestion or vomiting. It is contraindicated for those who are taking homeopathic remedies, babies, or those with serious respiratory problems where inhaling Menthol will cause temporary loss of breathing. It is considered a tonic stimulant, stupefying at elevated doses. It can cause trembling and agitation, and is considered an anticephalic.   —*Guide to [325] Essential Oils,* by Jeanne Rose

Lemon Mint *(Mentha citrata)*—A group of similar Mints which have the flavor of Lemons, Lime, and sour Oranges. With dark-green or bronze leaves, this group of Mints grows well next to sources of water. This Mint is used in the production of linalool.

Pennyroyal *(Mentha pulegium)*—First discovered in England, this plant has a strong, almost resinous flavor. It has hairy, 1/2-inch long, dark-green leaves, and is an excellent ground cover.

The essential oil contains mostly Pulegone, up to ninety percent, with Menthone and other components. The essential oil is often used for the manufacture of synthetic Menthol. Its properties include mucolytic, tonic, and stimulant. It is an emmenagogue when there is congestion in the pelvis. Often used to bring on the menses, has some use in menstrual difficulties. It has much value to repel insects on animals, and can be used diluted either in alcohol or vinegar as a rub to kill fleas, or the herb itself used in sleep pillows made of burlap for dogs and cats, to repel vermin. It is considered an oral toxin and uterine abortive, and many aromatherapists will not use this oil.

—*Guide to [325] Essential Oils,* by Jeanne Rose

Chocolate or Apple Mint *(Mentha suaveolens)*—An interesting type, with slight flavors of chocolate, apple or pineapple. A tall plant, it has round, fuzzy, gray-green leaves. It spreads less than most Mint plants.

Silver or Woolly Mint *(Mentha longifolia)*—This Mint has a silver, fuzzy leaf, and a light, variable flavor. It has oblong to elliptical-shaped leaves, 2–3 1/2-inches long, with white hairs. It grows wild in damp ground, and is also known as Horse Mint.

Chemical composition

Although the essential oils vary in composition, they all contain terpenes and alcohol menthol, which is present in both its free state and as esters. The varieties contain different flavonoid coloring matters, as well as triterpenoids. The oil is soluble in both water and alcohol, which is used in distillation. The oil consists of both solid and liquid portions, and all contain a hydrocarbon which prevents the crystallization of menthol. The Japanese Mint *Mentha arvensis* var. *piperescens* contains over ninety percent menthol.

Medicinal uses

The herb Mint has been used extensively for its medicinal properties for over three thousand years. It can be used internally as a tea, to make poultices or balms, or inhaled to make use of its high menthol content. Mint's medicinal properties include: stomachic, carminative, stimulant, calmative, diaphoretic, febrifuge, anesthetic, disinfectant, nervine, sudorific and vermifugal. The following afflictions are treated with Mint herb or essential oil:

Acne—A pinch of essential oils of Peppermint and Rosemary makes a good astringent in cleansing the infected area.

Bronchitis—Peppermint tea is excellent as an expectorant, as is inhaling the vapors of both Mint and Eucalyptus essential oils, the Mint for its high menthol content.

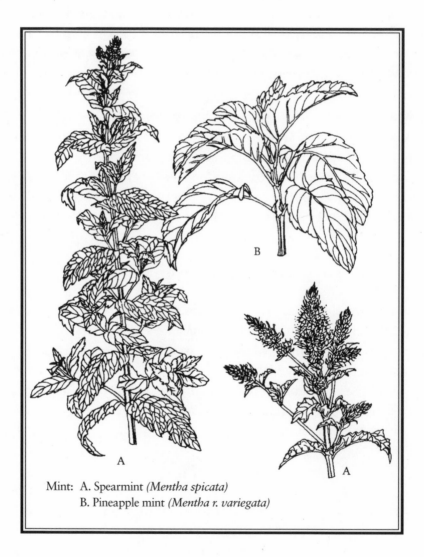

Mint: A. Spearmint *(Mentha spicata)*
       B. Pineapple mint *(Mentha r. variegata)*

Burns—Peppermint essential oil is used as a balm to rub on burns and sunburns, as its menthol cools the afflicted area.

Colds—The Flathead and Kutenai Indian tribes drank wild Mint or Spearmint herb teas to treat both the coughs and fevers associated with colds. Peppermint essential oil can also be added to oils and fats for a chest rub for associated respiratory diseases.

Dandruff—Peppermint essential oil mixed with essential oil of Rosemary and added to vinegar, is massaged into the scalp for relief. An added benefit is the coolness of the menthol, which promotes a positive psychosomatic response to the treatment.

Digestive ailments—An overall aid to most digestive disorders, Mint is especially beneficial in the treatment of flatulence, diarrhea, colic, retching and vomiting. Peppermint herb tea has been proven to stimulate the gastric lining, lessening the amount of time that food spends in the stomach. It is also said to relax the stomach, promoting burping. A poultice of Peppermint or Spearmint leaves over the stomach region also helps digestive distress. Peppermint also alleviates the amount of gas in the digestive system. Mint tea also helps to promote appetite.

Female afflictions—Spearmint can be used to treat strong menstrual cramps. In Near Eastern societies, it is used to increase sexual desire, suppress menstruation, decrease the milk supply of nursing mothers, and relieve the breast of curdled or congested milk.

Fertility—The Japanese and Arabs believe that Spearmint herb tea, or chewing several fresh leaves, helps to promote fertility in the male.

Headaches—Peppermint essential oil can be rubbed on the temples or in the affected area. The coolness of the menthol, along with the aroma, help in both minor and migraine incidents. The Lakota Indian tribe used strong Mint tea to treat all forms of headache.

Heart ailments—The Blackfeet Indians as well as other tribes chewed wild Mint leaves to treat chest pains and strengthen heart muscles.

Inflammation—Peppermint essential oil or a poultice containing Mint leaves can be used to reduce inflammation in muscle groups, joints, varicose veins. It is also a great treatment for gout.

Liver problems—Peppermint herb tea helps to promote the flow of bile in the digestive system, helping to cleanse the liver and gall bladder. It also may help in the reduction of kidney stones.

Nerve afflictions—Facial tics and sciatic nerve spasms are treated by rubbing Peppermint essential oil directly on the affected area.

Nervous system—All Mint teas have a soothing quality, and are used to treat nervousness, fatigue, nausea, vertigo, hiccoughs, palpitations, anger, confusion, depression and mental strain.

Rashes—Mint essential oil can be rubbed on poison ivy rash, diaper rash and athlete's foot.

Toothache—A drop of Mint essential oil can be used directly on the source of pain, to help alleviate the pain of both cavities and gum disease.

Travel-related afflictions—Inhaled from a handkerchief, Peppermint essential oil helps to alleviate the problems associated with jet lag, seasickness and motion sickness.

Viruses—According to laboratory studies, Peppermint essential oil has anti-viral properties against herpes simplex as well as other viruses.

Dangers

As in any use of essential oils, there are some points in which caution is needed:
- Never use Mint oils undiluted
- Don't use Mint oils at night; it may promote insomnia
- Avoid using Mint oils with homeopathic remedies; all Mint is considered an antidote

Culinary Uses

Mint has been used extensively in preparation of foods throughout the world. Though seldom cooked, Mint can be used to make teas, jellies, candies and gums. In the Middle East, Mint leaves are added to salads, for flavor, as well as high concentrations of vitamins A, C and carotene. Mint sauce is the basic accompaniment to roast lamb and veal, and is said to help in the digestion of the crude albuminous fibers of these immature meats.

Other Uses

Mints are used commercially in a wide variety of ways, which include:

Beverages—Spearmint is added to commercial teas and softdrinks to add flavor.

Dental-care products—All Mint is extensively used to flavor toothpastes and polishes, as well as gums and mouthwashes. It is used both to mask unpleasant flavors and as an antiseptic in such preparations.

Deodorants—Wild Mint is still used by Native Americans as both a deodorant and perfume.

Drugs—Peppermint is used to mask the taste of nausea-causing drugs.

Pest control—Pennyroyal *(Mentha pulegium)* produces a substance named pulegone, which has been used for centuries to dispel rats, ants, fleas, mosquitoes and other insects.

Working environments—Tests in both Japan and the United States confirm that the introduction of Mint essence into the atmosphere helps to increase worker proficiency, reduce the percentage of errors caused by workers, keep workers more alert, and improve the performance of routine tasks.

Conclusion

Mint is an extremely important substance in the use of aromatherapy. Its historical use of over three thousand years helps to support the health claims associated with its uses. It is a versatile, lively plant that can be found practically on your doorstep, and should not be overlooked when searching for natural remedies.

23

Essential Botany

Essential Oil Profiles of The Blue Oils and Lavender

Jeanne Rose

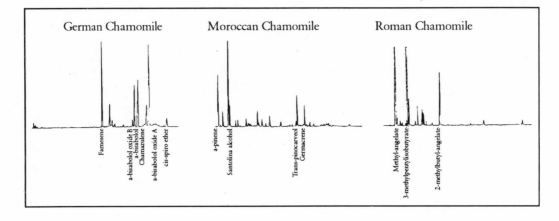

The Blue Oils

Chamomile, *Artemisia arborescens, Tanacetum annuum* and *Ormenis*

Since 1970, when I first started teaching aromatherapy courses, I was much intrigued by the blue and navy-blue color of some essential oils. Since that time I have studied and collected them, and only recently (1990) became aware of an oil called Ormenis, sold as Chamomile or Blue Chamomile. I had purchased it from various companies, and sometimes it was blue and sometimes yellow. This was very interesting, and I knew that there was definitely confusion amongst sellers and buyers of essential oils. I now wonder whether even some of the producers know what they are picking and distilling.

Recently Pamela Parsons wrote a detailed article describing some of the oils of the Compositae family labeled or sold as Chamomile. She discussed the Chamomile oils, other blue oils, their healing properties, specific applications, safety and perfumery usage. I found the article to be very exhaustive and complete. Parsons' article refers to many popular texts but lacks true taxonomic reference. She also says, "depending on which book or article you read, Blue Chamomile can mean two or more different plants entirely. Therefore, when I see something labeled or described simply Blue Chamomile, I am not amused." (Parsons, 1994) I agree with Parsons completely. After reading her article, it became apparent that there was much confusion regarding the genus Ormenis (Parsons called it "Ormensis") and I undertook to investigate this problem.

You can see from the following information that there are no hard and fast rules to giving common names to plants. Classifying and naming plant essential oils can also be a mess. Although many of the blue oils have similar uses, there are cases where it is important to know EXACTLY which oil you have or need. As with anything, the best way to clarify confusion is to do some research and experimentation. Especially, do talk to the various essential oil distributors and retailers, and get complete information about the oils you are purchasing, the Latin binomial, the part of the plant used, its country of origin and color to expect. Buy a small quantity of the same oil from two different sources, and compare color and scent. Remember that each year of growth, each harvest, each separate distillation will result in an oil with slightly different amounts of chemical components. The environment and individual ecology of a plant is important in the resultant essential oil. A year or two of great drought may result in a lower yield of essential oil but with improved or "stronger" components.

The fragrance of any particular essential oil varies from year to year and is totally dependent on the vagaries of "Mother Nature."

Ormenis/Chamæmelum

Naming • My first step in untangling the Ormenis mystery was to go to the California Academy of Science, visit the Botany department and examine their herbarium specimens of Chamomile and Ormenis. This Herbarium is one of the most prestigious in the world, and happens to be just five short blocks from my home. We looked up the reference for Ormenis in various books and periodicals, including *Flora Europæa,* Vol. 4, *Hortus Third, Economic Botany,* and in particular Cambridge University's, *The Plant Book,* by D.J. Mabberly. Imagine my surprise at the following entry: Ormenis (Cass.) Cass. = *Chamæmelum.* (Mabberley, 1989) Next we checked *Flora Europæa,* and found that Ormenis mixta was originally known as Anthemis mixta and is correctly called *Chamæmelum mixtum.* It is described as "*C. mixtum* (L.) All., loc. cit. (1785), a somewhat pubescent **annual** 10-60 cm, often much-branched, with divaricate branches . . . in cultivated fields, roadsides and maritime sands. Mediterranean region and S.W. Europe, extending northwards to W.C. France."(Tutin, Heywood, Burges, Moore, Valentine, Walters and Webb, 1976) The essential oil was not described.

The herbarium sample shows the plant to be a close look-alike to *Matricaria recutita* and almost identical to *Chamæmelum nobile.* This seemed to answer for me the question regarding the various confusing nomenclatures of Ormenis that I have seen in popular aromatherapy books (including my own *The Aromatherapy Book: Applications & Inhalations,* see page 78). It was apparent that aromatherapy books are using out-of-date nomenclature for plants that their authors never looked at.

To go further with this, please note that O. multicolis is a misspelling of O. multicaulis, which is a synonym of O. mixta, which is a synonym of O. mixtum. And O. mixtum is correctly identified as *Chamæmelum mixtum.*

Color • In taxonomy, plants' appearances are described, but the fragrance and color of the essential oil is rarely noted. I referred to Arctander's *Perfume and Flavor Materials of Natural Origin* for the fragrance and color of this particular plant: "This plant grows wild and is available in substantial quantities. Chamomile Oil, Moroccan is related to 'German Chamomile' botanically, but not at all resembling this plant is Ormenis Multicaulis, a good-looking plant, 90-125 cm high with very hairy leaves and tubular yellow flowers. . . .The plant is probably a native of northwest Africa, and evolved from a very common Ormenis species which grows all over the Mediterranean countries. . . . The oil of Ormenis Multicaulis *[Chamæmelum mixtum]* is a pale yellow to brownish-yellow, mobile liquid." (Arctander, 1960)

Arctander goes on to say that the lighter colored oils are obtained at the beginning of flowering and that towards the end of flowering the oil becomes darker and with a lower yield. "The odor of the pale oils, is fresh-herbaceous, slightly camphoraceous, but soon changes into a sweet, cistus-like and rich-balsamic undertone which is very tenacious and pleasant. . . ." (Arctander, 1960) [Note: This oil is *not blue.]* It blends well with Artemisia, Cypress, Labdanum, Lavandin, Lavender, Frankincense and others. "Chemically and olfactorily, the oil is distinctly different from the 'German' or the 'Roman' chamomile oils, *and cannot be considered as a replacement for them." [author's emphasis]* (Arctander, 1960)

Uses • What about the uses of *Chamæmelum mixtum*? Franchomme calls it "O. mixta and O. multicola Braun-Blanquet and Maire of mixed Ormenis flowers and other species of Ormenis called Moroccan Camomile" and lists the active principles and properties and indications as follows: "Active principles include a-pinene, terpene alcohols, 33% santolina alcohol, yomogi alcohol, camphor ketone and 1,8-cineol oxide terpene." *It presents the highest alcohol content of these three oils.*" The properties are anti-infectious, bactericidal against coli-bacteria, parasiticidal against worms and amoebae, a general tonic, neurotonic and aphrodisiac." It is indicated for problems of the liver and stomach, parasitosis, amoebic cysts, eczema, dermatitis, prostatitis, other sexual problems and disease, nervous depression and atherosclerosis. "No known contra-indications in physiological doses."(Franchomme and Pénoël, 1990)

Once again, please note that this is *not a blue oil*. And Guenther does not list an Ormenis species at all. (Guenther, 1976)

Chamæmelum nobile
Tea camomile or sweet camomile) Roman or English camomile.

Naming • "*C. nobile* (L.) All., F. Pedem. 1:185 (1785) (aka Anthemis nobilis L.). *Perennial;* more or less pubescent, decumbent, aromatic perennial (5-)10-30 c. Leaves 2- to 3-pinnatisect. Roadsides and damp grassland. W. Europe northwards to N. Ireland; formerly frequently cultivated for lawns, for ornament and for infusions and locally naturalized. Different from *C. mixtum,* which has most of the cauline leaves 1-pinnatisect, while *C. nobile* has most of the cauline leaves 2- to 3-pinnatisect." (Tutin, et al, 1976) Also called Roman Chamomile oil. [see also *Matricaria recutita.*]

Color • "Roman Chamomile oil is distilled from the ligulate florets. It is cultivated in England, Belgium, France, and Hungary for the flower head. Steam distillation takes place mainly in England. The oil is a pale blue, mobile liquid (when fresh) of a sweet herbaceous, somewhat fruity-warm and tealeaf-like odor. This odor is extremely diffusive but has little tenacity. The flavor is somewhat bitter, chemical or medicinal, but also fruit-herbaceous and warm." (Arctander, 1960) Steam distillation of the whole plant yields from 0.2 to 0.35% of oil. Upon exposure to air and light and on prolonged standing the light blue color of the oil changes first to green and later to yellow-brown. *They present the highest ester value of all essential oils, from 272 to 293.5.* The color is due to chamazulene and is present only in traces in Roman or English camomile. (Guenther, 1976)

Uses • "The properties are both positive and negative, antispasmodic, calming on the central nervous system, anti-inflammatory, antiparasitical against Giardia and lock-jaw. Indicated for neuritis, neuralgia, nervous tics, asthma that originates from nervous conditions, intestinal parasitoses, surgical intervention. Contra-indications: None known in physiological doses." (Franchomme and Pénoël, 1990) This oil is particularly good inhaled for insomnia or headache, and applied topically in cases of acne and skin irritation.

Matricaria recutita
Wild, German, Hungarian or small Chamomile

Naming • Called Matricaria chamomilla and correctly known as *Matricaria recutita* L. *Annual* plant. "The chamomile of commerce and the source of oil of Roman chamomile and chamomile tea is largely, if not exclusively, *C. nobile* which is cultivated as either a Roman double-flowered form or more frequently a German single-flowered form. . . . In most herb trade and medical literature, chamomile is referred to as M. chamomilla, which is incorrect. This binomial is a synonym of *M. recutita* L., the chamomile found throughout Europe, Asia, and many other parts of the world, often as a weed. It may be used to make a tea, but infrequently and mostly is used as a cultivated species of commerce. Because of nomenclatural confusion, therefore, the vast majority of nonbotanical references to chamomile in the literature, in pollen extracts made for immunotherapy, and in commercial sales is *not* to *M. recutita.* (M. chamomilla), but rather to *Chamæmelum nobile,* native only to southern and western Europe." (Lewis, 1992) "*M. recutita* L. [M. Chamomilla of auth., not L.] Sweet False Chamomile. Sweet-scented, much-branched, glabrous *annual,* to 2 1/2 feet; leaves to 2 3/8 inch long, 2-pinnatifid into linear segments; heads 1 inch across, receptacle conicle; disc flowers yellow, 5-lobed, ray flowers 10-20, white, reflexed, achenes 5-ribbed. Europe to west Asia; naturalized in North America." (Bailey, 1977)

Color • "High-grade [that is, whole or complete] Chamomile flowers are much too costly to use for essential oil production. For this purpose only lower grade [those that are broken], siftings and dust are employed in Hungary and Germany. Oil of Chamomile consists chiefly of high-boiling constituents, steam of high pressure is applied. Distillation of one charge requires from 7-13 hours . . . Certain constituents of the oil are soluble in large quantities of warm water and the distillation waters must be redistilled (cohobated). . . .The oil is deep blue liquid of strong and characteristic odor, and bitter aromatic flavor and more or less viscous. Under the influence of light and air the deep blue color of oil gradually changes to green, and finally to brown. The ester number is 3-39 and after acetylation 117 to 155 (not as high as Roman Chamomile oil). . . . The *most important constituent of the essential oil is an azulene named chamazulene as well as a component called bisabolol.* Bisabolol and chamazulene occur *only* in the morning and evening collections. Therefore, the plant must be distilled at these times. The content of chamazulene in the various Chamomile oils depends upon the origin and age of the flower material, and decreases during storage of the flowers." (Guenther, 1976) Chamazulene is formed during the distillation process and is highest in morning-distilled plants. "The oil is used as a flavoring agent in fine liqueurs and in perfume, to which it imparts pleasing and warm tonalities that are difficult to trace." (Guenther, 1976)

Uses • "Active principles are chamazulene, bisabolene, farnesene, sesquiterpenols, and others. The properties are tonic digestive, stomachic, anti-inflammatory, cicatrise, antiallergic, decongestive, antispasmodic and with hormone-like properties. It is indicated for dermatosis, infected sores, ulcers, eczema, dyspepsia, gastro-duodenal ulcers, cystitis, and menstrual difficulties like amenorrhea and dysmenorrhea." (Franchomme, 1990)

Generally speaking, we use *M. recutita* oil for severe skin problems, externally, as an anti-inflammatory, in a diffusor as an anti-allergenic; and the *C. nobile* for inhalation, asthma and oral uses. (Rose, 1994)

Chamomile CO_2 is one other product that we should mention. It is a thick, CO_2-extracted, solid, unctuous matter from Chamomile flowers *(M. recutita)* that contains all the natural parts of the flower plus the essential oil. It smells just like the fresh flowers, and could play an important part in your cosmetics and body-care products, whether they are home-made or for the professional market. I have made a hand lotion with this, using enough of the Chamomile CO_2 to scent the lotion with a delicious apple scent and then adding the essential oil to color it pale blue. Altogether a very aesthetically pleasing and beautiful product. The Chamomile CO_2 is available from Prima Fleur Botanicals. Cost: $42 per ounce.

Ormenis and Chamomile.

If you read *Shirley Price's Aromatherapy Workbook* regarding these three species, you will find that she recommends the Nobile Chamomile above all the others, and finds it has more uses.

Artemisia arborescens
sometimes called greater Mugwort.

Naming • "*A. arborescens* L., Sp. Pl. ed. 2, 1188 (1763). White-tomentose, aromatic **perennial;** stems 50-100 cm, woody below. Leaves 1- to 2-pinnatisect or the upper sometimes simple, petiolate; capitula 6-7 mm across, in a large, paniculate inflorescence. Receptacle hairy. Corolla glabrous. Mediterranean region, S. Portugal." (Tutin et al, 1976) This is a plant that I grow and have used. It is similar to *A. absinthium* and smells somewhat like it due to the presence of thujone. *If the plant and essential oil do not have this very characteristic odor of thujone it is NOT A. arborescens.*

Color • The flowers are distilled and the color is a deep navy-blue, even darker than *M. recutita*. The oil is almost viscous. The scent has a very characteristic scent of thujone.

Uses • "The active principles are the monoterpenes of limonene and sabinene, sesquiterpenes that include a very elevated level of chamazulene, dihydrochamazulene, monoterpenes that include *isothujone* of 30-45% [which gives it its characteristic odor], up to 18% camphor and other components. The properties are anticatarrh, mucolytic, anti-inflammatory, antiallergenic, antihistaminic, choleretique (increases bile production). It is indicated for bronchial catarrh and for asthma, problems of the skin and insufficient bile production." (Franchomme, 1990)

Comment • Here is an extreme example of an oil purchased from different sources, with two such different scents that *they cannot be of the same species*. It would be interesting to see just what species the producer had picked, distilled and sold to these companies.

Tanacetum annuum
sometimes called Moroccan blue Chamomile

Naming • *Tanacetum annuum*. L., "Sp. Pl 844 (1753). Ligules yellow *or* absent *(T. parthenium* has white ligules.) Greenish-pubescent **annual.** Stems 20-80 cm, branched. Leaves pinnatisect, the cauline 1-3 cm; segments linear, acute or acuminate, sparsely pubescent to glabrous. All florets hermaphrodite, tubular, 5-toothed. Achenes 5-ribbed. Cultivated ground and waste places. S.W. Europe." (Tutin et al, 1976)

Color • A very lovely, deep blue from the flowers. Oil not as viscous or thick as other blue oils.

Uses • "Active principles include monoterpenes with limonene as major component, sesquiterpenes of chamazulene up to 30% and dihydrochamazulene. The properties are anti-inflammatory, antiphlogistic, antihistamine, antiprurigenic, analgesic, nervous sedative, hypotensive, phlebotonique (blood), possibly thymus-stimulating and hormone-like. It is indicated for asthmatic crises (as it supplies theophylline, which is a bronchodilator), emphysema, irritating skin problems, allergic skin in adults and infants, abnormal reddening of the skin and cuperose skin, tubercular lesions, arthritis, neuritis, sciatica, muscular rheumatism, diabetes, hypertension, varicose veins, and leukemia (certain forms). Contra-indications: among certain women with endocrine imbalances." (Franchomme, 1990)

Tanacetum vulgare
sometimes called Common Tansy

Naming • *Tanacetum vulgare* L. [Chrysanthemum vulgare (L.) Bernh.]. Common Tansy, Gold-Buttons. Coarse, aromatic, subglabrous, rhizomatous *perennial,* to 3 feet; leaves pinnate, to 4 3/4 inches long, lfts. toothed or incised, punctate; heads many, flowers all tubular, golden-yellow. Europe, Asia; Widely naturalized in North America. (Bailey, 1977)

Color • Oil of Tansy has a strong, aromatic odor and very bitter taste, and is "a liquid of peculiar, aromatic odor and yellowish color which turns brown under the influence of air and light." (Guenther, 1976) It is also occasionally a very pale, watery blue.

Uses • There is *no* aromatherapy use for this oil, which contains a toxic amount of "ketone content, calculated as thujone of 50-67.3%." (Guenther, 1976) Used medicinally to rid the body of worms and other parasites, under medical supervision.

Other Blue Oils

During this investigation of "The Blue Oils," and because I have been involved in organizing the growing of essential oil plants in the Pacific Northwest, specifically California, for the express purpose of encouraging distillation here of aromatic plants as an industry, I was able to look at and smell many oils that had been recently distilled in Oregon. I will not go into detail about their naming and uses, and will only briefly name a few of these oils.

Artemisia arborescens was a luscious, deep-blue, indigo-colored oil with the characteristic scent of thujone. This sample had been analyzed as having a 20% azulene content.

Artemisia douglasiana (A. heterophylla) is a clear royal-blue, with a sweet sage-like odor. With this color of azulene and knowing the Native American uses of the

plant, I would think that this California and Pacific Northwest species will ultimately find wonderful uses in the body-care industry, especially for serious skin
conditions and externally for rheumatism or headache.

Tanacetum vulgare cv. Goldsticks. This essential oil is a very pale sky-blue, with a
hint of thujone odor. I do not feel that it has any external applications in the body-
care industry, or use in aromatherapy.

Artemisia ludoviciana var. latiloba (White Mugwort) is a watery blue in color,
very perky-scented, with sage and eucalyptus overtones. According to the Native
Americans, the herb was used as a tea to expel a dead fetus, among many uses,
and externally to remove tumors.

Two other oils with a pale blue color were *Daucus carota,* which is commonly
called Queen Anne's Lace (wild Carrot) and Chinese Celery. The oils of *Aralia californica* leaves and flowers, and *Conioselinum pacificum,* with their pale colors,
almost green in hue, do not fall within this short article.

Conclusion

It is obvious that people who sell aromatherapy essential oils are not always careful
about the naming of their product, or the correct spelling of the binomial. Where
are the spell-checkers and editors? The confusion seems to lie in a lack of integrity
by the persons who pick, distill and package the original product and sell misla-
beled product to distributors who pass on their errors to retailers. By examining all
of these oils, one can see which were the old and improperly stored oils, and even
last year's distillation, by the color: brownish-yellow for Ormenis and greenish-
black for azulene-containing oils. Sometimes it is a disadvantage for the essential
oils to be sold in brown bottles, because the consumer cannot judge the age and
quality of the oil by the color. My suggestion is that knowledgeable consumers
carry around a bit of blotter paper and take a small sample of these expensive oils,
examining them carefully for color and scent before purchase. Also, the consumer
must take some responsibility, learn the Latin binomial and make sure essential oils
are labeled completely before they buy them.

It appears that some of these samples of essential oils were sold as either
Artemisia arborescens or Blue Moroccan, when in fact they were actually *Tanacetum annuum,* which has much different uses and in general is *not* a viable substitu-
tion. Consumers must educate themselves, learn to understand and use the correct
Latin binomials and demand that this name be on the oils they purchase.

When it comes to the expensive essential oils, it pays to call around for pricing. Only order oils from those companies that will tell you the common name, *Latin name,* condition of the oil you want and the color, particularly with the blue-colored oils. These show age and oxidation with a change in color from blue to greenish-black, or from pale yellow to yellow-brown.

Analyze the chart and read the text again for the key differences in these oils.

Definitions:

1. *herbarium:* a collection of dried plant specimens systematically arranged for botanical reference
2. *Herbarium:* the place where a collection of dried plants is kept
3. *pubescent:* covered with soft, fuzzy hair
4. *divaricate:* having branches spread widely apart
5. *taxonomy:* study of general principles of scientific classification
6. *decumbent:* a plant stem or shoot reclining on the ground but with ascending apex or extremity
7. *pinnatisect:* cleft, having similar parts arranged on opposite sides of an axis, as a feather, to or almost to the midrib
8. *cauline:* growing on the upper portion of a stem
9. *ligulate:* furnished with a flattened, strap-shaped corolla in the ray flowers
10. For other definitions, kindly consult your botany text or *How to Identify Plants* by H.D. Harrington, Swallow Press, Chicago, IL, 1957

Note: The botanical descriptions in this article are not complete. If you are interested in a complete description, please refer to a taxonomy text. It would also help if all persons who consider themselves experts in aromatherapy have a basic understanding of botany and taxonomy.

The Blue Oils©

Latin Name	Other Names	A/P*	E.O. Color**	E.O. Aroma	Major components	Essential Oil Uses
Chamaemelum mixtum	Ormenis multicolis Ormenis multicaulis Ormenis mixta Ormenis mixtum Anthemis mixta Ormensis spp. Moroccan Chamomile	A	golden yellow	spicy-fruity	alcohol	All problems of liver & stomach including parasites; Serious skin disease
Chamaemelum nobile	Tea chamomile Sweet Chamomile Roman Chamomile English Chamomile Anthemis nobilis Nobel Chamomile	P	very pale blue to clear	sweet, herby, no tenacity	esters	Asthma and oral uses Best for all uses
Matricaria recutita	Wild Chamomile Small Chamomile Matricaria chamomilla German chamomile Hungarian Chamomile Sweet False Chamomile	A	deep blue	fruit & toasted nuts	azulene bisabolene bisabolol	Anti-inflammatory, All skin care
Artemisia arborescens	Greater Mugwort	P	deep blue	Wormwood-like	thujone & azulene	Anti-catarrh; Skin-care
Tanacetum annuum	Moroccan Blue Chamomile	A	deep blue	toasty odor & warm flavor	azulene limonene	Hormone-like; Skin; Asthma
Tanacetum vulgare	Common Tansy (many chemotypes)	P	yellow to very pale watery blue	Wormwood-like	up to 60% thujone	NO USE IN AROMA-THERAPY
OTHERS	SEE TEXT					

*A=Annual   P=Perennial

**Oxidation changes the chemical composition of the essential oil. If any of these oils are greenish-black when they should be deep blue, it indicates oxidation, age, and the existence of free radicals, and they should not be used for therapy. Furthermore, if the clear to yellow oils appear deep yellow to deep brown, they too have oxidized and are too old to use therapeutically.

Lavender

Recently, I have been made aware of the almost universal confusion regarding the genus *Lavandula*. This short article is to help clarify the issue as well as describe the two major Lavender oils, called Lavender and Lavandin.

"**The Botanical Species.** First of all, we must know the exact botanical species of the plant used for distillation. The name 'Lavender essence,' for instance, is inadequate because there are many species of Lavender, not just one. Each one has its own aromatic features, and a specific essence is found in its tissues.

"A properly defined botanical species gives the name of genus in Latin, followed by a qualifying adjective, and sometimes the variety if such exists. *Lavandula*, then, is not a species but a genus which covers various types of Lavender. *Vera, spica, stoechas, hybrida* are the qualifying adjectives which individualize each of these Lavenders. Var. and CT indicate the varietal forms of a species. While var. indicates a varietal form based on appearance, CT indicates a varietal form based on chemistry.

"The association of the genus and the adjective defines the botanical species; *Lavandula angustifolia* vera (in English: Wild-grown Lavender) [the 'vera' signifying that it is wild], and in *Lavandula x hybrida* we need to mention the variety, because there are many of them. There is *Lavandula angustifolia* vera var. Fragrans, which is of wild origin, for instance, or var. Maillette, which is a cultivated clone.

"For Lavandula hybrida, a cultivated species, the correct name is *Lavandula x intermedia*. There is the var. Abrialii (becoming less common), the *var. Super* and the *var. Grosso,* which is the most prevalent.

"The name of the variety narrows down the description of the botanical species and its origin. We'll see that the description 'wild' or 'cultivated' is of importance as far as the quality of the obtained product is concerned." (From *Les Cahiers de l'Aromatherapie Records,* No. 1, Sept, 1995)

Briefly, true Lavender is *Lavandula angustifolia,* which has also been called, in the past, Lavandula Vera and Lavandula officinale. These three names are really just synonyms of the true Lavender. They are all the same plant. This is the so-called legendary "English Lavender," which has been employed in perfumery for its fresh, clean scent. The scent is very distinctive, very soft, and sweet, with no camphoraceous overtones.

All forms of *L. angustifolia* will produce essential oil. Some of these varietal forms produce a sweeter oil than others. Currently, my favorite smell of Lavender comes from *Lavandula angustifolia* cv. Delphinensis and L.a. cv. Maillette. I also have a new Lavender called L.a. cv. Sachet that I am told produces a lovely sweet oil. This Lavender has been developed in Oregon for that particular climate.

The AOC* has been applied to Lavender produced solely from *Lavandula angustifolia* grown on the limestone foothills of the Alps at a higher altitude than 800 metres and with a Mediterranean climate, distinguished by sunny days and short nights. 25 kilograms per hectare is the maximum quantity permitted, all of which is produced solely by steam distillation. Batches are approved after the identity and purity has been established, and most batches submitted are approved.

There was much debate and heart-searching as to whether in today's world this system may have outlived its validity. For instance, how can an "AOC" be applied to a Camembert cheese produced from livestock from Denmark fed with fodder from Britain, which happens to be produced in Normandy? With modern technology and expertise, just how important are these imponderables associated with "Terroir(e)." The Australian wine producers were not mentioned (the "enemy" was clearly the Californian wine growers), but their expertise is being made available to other countries (even France?) to maximise the production of good quality wine. How does this fit in with this concept of "Terroir(e)"?

Turning to essential oils, is there really a unique product in French Lavender with the AOC accreditation? How does it relate to other standards such as AFNOR, ISO and Pharmacopoeial monographs? The belief in "Terroir(e)" was confirmed but. . .

Terroir(e) = territory   —From *The Aromatherapist*, Feb. 1995

All types of Lavender will produce essential oil if you take the time to distill them.

Other Lavenders are *Lavandula dentata*, the so-called "French Lavender." This is native to drier regions, such as Spain and Gibraltar. It is an attractive bush, with many-toothed leaves topped by flowers that emit a sweet, fresh scent.

Lavandula latifolia is a handsome plant with tomentose leaves on a shrub-like plant. The flowers are a lavender color on long stems. This plant is suitable for

---

*AOC is the Aromatherapy Organizations Council. It is the main umbrella body for aromatherapy in the UK and represents the collective voice of the therapy when liaising with government or other authorities.

making lavender wands and lavender baskets, but the scent is not sweet and actually rather harsh.

Lavandula multifida is a unique plant, low, lacy foliage with purple flowers in pairs or groups. The scent is pungent and not suitable as perfume.

Lavandula pinnata is called the "Fern Lavender." It has a very strong pine scent with deep blue flowers.

Lavandula spica is considered one of the most fragrant varieties with tall greyish foliage and profuse flowers that are ornamental and perfect for lavender wands and lavender baskets as well as for drying for baths, potpourris and other special projects.

Lavandula stoechas is dwarf, with profuse, fat flowers that are dark purple. The spikes are broad and square, like "purple corn cobs with a lilac topknot."

Our most important Lavender for producing oil for the trade is *Lavandula x intermedia*, also called *Lavandula x hybrida*. This is a cross of two plants, *Lavandula angustifolia* and *Lavandula latifolia*. The important varieties are *L. x intermedia*, Abrialii, Super, and Grosso. Grosso is not gross but was named after a Frenchman named Grosso. "Provence" is a commonly used name for a landscape Lavender, but it is not an essential oil producing plant.

These three cultivars mentioned above produce the essential oil that is called Lavandin. And Lavandin is the product that most of us are used to and have smelled all these years. Lavender 40-42 is not a natural product but a product concocted from combinations of essential oils of Lavender to artificially produce one with components of linalyl acetate and linalool that approaches 40-42%.

Lavandula x intermedia cv. Super has good linalyl acetate, and *Lavandula x intermedia* cv. Abrialii has good linalool. *L. intermedia* cv. Grosso represents 90% of the French production of Lavandin including the plants in Provence. One can produce 1 kg. of essential oil from 35-50 kg. (75 to 110 lbs.) of Lavender tops.

Lavandula x intermedia "Provence" is NOT the famous Lavender developed for the perfume fields of Provence in southern France. What is called Provence is simply an American plant developed to look like the plants in Provence. It is cherished for its wonderful intense scent, but does not produce a quality oil high in linalool and linalyl acetate. It actually produces an oil that is very high in cineol and borneol, with some camphor and very little linalyl acetate.

L. x intermedia "Provence" CT cineol, borneol. The US-grown Lavender has high levels of cineol and borneol. It can be used to decongest the lungs and bronchii, as an expectorant that stimulates the mucus glands. It could also be a powerful immune system modulator and possibly may help those with bulimia. A general tonic for the system, for chronic infections and general fatigue. *Caution:* This oil can only be used by inhalation. External use will cause skin burning.

There you have it.

True Lavender oil (Sweet Lavender) has a fine, sweet, soft fragrance useful for inhalation and application therapy, while Lavandin oil is used for industry as well as therapy.

You must smell all of these oils separately and then sequentially to truly understand the uniqueness and individuality of each oil.

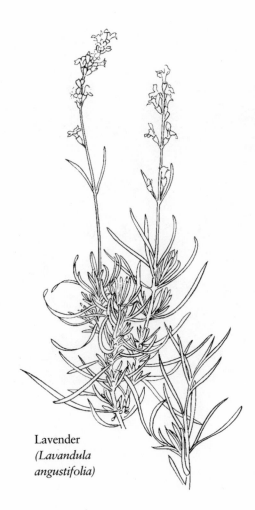

Lavender
*(Lavandula
angustifolia)*

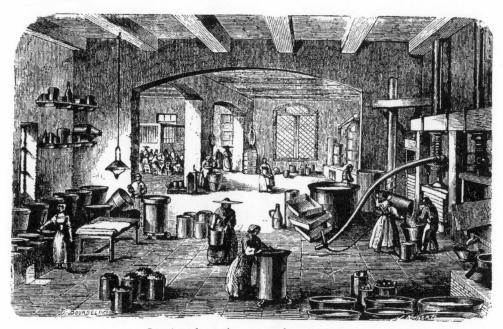

Interior of a perfume manufactory at Nice

V

Case Studies

24

Planting Aromatherapy Seeds

Elizabeth Jones

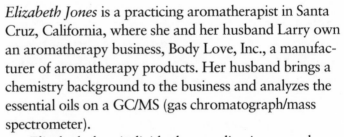

Elizabeth Jones is a practicing aromatherapist in Santa Cruz, California, where she and her husband Larry own an aromatherapy business, Body Love, Inc., a manufacturer of aromatherapy products. Her husband brings a chemistry background to the business and analyzes the essential oils on a GC/MS (gas chromatograph/mass spectrometer).

Elizabeth does individual counseling in aromatherapy. She teaches at two local colleges, and does voluntary aromatherapy work at a local convalescent hospital. She is currently writing a book on women and aromatherapy.

Labiatae

*A*romatherapy has become the fragrant lens through which I can express all that I hold dear. It offers an opportunity to provide physical healing to the body, balance to human emotions, and a window to the spiritual nature. In teaching it I can stimulate people's olfactory sense gently with Lavender *(Lavandula spp.)* or boldly with Juniper *(Juniperus communis)*. The essential oils calm our emotions, expand our minds, clear up infections, and sprout new spiritual awareness.

Education has always been an exciting path for me. I once was the head teacher at a primary school for five-to eight-year-olds, providing everything from math and science to art and sports. Later I taught art and English to high-school students. Now I have found the subject I was born to teach. It brings me great joy, after being an herbalist for twenty-five years and creating a business thirteen years ago that manufactures aromatherapy products, to directly share my fascination with plant energy.

I am fortunate to be a teacher of aromatherapy at two colleges dedicated to the healing arts. I find it very rewarding to offer a ten-week (thirty-hour) class. The students are mostly women who are personally committed to healing themselves and others. Many of these are massage therapists, acupuncturists, psychotherapists, caregivers for the elderly, and last, but best, mothers. They love the enhanced healing power that comes from adding essential oils to their personal lives, and then their professional routines.

I include three to four essential oils in each class. We cover many aspects of aromatherapy including the history, the fundamental chemistry and extraction methods of the oils, and how they interact with different body systems. I teach reflexology, and we spend several sessions applying the oils to selected reflexology points, such as Peppermint *(Mentha x piperita)* to the stomach and intestinal meridians. As the class unfolds, the students begin experimenting with single oils, and eventually blending fragrant synergies for family, friends, and clients.

I am always amazed at the creativity that blossoms in each class as the students discover the beauty of the fragrances, and how beneficial each oil is in its unique reactions in the body and mind. At first there are some doubts to overcome at how something so natural and unrecognized in society could actually be so powerful. Yet there is always an intuitive acknowledgment that oils extracted from plants can create healing changes on a physical and emotional level. As everyone begins sharing their experiences, there is soon a large collection of data as to how certain oils positively affect the circle of people surrounding each student.

When a seed is planted and a sprout emerges, we can only water and feed it. We cannot tell it which way to grow, where to flower, or when to seed. These processes which are beyond our control are gifts to the gardener from Nature. They let the gardener know that other forces are at work, and that she is not nursing the seeds alone. As a teacher, it is a great pleasure is to watch the unpredictible growth and flowering of my students, and it is a wonderful gift to see my students plant their own seeds, and to watch our aromatherapy garden expand with a life of its own. I would like to share with you a bouquet from seeds that I have planted.

Jacqui is a mother of two small sons, four months old and two-and-a-half years old. She described her youngest as having respiratory problems ever since she brought him home from the hospital. Her doctor told her that his nasal passages were slightly underdeveloped. It was a few days before Thanksgiving, and he had contracted a bad, upper-respiratory type of cold. She was a bit overwhelmed with Thanksgiving dinner preparations, and since she had little time to devote to Andrew, she decided to try aromatherapy to clear it out of his system as soon as possible.

She made a blend of the following oils:

Eucalyptus Oil *(Eucalyptus globulus)*	5 drops
Tea Tree *(Melaleuca alternifolia)*	5 drops
Thyme *(Thymus vulgaris)*	4 drops
Sandalwood *(Santalum album)*	3 drops
Roman Chamomile *(Chamamaelum nobile)*	3 drops

She mixed the essential oils in a Sweet Almond oil base.

Jacqui purchased a steam vaporizer and used the recommended amount of medication by the manufacturer, substituting the essential oil blend for the Vick's medication that had Camphor, Eucalyptus, and menthol in a seventy-four percent alcohol base. She let the vaporizer run all night and the next morning her son's breathing seemed a little better. She decided to give him an all-over body massage with her special new massage oil.

"Andrew really enjoys having his body massaged, and the oils take almost immediate effect. He seems to calm down within a few short moments. He doesn't have any resistance to the smell of the oils. When I massage Andrew with the essential oils, I massage his entire body, and I also massage the reflexology points on his feet. This seems to have the most immediate effect on him. He generally goes to sleep within five minutes or so after I have done this. I feel his immune system is getting just what it needs right now."

By that afternoon, Andrew showed a dramatic increase in his ability to breathe through his nose. The cold never did manifest in his chest. Jacqui believes that the essential oils had a great deal to do with Andrew's quick recovery. Her Thanksgiving was a success, and her baby was well enough to greet all of the relatives.

Jacqui repeated this aromatherapy respiratory treatment with her toddler a few weeks later. He too responded very well, and seemed to enjoy the smell of the respiratory blend. She remarked, "This particular blend has definitely proven itself invaluable as an aid to my children with their colds."

Cyndi is a student who immediately took to using the essential oils. She commented that she felt as if she were home—as if she had been around the oils before, as if these fragrances had been passed down through time to her. She relates to them in the tradition of Cleopatra and Theodora. She trusted her ability to make blends and choose the right oil in the very beginning of class. It was love at first smell!

Cyndi was intelligent and interested in the other students, but she seemed nervous and restless in the first classes. She had grown up in a family where her mother was both physically and mentally ill, and unavailable to her. Cyndi and her sister were forced to live with a British family that was extremely rigid and methodical. It is as if Cyndi's creativity had been boxed and sealed up, leaving her anxious and unstable. In truth, she seems to have great intuitive abilities, and now she is a visual artist, a fiber artist. The essential oils are enhancing her efforts to heal and integrate her emotional states.

The setting for her aromatherapy treatments is the bathroom. The entrance is through a beaded curtain, into a room with delicate flute music playing. A candle is the only light, and the smell of Bergamot *(Citrus bergamia)*, Lemongrass *(Cymbopogon citratus)*, and Lavender *(Lavendula angustifolia)* hover enticingly above the water in the tub. It is a place where she can leave the material world and cares behind, stepping into a quiet mode of peace and transformation. Cyndi can access her feelings and intuitive state, and receive flashes of insight into her life. She often chooses the essential oils of Cedarwood *(Juniperus virginiana)* and Frankincense *(Boswellia carterii)* for their ability to open her mind to her higher self. The Cedarwood provides a calm strength, and the Frankincense offers spiritual awareness and a sense of letting go of the heaviness of the past. Sometimes she also chooses Patchouli *(Pogostemon patchouli)* or Vetivert *(Andropogon muricatus)* to receive a sense of grounding.

There in the quiet, she can honor the deep feelings that she has, listen to the different voices of her personality, and access the higher self who can guide and harmonize the various parts of her psyche. She says that, thanks to aromatherapy, she is beginning to trust who she is.

She also uses the oils in an aroma lamp in the room where she does her artistic work. She spontaneously creates blends for her different emotional needs like Clary Sage *(Salvia sclerea)* when she feels blocked, or Lemongrass *(Cymbopogon citratus)* to get things going, or Jasmine *(Jasminum grandiflorum)* to feel a little wild. For her, Cedarwood evokes a higher presence. A typical formula:

Clary Sage *(Salvia sclerea)*	4 drops
Grapefruit *(Citrus paradisi)*	5 drops
Cedarwood *(Cedrus atlantica)*	3 drops

She says the long-term effects of taking baths and using the oils via inhalation is that she recognizes when she is in a chaotic state with the old nervous, fidgety, conflicting energy. She is aware of her former diverse mood swings, and creates the serene space to dispel them. She says she doesn't feel so fragmented and alienated from herself. She is more comfortable, more balanced, more in a state of inner peace.

Her dream is to someday have a space with a sacred garden and a large bathtub, where she can provide the setting for others' transformative baths. Her talents and ability to heal with the oils would greatly lend itself to a business called Cyndi's Sacred Baths.

Laurel has been a massage therapist for ten years and practices Swedish and acupressure massage techniques on her clients. After taking my aromatherapy class, she added essential oils to every client's massage. She has a large and effective practice due to her innate healing abilities, and she says her practice has grown since she began using the aromatics. She claims that, almost without exception, people love the oils. She related two examples:

A man came to her in a state of rage over stress from work, his marriage, and settling his father's estate. He seemed very stressed, tight and angry. As with all her clients, she asked him how he was, physically, emotionally, and spiritually. As the client talked, she chose the oils she thought would be best. She made a blend of the following oils:

Melissa *(Melissa officinalis)*	3 drops
Rose *(Rosa damascena)*	5 drops
Ylang-Ylang *(Cananga odorata)*	6 drops
Roman Chamomile *(Chamamaelum nobile)*	3 drops

She poured out one ounce of vegetable oil in a dish, added the essential oils, and mixed it with her fingers. She began the massage by applying the blend to the neck, shoulders, and then feet of her client in the beginning of the massage. The essential oils were on her hands throughout the massage.

Almost immediately after the massage, the client stated that he felt more relaxed and emotionally uplifted. She said he left seeming human again, because when he arrived he was like a raging animal. He later told her that the soothing effect had lasted for some time.

Another of Laurel's clients was suffering from great migraines and allergies due to an inability to feel or acknowledge her emotions. She tried chiropractors, acupuncturists, and psychotherapists. Laurel saw her once a month for a year without much change. Then one day she tried an acupressure treatment with the following blend:

Marjoram *(Origanum majorana)*	4 drops
Melissa *(Melissa officinalis)*	3 drops
Lavender *(Lavandula angustifolia)*	7 drops
Basil *(Ocimum basilicum)*	4 drops

The woman left, feeling nauseated as she drove home. About one-half hour after she left Laurel's, she suddenly had a window of clarity. Her thinking became sharp as a bell, and the migraine passed. For the first time she realized that she could get through a migraine without any pharmaceutical drugs. She continues to improve, and the migraines are less and shorter. Laurel has switched back to Swedish massage, and changes the blend to fit her client's needs.

Laurel also finds that her own health has improved. For example, the other three members of her family were sick during the Christmas season, but as long as she gave aromatherapy massages, Laurel stayed well. She also appreciates the fact that using the essential oils allows her to communicate with her clients on many levels and in a deep, holistic way. She says most people remember the oils she used the last time, and often want to repeat one or two. Some of the more confident ones, on arrival, go right to her oils, and pick out the essential oils they want that day. She says that aromatherapy has enhanced the healing experience for everyone.

Another charming student is Shanti, who was born in New Zealand. She is the follower of a yogi named Kaliji, who founded a fine yoga school, the Tri-Yoga center, where Shanti works as a yoga instructor. Since taking the aromatherapy class, she includes blends of oil in aroma lamps in her yoga classes. She feels that this is in the tradition of great Hindu saints, who often manifest their presence in the aroma of Sandalwood. She is truly delighted with the essential oils. Due to her giving and loving nature, she finds creating a blend for someone in the school is one of her greatest joys. Her "inspiration and wisdom come from the grace of guru Kaliji."

At the Tri-Yoga center, Shanti often uses the following oils:

Frankincense *(Boswellia carterii)*   4 drops
Neroli *(Citrus aurantium)*   6 drops
Sandalwood *(Santalum album)*   7 drops

She places the oils in an aroma lamp for the spiritual upliftment of everyone at the center. This blend slows down the breath (Frankincense), so in meditation or quiet yoga postures more focus can be given to the breathing process. The Sandalwood *(Santalum album)* has a calming, centering effect on a racing mind and body. Since it is a sacred oil of India, she always includes it expressing the awareness that it comes from an endangered tree that must be used sparingly.* Neroli *(Citrus aurantium)* lifts the person too immersed in the material world to the place where the higher self can be contacted. All of these oils have an affinity with the crown chakra, and all are very useful for a yogi seeking a spiritual path.

Shanti is about to blossom into an aromatherapy business with a partner. Her goal is to design, have manufactured, and sell aroma lamps that really work, so that other schools and individuals can enjoy the benefits of the airborne molecules of the oils.

Aubrey works at a health spa as a massage therapist and æsthetician. She is so inspired by the essential oils that she often teaches classes at a local beauty college on the subject. She takes them with her on travels, and administers them—usually a single oil—to people as she passes by.

Aubrey has a client at the spa who has suffered from depression for over ten years. He claims he inherited this condition from his father. He also had a stressful job at a computer company, which he recently left. Aubrey has massage sessions weekly with him. She has begun to use essential oils in these sessions, and is seeing some real improvement in his emotional state.

---

* A good substitute for Sandalwood is Vetivert.

She uses the following blend:

Clary Sage *(Salvia sclarea)*
Orange *(Citrus sinensis)*
Bergamot *(Citrus bergamia)*

She gives him an hour-and-a-half massage with the above oils mixed into a vegetable-oil base. After three sessions he became a lighter, happier person. He used to come in with a "crinkled brow" and heavy, bent shoulders. Now he is standing more erect, joking with some of the other women that work there, and beginning to open up. She is delighted with the change in his personality. Aubrey shows real promise as a dedicated aromatherapist.

* * *

There are many other women I could include here, who are equally vital in the healing arts with aromatherapy. I hope the vignettes above are inspirational to women everywhere. As the catalyst for introducing the use of essential oils, I am profoundly honored to know these women, and amazed at their diverse and sincere creativity. I am encouraged to continue teaching, making blends myself, doing individual aromatherapy counseling, and developing new products.

The needs of our time elicit a deep response in the feminine psyche to utilize our innate healing abilities. The imbalances we see projected everywhere rally those of us fortunate enough to know about the fragrant palette to dedicate the essential oils to restoring health. As we seek guidance from a higher power within, aromatherapy becomes truly meaningful as a healing modality.

25

Aromatherapy and Health in the Theatre

Lucy Scott

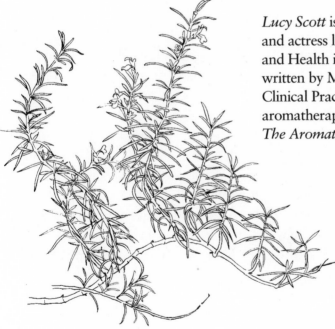

Rosemary
(Rosmarinus officinalis)

Lucy Scott is an aromatherapy practitioner and actress living in England. "Aromatherapy and Health in the Theatre" was a dissertation written by Ms. Scott for the Shirley Price Clinical Practitioner's Diploma, an advanced aromatherapy course. It was first published in *The Aromatherapist*, Vol. 2, No. 1.

Then, were not summer's distillation left,
A liquid prisoner pen in walls of glass,
Beauty's effect with beauty were bereft,
Nor it, nor no remembrance what it was
But flowers distilled, though they with winter meet,
Leese but their show; their substance still lives sweet.
Sonnet, William Shakespeare

*A*romatherapy provides interesting work, a sense of security, and the wonderful feeling of being able to help others. The job of an actor, although it may provide artistic satisfaction, is very hard work requiring a competitive spirit and vast quantities of patience and calmness; and it is, on the whole, a very unstable way of making a living. As both an aromatherapist and an actor, I can see how well these two professions may unite.

On the one hand, I work with a body of actors who are well aware of the stresses of their work, and on the other I am a therapist who is aware of how to help. In dealing with mainly emotionally based problems, a gentle complementary medicine like aromatherapy is preferable to the stronger measures of allopathic medicine.

After completing part of my aromatology course with Shirley Price, I moved to The Crucible Theatre in Sheffield to begin work on a new play. It seemed an ideal time to carry out a study of the level of health and stress in the acting world, and the ways in which aromatherapy could help.

What is Health?

Total health is not merely absence of symptoms, but also includes feeling physically well, being self-reliant, having the ability to adjust to change, having a sense of responsibility for yourself, developing an insight into your own feelings and actions, and cultivating a degree of self-worth which can stand on its own without the good opinion of others.

What is Anxiety and Stress?

Anxiety is fear of the unknown. When we are afraid or excited, there are chemical changes in our bodies that increase the energy levels and enable us to respond to the danger or stress, such as working spontaneously and freely in rehearsals or running for a bus.

The sympathetic division of our autonomic nervous system is responsible for our body's prompt reaction. It prepares us for physical activity by stimulating the heart rate, blood-pressure, breathing, and perspiration. It is also responsible for releasing glucose from the liver for energy, stimulating mental activity, and inhibiting digestion. This system is referred to as the "fight or flight" system because, as it increases the physical activity of the body, it prepares the person either to stand and face a threat or leave as quickly as possible!

The trouble starts, however, if we cannot switch off the extra energy when it is no longer needed. This is when the parasympathetic division of the autonomic nervous system should "kick in," after the crisis is over. This system stimulates vegetative activities such as digestion, defecation, and urination. At the same time, it slows down the heart rate and respiration. When there is anxiety the body fails to adjust, and we feel "wound up." It would be like leaving the car engine running twenty-four hours when you only need it for two short trips. In the same way as the petrol is wasted and runs out, our energy is wasted, our nervous system depleted, and we eventually become ill.

Stress is anxiety and anything else that disturbs the normal balance of mental and physical health, causing us to "keep the car running."

Acting

Anxiety is part of the life of all human beings, and performing artists suffer more than their fair share of it. Many anxiety-producing factors converge to make performance one of the more stressful occupations: the competitiveness of the field, the desire to give a "perfect" performance, being under close critical observation by audience and critics, and the need to have complete control over the very psychobiological processes that are most impaired by anxiety (muscular coordination, concentration, and memory).
—From "Anxiety and How to Control it"—a paper by P. Lehrer

A career in acting is accompanied by many stressful circumstances from both internal and external influences. Throughout a career, often many times a day, an actor may experience insecurity, feelings of worthlessness, and performance nerves. These emotional strains are often pushed to their limits by constant rejection, tough competition, and public criticism. Living away from home, actors may be prone to loneliness and homesickness, and must cope with the strains of maintaining long-distance relationships. Relationships with other actors, directors, and stage technicians can become strained and a career in acting requires patience and a sense of humor. Such factors, combined with long hours of physical work leave many actors in a state of emotional and physical exhaustion. Perhaps even more troubling to the actor are the periods of "resting" and almost every actor can count on an unstable salary.

After that depressing description, you may wonder why anyone decides to carve themselves a career in acting! There are, of course, many wonderful and fulfiling sides, particularly on a creative level. I am listing the drawbacks so that you can see what a demand there is for a helping hand.

The aim of my study was to find out the best, simplest, and most practical ways that aromatherapy can be useful to an actor. I have also listed some less expensive alternatives to some of the exotic oils, so as to make them more affordable for the poorly paid actor at the end of this article!

I began my study by distributing sheets of paper to the volunteers, which listed questions about their current state of health, medical history, how they coped with stress, etc. I knew this part would not be a problem, as actors generally love to talk about themselves!

Once the questionnaires were answered and gathered, I began mixing appropriate oils and creams at night, and the next morning distributing them before rehearsals with brief instructions on how to apply them. The results slowly filtered back to me over the next eight weeks. I was not able to do in-depth case histories, as there was insufficient time, but I am going to arrange my results under various headings.

> Ophelia: *There's rosemary, that's for rememberance;*
> *pray love, remember*
> *Hamlet,* William Shakespeare

Insomnia

The initial problem I discovered was that many of the actors had problems adapting to their new "home." Their sleep was disturbed by the pressure of learning lines and meeting a large company of new faces. One young actress found that her sleep was light, and she would wake up in the middle of the night with her arms stretched upwards toward the ceiling. She said her dreams were vivid and sometimes distressing. Under stress, this actress developed small patches of eczema. I mixed her a small bottle of four essential oils mixed in equal proportions:

Salvia sclarea (Clary Sage)—useful where muscular tension arises from mental or emotional stress—warming and relaxing in the bath; no alcohol to be taken with this, as the two together may create vivid dreaming.

Lavandula angustifolia (Lavender)—anti-inflammatory, anti-irritant—blends well with *Salvia sclarea* (Clary Sage)—sedative properties—calming, soothing, and may be used on delicate or sensitive skins.

Chamaemelum nobile (Roman Chamomile)—anti-inflammatory—excellent, gentle sedative.

Styrax benzoin (Benzoin)—sedative—warming to the body—delicious vanilla ice-cream odour!

She put 4 to 6 drops in her evening bath, then a few more drops on a handkerchief which she left on her pillow that night. The next day she informed me that the effect was instant. She knew she had slept deeply, as she woke up in the same position in which she had fallen asleep. She also felt very refreshed. She continued to use these oils in her bath for the next three weeks of rehearsal, to good effect. The eczema on her legs also reduced, but I cannot say if it was due to the oils or the slow lifting of pressure as the work progressed.

Another actress in her middle years also had difficulty sleeping. As the years have passed she has been finding it increasingly difficult to live away from home, particularly the feelings of guilt and sadness at leaving behind her husband. I mixed essential oils of *Salvia sclarea* and *Lavandula angustifolia* also, and again in equal proportions. These oils are a synergistic blend and have balancing properties. I asked her to use them in an evening bath and tell me what effect they had on her. She loved the smell, and found they had a very relaxing effect on her mind and body just before going to bed, so she also felt very refreshed at the start of the day.

> Arkadina: *You're not looking after yourself, not taking any medicine. It's not right.*
>
> Sorin: *I'd be delighted to take medicines, but the doctor doesn't want to give me any.*
>
> Dorn: *Taking medicines at sixty!*
>
> Sorin: *Even at sixty you still want to go on living.*
>
> Dorn: *(Irritated) Huh! Well . . .take some valerian drops.*
>
> *The Seagull,* Anton Chekhov

Circulation

We were in Sheffield during a particularly cold spell, and because of its high location we were subject to much ground-freezing weather and snow. This highlighted a common problem, particularly among the women—poor circulation. Our rehearsal space was an enormous, linoleum-floored room with adequate heating, but as many hours of the day were spent sitting, concentrating, and being attentive and still, those with sluggish circulation quickly began to feel the cold.

For two actresses I mixed 15 drops of Shirley Price Aromatherapy circulation mix into 30 ml. white lotion. The oils in the mixture are *Piper nigrum* (Black Pepper), *Juniperus communis* (Juniper), *Rosmarinus officinalis* (Rosemary), and *Styrax benzoin* (Benzoin).

The first three oils have rubefacient qualities, and stimulate circulation locally in the area to which they are applied. They cause capillaries to widen, so a greater volume of blood can flow through them. *Rosmarinus officinalis* is a valuable stimulant where there is general sluggishness. *Juniperus communis* is a good tonic and diuretic. The fourth oil, *Styrax benzoin,* as well as being a fixative, has the ability to "melt away" blockages, so it helps warm and tone the heart and circulation.

Every morning, preferably after a bath, they would rub the lotion quite vigorously into their feet, calves, and thighs. One young actress rubbed this mix into her legs after her evening bath just before going to bed. She said that as well as having glowing warmth in her legs, she also had very energetic, vivid dreams. She didn't mind the dreams but changed to morning-time application, and her legs, hands, and feet stayed much warmer during the morning rehearsals, without the vivid dreaming at night, which may of course have been due to a different cause.

One older actress suffered from poor circulation as well as aching varicose veins and low blood pressure. Varicose veins can develop as a result of a poor circulatory system and, particularly in this example, through prolonged periods of standing. I mixed these oils into 30 ml. white lotion:

Cupressus sempervirens (Cypress)	5 drops
Citrus limon (Lemon)	6 drops
Thymus vulgaris (Sweet Thyme)	4 drops

I chose *Cupressus sempervirens* as it would help to strengthen the veins. Its qualities help to contract the capillaries. When massaging the cream lightly into her legs she was to apply it above the affected area of the vein and not below it (the foot end) as it would only increase the pressure in the vein. *Citrus limon* has a tonic effect on the circulatory system. *Thymus vulgaris* helps circulation, raises low blood pressure, revives body and mind, and is reputed to stimulate the brain and improve the memory. This actress admitted to becoming slower at learning her lines, so I thought this last oil would be helpful. (I also gave her *Rosmarinus officinalis* on a handkerchief to smell throughout the working day.) She found her lotion very stimulating and refreshing. There was no immediate improvement with her varicose veins, but the aching feeling seemed to subside a little. The *Rosmarinus officinalis* cleared her head and made her feel much sharper.

Maximize the Placebo Effect!

There is great comfort to be found from taking care and indulging yourself a little with creams, bath oils, and aromatic delights, particularly when living away from home. As well as the good effect of the oils, there is also the psychological one. After all, the healing process must involve the power of the mind. If there is confidence and faith in a certain type of medicine, it is even more likely to work. The placebo effect will change the body chemistry.

I always hand over the oils promoting their natural healing qualities and beautiful aromas, and the clients look forward to using them. They know the oils will benefit them, and the result is that they do. So essential oils and human psychology are a wonderful synergistic blend as well!

> *Yet marked I where the bolt of Cupid fell,*
> *It fell upon a little Western flower,*
> *Before milk-white, now purple with love's wound:*
> *And maidens call it "love-in-idleness"*
> *Fetch me that flower; the herb I show'd thee once.*
> *The juice of it on sleeping eyelids laid,*
> *will make or man or woman madly dote*
> *upon the next live creature that it sees.*
> *A Midsummer Night's Dream*, William Shakespeare

Headaches

Four members of the company suffered from regular headaches. There are many reasons for headaches: everyone was under some sort of pressure; one had inherited migraine and had too much red meat and wine in his diet; another was constantly playing the loud, quick-witted entertainer, and his way of coping with pressure was to behave in an even more extroverted fashion until he ended up with what he called "a corker"; another was completely the opposite—she found it hard to express her frustrations and would become quieter and quieter while the pressure in her head became stronger and stronger. Everyone in the company had the added pressure of performing perfectly to a large crowd every night.

I looked in several aromatherapy books, and out of the great range of analgesic oils, those which seem to be most effective are *Lavandula angustifolia* and *Mentha x piperita.*

> Lavender has the ability to enhance the action of other oils when it is used in blends. Lavender is a sedative, Peppermint a stimulant and many commercial headache remedies combine a stimulant with one or more analgesics. This is because many of the painkilling drugs have a slightly sedative and sometimes even a depressant effect, and the stimulant is included to counteract this. By using Lavender and Peppermint, a similar effect is produced without the dangers inherent in synthetic drugs.
>
> —From *Aromatherapy An A-Z*, by Patricia Davis

I mixed *Lavandula angustifolia* and *Mentha x piperita* equally, giving a separate bottle of *Rosmarinus officinalis* to two actors whose headaches stemmed particularly from mental stress. This oil helps to clear the head and relieve pain, especially if the headache follows a period of mental effort. I directed the four "sufferers" to rub the mixture, neat, onto the temples and forehead at the onset of a headache.

The results from two actors using *Lavandula angustifolia* and *Mentha x piperita* mix topically, and *Rosmarinus officinalis* on a handkerchief, were extremely positive. They came back to me a week later to say that each time they had applied the oil, the pain of the approaching headache had lifted. This happened every time they used the oil, and they excitedly decided to replace their usual remedy of aspirin with this mixture. The migraine sufferer only had mild headaches that the oil helped to clear, but no migraine during our time in Sheffield.

Nerves and Stage Fright

Can you imagine how appalling it must feel to walk from the safety and darkness of a backstage area into the glaring lights of a stage? To be surrounded by a large audience who have paid good money to be entertained? You may be sweating with fear but you must appear relaxed, responsible, and pretend that a thousand people are not looking at you—and God forbid that you should forget your lines! Your body can become flooded with adrenaline, and it can be the easiest thing to forget anything you ever rehearsed!

Acute stress may produce changes that affect the respiratory system. Breathing may become stiff and inexpressive.

> The most commonly used modern technique for treating the physiological components of anxiety is taking tranquilizers. Tranquilizers are by far the most commonly prescribed of all drugs. However, tranquilizing medication is difficult to regulate, and it often has undesirable side effects. Often it takes too much anxiety away, so that the performer no longer 'cares' enough to give a good performance. Alternatively, it may not be strong enough to block a panic attack. Also, if taken regularly, most tranquilizing medication is addictive, physically as well as psychologically. As we become less able to predict and control our emotions without the use of drugs, we become increasingly anxious and more drug-dependent.
>
> —From "Anxiety and How to Control It"—a paper by P. Lehrer

On the first-night performance, as audience and members of the press began to gather in the foyer, three members of the cast asked me if there were anything I could provide to help their nerves. I let them smell several oils and then choose an oil they thought might suit them for this purpose. One actress, whose nerves affected her stomach and bowels the most put a few drops of *Citrus aurantium amare flos* (Neroli) on her wrists. Another liked the comforting smell of *Cinnamomum zeylanicum* (Cinnamon leaf), so I put a burner in her dressing-room containing this oil, adding a little *Citrus bergamia* (Bergamot), as it is a fruity, comforting oil and good for anxiety. The last actor chose *Salvia sclarea*, so I dotted this oil onto his wrists so he could always have the aroma nearby.

They inhaled these different smells deeply during the nerve-wracking hours before the show. Deep breathing has a direct effect on the cardiovascular system and can produce, temporarily, a lesser state of panic. I suggested that they smile, too, as changing the pattern of facial muscle tension appears to have some effect in actually changing the emotions that people feel.

"Ladies and gentlemen of the 'Mansfield Park' company, this is your Act I beginners call"—words that can instill fear into the heart of even the most confident actor! We stand in the darkness backstage, ready to begin.

At the end of the play, actors dash off stage in the most elated mood. Everything had gone well on this first night, and the piece had been received with much applause. The "Neroli" actress had found the oil very soothing at her weakest moments of nerves, and very settling on her stomach; the "Clary Sage" actor found his oil almost too much. He described it as "seeping into my head, making me feel . . ."

"Euphoric?"

"Yes! Euphoric. I felt rather too light-headed for my liking."

He had not felt quite as centered and in control as he would have liked, so we decided that drops on a handkerchief would be better if he wanted to use it again. The "Cinnamon/Bergamot" actress loved the relieving and nurturing quality of these oils. The Cinnamon leaf particularly reminded her of home and her mother's kitchen. The next day she bought her own burner and oil, sometimes exchanging the Cinnamon for Clove bud and Lemon oil. It made me realize that oils are very personal, and the same oils cannot always be applied to different people for the same conditions.

Overindulgence

It is a quite normal practice for actors to go out to a pub or restaurant at the end of a show and enjoy a large meal at midnight! This is fun and exciting once in a while, but some actors continue to do it on a regular basis. One actor described it as his way of relieving tension. If he was at all "wound up," he would eat and drink for comfort.

He regularly suffered discomfort in his liver and large intestine. He had constipation just as regularly, too. He told me that when he was a boarding-school boy he had trouble defecating. The communal toilets there had no locks on the doors, and he had always been fearful of someone bursting in on him. Even now, if he is working or on holiday, away from the comfort and privacy of his own bathroom, he may not go to the loo for two weeks.

This condition is a perfect result of anxiety. I let him choose from my collection of sedative oils. He liked the smells of *Citrus begamia* and *Cedrus atlantica* (Cedarwood), so I mixed them equally together and told him to put 4 to 6 drops in his evening bath to help relax him. Then for his indigestion, constipation, and liver I mixed:

Rosmarinus officinalis (Rosemary)	20 drops
Mentha x piperita (Peppermint)	15 drops
Cupressus sempervirens (Cypress)	10 drops
Citrus limon (Lemon)	15 drops
Juniperus communis (Juniper)	10 drops

I chose these oils because they all have hepatic qualities. *Rosmarinus officinalis* stimulates the production and flow of bile, and is a general liver tonic. *Mentha x piperita* benefits the liver and digestive system as a whole. *Cupressus sempervirens* and *Citrus limon* help a congested liver, and *Juniperus communis* aids detoxification.

I told the actor to prepare a warm compress, put 4 to 6 drops on it, and place it on the liver for relief. I advised him to drink Peppermint herb tea, which strengthens the liver and is calming on the stomach. I also showed him how to carry out an abdominal massage with the oils for constipation, and told him to make sure his fiber intake was high.

He found the bath oil very refreshing and relaxing, the five-oil mix on a warm compress very relieving to his liver, and the Peppermint tea calming and cleansing. After his bath he would carry out an abdominal massage; he claimed this was quite uncomfortable at first, as he felt blocked and bloated, but after a few days of self-massage the blocked feeling began to ease a little.

The result from this is that the oils provide temporary relief before he begins to indulge again. He is, at least, aware of his reasons from overeating, so it would be his choice to try and stop the cause of his indigestion.

This paper shows the result of my eight-week work with these actors. It is not the result of case histories concentrating on one problem for a long time, so the results are not complete. I hope to make an actor aware of the qualities of essential oils and their applications so that whatever remote part of the country they are in (or even working abroad), they will feel confident to be able to help themselves.

There is enormous fulfillment in suspending reality for an audience, being able to manipulate and entertain them. You can feel on top of the world when they respond exactly as you had wished, and the final applause at the curtain call provides instant gratification and recognition of your work. After a show an actor can feel the same elation and physical exhaustion as that of an athlete who has just completed a long-distance run. Being aware of your limits, your health and well-being, however, will help to create a happier, more relaxed self and perhaps an even better actor. I am sure that aromatherapy can go a long way to help achieve that.

> Oberon: *I know a bank where the wild thyme blows,*
> *Where oxlips and the nodding violet grows,*
> *Quite over, canopied with luscious woodbine,*
> *With sweet musk-roses, and with eglantine.*
> *There sleeps Titania sometime of the night*
> *Lull'd in these flowers with dances and delight.*
> *A Midsummer Night's Dream*, William Shakespeare

A List of Less Expensive Essential Oils and Suggested Alternatives to the More Expensive Ones.

Styrax benzoin—soothing and stimulating and three times less expensive than *Commiphora myrrha* (Myrrh) and four times less expensive than *Boswellia carterii* (Frankincense); for sedative qualities it is five times less expensive than *Rosa damascena* (Rose) and nine times less expensive than *Jasminum officinale* (Jasmine).

Melaleuca leucadendron (Cajeput)—less expensive than *Eugenia caryophyllata* (Clove bud) to dull the pain of toothache.

Cedrus atlantica (Cedarwood)—similar "masculine" odour and three times less expensive than *Santalum album* (Sandalwood).

Foeniculum vulgare (Fennel)—less toxic, from the same plant family and less expensive than *Pimpinella anisum* (Aniseed).

Lavandula angustifolia (Lavender)—stimulating the growth of healthy new cells it is eight times cheaper than *Citrus aurantium amara flos* (Neroli)—this oil is enhanced in action by being blended with other oils.

Citrus reticulata (Mandarin)—in calming intestine, is six times less expensive than *Citrus aurantium amara flos* (Neroli).

Citrus aurantium var. sinensis (Sweet Orange)—overlaps *Citrus aurantium amara flos* (Neroli) in many qualities—anti-depressant, sedative.

Pogostemon patchouli (Patchouli) in fungicidal qualities, treating skin conditions and cell regeneration, is nine times less expensive than *Citrus aurantium amara flos* (Neroli).

Mentha x piperita (Peppermint)—is two times cheaper than *Rosmarinus officinalis* (Rosemary); for "cephalic" qualities to help clear thinking is two times less expensive than *Ocimum basilicum* (Basil).

Citrus aurantium var. amara fol. (Petitgrain)—resembles *Citrus aurantium amara flos* (Neroli), although less sedative—and is nine times less expensive.

Rosmarinus officinalis (Rosemary)—for clearing the head and mental fatigue, is a less expensive alternative to *Ocimum basilicum* (Basil).

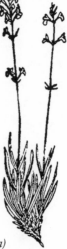

Lavender *(Lavandula angustifolia)*

Use of Oils for an Actor

Problem	Oils
Headaches	*Lavandula angustifolia* *Mentha x piperita* *Rosmarinus officinalis*
Insomnia	*Lavandula angustifolia* *Salvia sclarea* *Chamamælum nobile* *Styrax tonkinensis*
Long, tiring car journeys	*Ocimum basilicum* *Mentha x piperita* *Rosmarinus officinalis* *Pelargonium graveolens* (Geranium)
Nervous tension (women)	*Citrus bergamia* *Chamamælum nobile* *Pelargonium graveolens* *Rosa damascena*
Nervous tension (men)	*Citrus bergamia* *Cupressus sempervirens* *Lavandula angustifolia* *Cedrus atlantica*
Poor concentration (weak memory)	*Ocimum basilicum* *Mentha x piperita* *Rosmarinus officinalis*
Loss of voice	*Cupressus sempervirens* *Lavandula angustifolia* *Citrus limon* *Thymus vulgaris* *Cinnamomum zeylanicum*
Bad breath (stage kissing!)	*Mentha x piperita* *Rosmarinus officinalis*
Performance stress	*Citrus bergamia* *Coriandrum sativum* (Coriander) *Citrus aurantium fol.* *Rosmarinus officinalis* *Citrus limon* *Zingiber officinale* (Ginger) *Citrus paradisi* (Grapefruit) *Styrax tonkinensis* *Rosa damascena* *Salvia sclarea*

26

Doctor Predicts Human Eggplant . . . But Essential Oils Save the Day!!

Sheryll Ryan

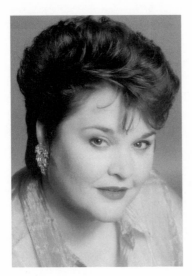

Sheryll Ryan is a recovered computer engineer who used aromatherapy to maintain a modicum of sanity while dealing with corporate America. During her mad-scientist phase, she read every book that she could obtain, took classes from Kurt Schnaubelt, Jeanne Rose, Michael Scholes, and every aromatherapist she could find in the Texas area. All friends and family and a few hapless strangers were pressed into service as guinea pigs for testing her blends.

In 1993, she began teaching introductory and advanced classes, and has recently begun consulting for several large companies in the health and beauty industry. Sheryll is the District Director of the West Region of NAHA.

everal months ago a friend was in an auto accident from which she should have emerged bruised to the color of a very ripe eggplant—or so the doctor predicted. She was not wearing a seatbelt, and her BMW was totaled, sent to an untimely burial at the local junkyard. The story has a happy ending, however, because she now has a shiny new Beemer and a pretty incredible recovery to boot.

I was with Diane in the emergency room, and was witness to the doctor's assessment: massive bruising, lots of pain, and a need for mass quantities of ibuprofen. The emergency room bill for $600 was probably the worst of the pain! Her two roommates and I took her home, put her to bed, and adjusted our wings (ministering angels, you know . . . wings always need adjusting).

I carefully hid all Advil, and instead made an anti-inflammatory and relaxing blend of Lavender *(Lavandula angustifolia)*, Everlasting *(Helichrysum italicum)* and German Chamomile *(Matricaria recutita)*. A high concentration of Lavender in the blend served as a carrier, rather than a fatty oil, to allow for maximum penetration into the skin. German Chamomile was chosen for its high bisabolol content, which is known to reduce inflammation.

A second blend of Hyssop *(Hyssopus officinalis)*, Spike Lavender *(Lavandula latifolia)* and Marjoram *(Origanum majorana)* was alternated with the first blend to reduce bruising. Because Everlasting and Hyssop are considered somewhat toxic, care was taken to use small doses of these oils. Some of the literature suggests that Everlasting is more effective in small doses and, a "less is more" approach is advocated.

Every four hours, approximately ten minutes apart, we applied each blend, over Diane's left side, covering every area that appeared to have hit the side of the car. She would then fall back to sleep until the effect of the oils wore off and the pain intensified. During the next two days she took no aspirin or ibuprofen, and experienced pain only occasionally. Within seventy-two hours she was out of bed, and being driven to appointments. Remarkably, she had no bruises!

Five days after the accident, Diane led a women's retreat, fully participating, able to dance and exercise. The only eggplant to be seen was the one in the vegetarian casserole. Despite the dire predictions of massive bruising, Diane had no bruises. She eventually experienced some stiffness and soreness internally, primarily because she stopped using the blends, believing herself to be back to normal. She has since seen the light and now carries an aromatherapy travel kit and stocks her medicine cabinet with essential oils and herbals.

27

Aromatherapy Institute Case Studies

Maria Dolores Gonzalez

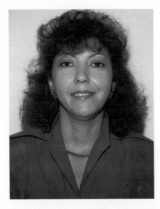

Maria Dolores Gonzales is an aromatherapist, licensed aesthetician and founder of the Aromatherapy Institute in Dallas.

A native of Spain, she became an aromatherapist while living in England, and trained under world-renowned aromatherapist Shirley Price. She did post-graduate studies under Professor Pierre Franchomme of France, an advanced researcher on medical aromatherapy, Kurt Schnaubelt of California, and Martin Watt of England. She is an accomplished aesthetician trained in Spain, with over eighteen years of experience.

Maria Dolores founded the Aromatherapy Institute of Dallas in 1991, upon returning to the United States. In addition to her practice, she has developed her own product line, and has created a series of aromatherapy training and educational courses ranging from introductory to technically advanced classes for the professional. Through her institute she also provides workshops, presentations and lectures on a regular basis.

The following pages present two case histories of clients whose conditions responded favorably with the application of essential oils.

Asphyxiated Skin, Broken Capillaries, Stress

Case History Number 1: Kareen

Age: 45

Complaint: Asphyxiated skin, broken capillaries (couperose), stress

Oils: Roman Chamomile *(Chamamælum nobile)*

German Chamomile *(Matricaria recutita)*

Cypress *(Cupressus sempervirens)*

Bergamot *(Citrus bergamia F.C.F.)*

Everlasting *(Helichrysum italicum)*

HO *(Cinnamomum camphora)*

Lavender *(Lavandula angustifolia)*

Petitgrain *(Citrus aurantium* var. *amara)*

*K*areen is forty-five years old, owner of a marketing company, married, and the mother of two children, ages eleven and fourteen.

An examination of her face and neck revealed an inflammation of the skin, with small red bumps underneath the surface, similar to grains of sand to the touch. Broken capillaries were predominant on her cheeks and both sides of her face. Redness and sensitivity aggravated the situation, and her forehead was extremely dry.

Her diet is healthy and leans to the vegetarian side. According to Kareen, her skin problem started a year earlier when she got some sort of parasite after returning from her holiday.

The demands of her job and family responsibilities resulted in stress and depression, which was evident in the appearance of her skin.

Kareen was also suffering from constipation, and I suspected a correlation between that complaint and the condition of her face and neck. She was already undergoing homeopathic treatment for a clogged ileocecal valve.

I initially gave Kareen a weekly treatment using both Cypress and Roman Chamomile oils with water, in compresses. The Cypress oil was used to strengthen the capillary walls, and the Roman Chamomile to reduce inflammation and redness. A soft lymph drainage massage was performed with German Chamomile for its anti-inflammatory and bactericidal effect. A Calendula and St. John's Wort carrier oil was used.

For home treatment, I suggested a skin-care program I prepared especially for her case. The treatment consisted of a light cream cleanser with Roman Chamomile and Lavender, which is antiseptic and cytophylactic. A skin freshener made with floral water of Rose and Lavender, and a light aqueous cream moisturizer with essential oils of Cypress and Roman Chamomile, completed the home treatment.

To address her stress and depression symptoms, I made an aqueous light cream, adding Bergamot oil for its balancing effects and to help rebuild strength and self-confidence. HO oil *(Cinnamomum camphora* from China) was added for its calming effects on the nervous system, and Petitgrain *(Citrus aurantium)* served to relieve stress and depression. I instructed Kareen to use this preparation twice a day, by first inhaling its aroma and then applying the lotion to the back of her neck, shoulders, and feet.

Kareen came for treatment every week during the first month, then treatment was reduced to every other week during the second and third month. For each session, I alternated the oils I used during the initial treatment and added Everlasting, a cicatrizant, and Lavender for its antiseptic and cytophylactic effects.

Kareen reported a remarkable improvement in her skin within the first three days of the initial treatment, and her skin was less sensitive and inflamed after each session. With the continued use of the stress-relief blend, Kareen reported feeling more relaxed and calm when performing her job.

Kareen's skin continues to improve. Her skin is no longer asphyxiated, and the red bumps underneath the surface of the skin have dissolved. The inflammation is gone, capillaries are less noticeable, and the redness on the face and neck has decreased considerably.

Infertility, Insomnia, and Depression

Case History Number 2: Jaci

Age: 42
Complaint: Infertility, insomnia, depression
Oils: Basil *(Ocimum basilicum)*
              Clary Sage *(Salvia sclarea)*

Juniper *(Juniperus communis)*
Neroli *(Citrus aurantium amara flos)*
Peppermint *(Mentha x piperita)*
Rose Otto *(Rosa damascena)*
Sandalwood *(Santalum album)*
Rosewood *(Aniba rosaeodora)*
Ylang-Ylang extra *(Cananga odorata)*

Jaci came to me as a result of a gift certificate because a friend thought aromatherapy could help her.

She was extremely depressed and experiencing insomnia, and was going through the extremely emotional experience of attending counseling in an attempt to work through past family issues.

She has a twelve-year-old daughter from a previous marriage, and no children with her second husband, even though they had been trying to conceive for the past five years without success.

A reflexology treatment showed areas of tenderness relating to the adrenals, pituitary, solar plexus, and ovaries. I used Rose Otto in her first session for her psychological pain and to strengthen her inner being. I added Neroli to counteract adrenal exhaustion and relieve stress and depression. In addition, I included a small amount of Clary Sage for its euphoric, relaxing, and sedative effects on the nervous system. The essential oils were added to a vegetable oil base and applied for a body massage.

Jaci felt more relaxed after this initial treatment, and asked what she could do at home to experience the relaxation and sense of well-being that she felt after the treatment. I suggested a bath therapy with Bergamot and Geranium. Her daily bath included four drops of Bergamot and six drops of Geranium.

Jaci came for another treatment three months later. She reported that after her previous session she felt better, slept better, and felt more uplifted and in control of herself.

For this second session I used Rosewood, a tonic and stimulant useful for depression; Basil for mental fatigue and as a general tonic; and Juniper to promote clearing of the body and spirit. I blended the oils in a carrier made of Jojoba and Calendula.

I added a body cream blend with Rose Otto and Neroli as part of her daily home treatment.

Jaci continued coming for regular aromatherapy treatments. She reported that she felt more confident in herself, her depression was subsiding, and that she could handle her counseling sessions with greater strength.

She came for a treatment just before having one of her counseling sessions in which she planned to face some of her relatives. I used Ylang-Ylang to help her overcome anxiety, anger, and fears, and Sandalwood to soothe a nervous cough. I later learned from Jaci that the counseling session she had prepared for went very well. She felt more in control of her emotions, did not feel the need to cry, and throughout the session she felt relieved and content.

The combination of Ylang-Ylang and Sandalwood was one of Jaci's favorite blends, and therefore became part of her daily home treatment. A blend of six drops of Ylang-Ylang and nine drops of Sandalwood per ounce of vegetable oil was applied daily on her back, lower abdomen, and the bottoms of her feet.

Jaci's condition has improved tremendously since the initial aromatherapy treatment. Aromatherapy has helped her to relax and be herself. Seven months after her initial treatment, Jaci announced with great happiness that she had just learned she was pregnant, and I was the first to know! When she consulted her doctor and mentioned the aromatherapy treatment, her doctor agreed that finding a way to relax the body and mind gave nature an opportunity to do the rest.

I continued to see Jaci throughout her pregnancy. Peppermint oil *(Mentha x piperita)* was suggested by inhalation for her first-trimester nausea (morning sickness), which helped her tremendously. To avoid stretch marks after the third month of pregnancy, I prepared a cream blend with Jojoba, Calendula, Rose Otto, and Neroli to be massaged into her belly.

The big day was approaching. To help her through labor, I used Rose Otto and Clary Sage in an oil base, applied on the lower abdomen and back. I also suggested inhalation of Lavender oil to keep her calm and relaxed. Jaci had a healthy baby boy through a Cæsarean section. She said that using the oils helped her to recover quickly, and she did not retain any stretch marks. Her little boy is now two years old and has been an aromatherapy baby since birth.

28

Memory Loss and Alzheimer's Disease

Deanna Wolf

Deanna Wolf, Texas Regional director for NAHA, has been involved in aromatherapy for the last 4 years. Deanna's interest in aromatherapy began as she sought a natural approach to her daughter's medical problems. Essential oils have helped her daughter's OCD and surgical scars, and other family member's conditions.

Although her college work was in data processing, Deanna is constantly studying plants and their many uses with teachers such as Jeanne Rose, Michael Scholes, Marcel LaVabre, and Kate Damian.

Troy, Texas is home to Deanna and her family, where she continues spread word about benefits and educational aspects of aromatherapy. In Troy she is known fondly as "The Oil Lady," especially by the young ones.

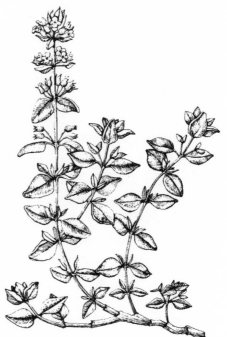

Thyme *(Thymus vulgaris)*

Condition

An eighty-six year old female presented with signs of forgetfulness, continuously repeated conversation, and emphysema. She was otherwise in good health. She was taking Prozac for depression and Meclazine for side effects of Prozac. She moved into our home to live, off and on, from May to November. She was confused by the new home and surroundings.

Diagnosis

Signs of possible dementia or Alzheimer's.

Treatment

Essential oils of Rosemary *(Rosmarinus officinalis)*, Peppermint *(Mentha x piperita)*, Basil *(Ocimum basilicum)*, and Ginger *(Zingiber officinalis)* were used for memory. She had a preference for Basil and Rosemary. For breathing, essential oils of Eucalyptus *(Eucalyptus spp.)*, Pine (species not given), and Douglas Fir *(Pseudotsuga menziesii)* were used. Eucalyptus and Pine were favorites. Herbal wreaths and pillows were used in her bedroom and around the house. Electric and candle diffusors were used. Her clothing was washed in the oils, and a Lavender wreath was hung above her bed to promote sound sleep.

Her diet was supplemented with vitamin B-12. Gingko biloba was added to her morning juice, and fresh herbs were used as much as possible in cooking.

Respect for her as an elderly and dignified person was shown. The family stressed that it was not shameful for her to be confused, and that her happiness was most important. She was encouraged to help with chores, and with conversations of the past and present. Her opinions were sought on different matters. Trips to the grocery store and walks with pets were favorite pastimes.

Results

By September she repeated herself less often, and remembered where her bedroom and clothing were to be found. Members of the family remarked that she seemed content and less confused. Neighbors noticed a difference in her behavior. Each week she showed progress. She soon began to ask for the oils, and want to make sure that they were nearby. Her frustration level diminished, since she was less confused. She helped the children with their homework, and was jubilant when she was correct.

In November, a fire destroyed my husband's business, which forced me to work outside the home. Since we could no longer care for her, her children had her committed to a nursing home, where they encourage her to participate in activities. Her memory has lapsed since then. The doctors have taken her off the medications.

At Christmas she knew which packages were ours because of the scent. She remembered using the oils, and was able to identify them. Memories of her time with us was acknowledged.

Editor's Notes About Alzheimer's Disease

Known as the "disease of the century," Alzheimer's disease is considered an irreversible and progressive disease of the brain, and may affect up to two million Americans. The risk of developing Alzheimer's increases with age, and is the most common cause of mental deterioration late in life. As life expectancy continues to increase, an epidemic of Alzheimer's is a serious possibility. The cause is unknown, and no cure currently exists.

The process of gradual mental deterioration due to structural deterioration of the brain (dementia), of Alzheimer's disease is traumatic, not only for the victim, but also for family and friends, leading Alzheimer's to be called the worst of all diseases. The only definitive diagnosis is determined through examination of brain tissue during autopsy. Initial symptoms of the disease are subtle and vary with individuals. Memory impairment is one of the earliest symptoms and may later be accompanied by symptoms such as aphasia (language impairment) and apraxia (impairment in motor abilities), and personality change. Progression of these symptoms is a distinguishing characteristic of Alzheimer's. In advanced stages of the disease, the victim becomes nonverbal, unable to move, unable to perform any normal daily activities. Stiffening of muscles to the degree that the patient is bent into the fetal position and impaired swallowing, seizures or muscle jerks are also possible in advanced stages. Ultimately, the patient may live from months to years totally dependent on others for all aspects of daily care. Total duration of symptoms from onset to death vary with individual, the average duration being recorded as approximately nine years.

Treatment focuses on addressing potentially treatable symptoms such as insomnia, restlessness, and depression. Involvement in support groups, family support, and counseling are considered important variables in treatment.

Source of Information: *The Alzheimer's Caregiver: Strategies for Support* Edited by Kathleen O'Connor and Joyce Prothero. Seattle: University of Washington Press, 1987.

29

Parkinson's Disease Project

Is Aromatherapy an Effective Treatment for Parkinson's Disease?

Shirley Price

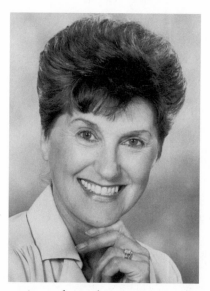

Shirley Price always had a keen interest in natural therapies sparked initially by her father, who was a strong believer in natural healing. She taught primary school, then trained as a beauty therapist and ran a successful health-and-beauty salon for nearly twenty years. She studied aromatherapy, reflexology, orthobionomy, shiatsu, and Touch for Health. With her husband, Len, she began to construct a specialized massage technique using lymphatic drainage methods that were not widely taught at the time.

She founded the Shirley Price International College of Aromatherapy in England in 1979, and has become what is believed to be the biggest school in the world, with about two-thirds of trainees from the nursing profession. She has written five books, the latest of which is *Aromatherapy for Health Professionals*.

$\mathcal{M}$y view that aromatherapy could help to improve the quality of life of a Parkinson's Disease sufferer was shared by several therapists with Parkinson's Disease clients who had shown improvements in movement ability and reduction of side effects such as insomnia and constipation after use of essential oils.

I have a very dear friend with Parkinson's Disease, and offered him complimentary treatments, but sadly he and his wife did not want to try them because they felt such treatments would not help. I have never been one to be discouraged, and I wanted to prove that my suggestions would help, in the hope that my friend would accept treatment. Actually, I have to thank him for not wanting me to help him, as the resulting research has helped many people overall.

I decided to ask in my newsletter, *AromaNews,* if there were any therapists who would be willing to give their time to my Parkinson's Disease Project free of charge—to give an hour's treatment eighteen times over a period of nine months—if I donated the oils for the treatment and for home use by the client. The response was wonderful, and soon we had twenty therapists and twenty Parkinson's Disease sufferers beginning Project Number One. We set up three separate Parkinson's Disease trials within our overall project (each with twenty people) and the results of all three follow.

Pre-requisite conditions for those participating:
(a) permission from their doctor to take part
(b) willingness to perform home treatments

Nature of Part One of Project

Stage One: Each volunteer was given a body massage once a week for twelve weeks, by one of our trained volunteer aromatherapists. Each client, or their caretaker, also applied a lotion containing essential oils daily for three months, and was given the same blend of essential oils to use in the bath once or twice a week. Weekly reports were kept by both client and therapist, followed by a summary.

Stage Two: Each client received a massage once a month for six months, and applied the lotion every other day. This change of routine was undertaken to establish whether the lower number of treatments and applications sustained any improvement shown in the first three months.

Essential Oils Used for Stages One and Two

Salvia sclarea (Clary Sage): relaxant, nerve tonic, antispasmodic. To relieve stress, and for general relaxation.

Origanum majorana (Sweet Marjoram): relaxant, nerve tonic, analgesic, antispasmodic. To relax muscles (relieving any pain) and reduce anxiety and insomnia. Also a good digestive oil.

Lavandula angustifolia (Lavender): relaxant, analgesic, antispasmodic. To relax muscles (relieving any pain) and relieve anxiety and insomnia.

The essential oils were used in equal proportions in a 1/2 percent dilution (i.e., 10 drops of each in 100 ml. of carrier). 6–8 drops undiluted oils were used in the bath.

Project One Report

Of twenty clients, only ten actually completed the entire nine month schedule. One stopped after three months of weekly treatment because there was no improvement in the general symptoms, including lack of use of left-hand side, and speech problems in times of stress. However, this woman admitted to sleeping better and having fewer leg cramps during the three months of treatment, so something was apparently gained.

One client transfered to our Phase Two trial; one, unfortunately, passed away two weeks after commencing the project. Two had hospital visits that broke the routine, and the rest had to drop out after two or three weeks either because they or the caretaker could not apply the lotion every day or they could not manage the strict routine.

The ten people who completed the project were on varying strengths of medication with several different brands of tablets: Sinemet [6], Selegiline [5], Madopar [4] (two of these four were on a weaker Madopar as well), Eldepryl [4], Artane [2], Revanil [1], Disipal [1], and Amantadine [1].

Some individuals were taking the following to cope with side effects: Amitriptyline (depression), Cemmetrol (unknown), Clonazepam (epilepsy), Motilium (nausea), Bromocriptine (dry mouth), Capoten (hypertension), Allopurinol (gout), Propanodol (high blood pressure) and Dothepin (depression).

Symptoms presented by more than one person: Body tremors [7], face tremors [3]; slurred speech [5]; stiffness [5]; difficulty walking, inability to stop shuffling [4]; muscle or joint pain or cramp [4]; low energy [3]; poor balance [3]; sleeping difficulties [3]; lack of limb control [3]; falling [3]; weakness in limbs [2]; hypertension [2]; loss of memory [2]; speech problems [2]; anxiety [2]; immobility, rigidity [2].

Singly presented symptoms: depression; loss of smell, sight, and hearing.

Side effects presented by more than one person: insomnia [4]; constipation [4]; headaches [2]; dry mouth [2].

Singly presented side effects: nausea, nightmare, difficulty in swallowing, memory loss, bad taste in mouth.

Stage One
(twelve weekly treatments and twice daily application)

Improved muscle strength, more active [5] (one can now use Hoover again); improved sleep [5] (one without serious problem said sleep improved); reduced pain [4]; improved energy [3]; less constipated [3]; improved mental attitude [2]; improved speech [2]; reduced anxiety [2]; diminished tremors [2]; no headaches [1]; improved circulation [1].

Stage Two
(six monthly treatments and applications every other day)

- Seven maintained improvements and generally felt more energetic (one still became depressed, and one slowed down in improvement during the first two weeks but recovered after that);
- One slightly deteriorated during first month, but still felt better than before treatment commenced, effects lasting on average four to six days;
- One had slight lessening of improvements—therapist feels once weekly needed—client says he feels no worse and that the overall result is positive;
- One improved for two to three days only after each aromatherapy treatment—client would like twice weekly treatment. However, overall shaking diminished.

Summary

Overall, massage and essential oils have helped movement in most participants and the side effects of constipation and insomnia were reduced in all who presented them, two coming off their medication for this and one having no more nightmares. Only two seemed not to maintain their improvement on one treatment a month, and would perhaps have been best left on a weekly or fortnightly treatment.

I am only an amateur regarding the procedure of setting up a project for research purposes, and have since met Dr. David Stretch, an expert in the field, who is very interested in the Parkinson's Disease Project. I am currently working with

Symptoms Presented and *Side Effects*	A	B	C
Tremors, body	7	4	3
Tremors, face	3	1	–
Slurred speech	5	2	2
Stiffness	5	5	5
Shuffling, unable to stop	4	3	2
Immobility—rigidity	2	2	2
Falling	3	–	–
Low energy	3	3	3
Poor balance	3	3	2
Muscle/joint pain	4	4	4
Weakness in limbs	2	2	2
Anxiety	2	2	2
Depression	2	1	1
Loss of memory	2	N	
Loss of smell	1	N	
Sight and hearing loss	1	N	
Insomnia	4	5**	5
Nightmares	1	1	1
Constipation	4	3***	3
Headaches	2	1	1
Poor circulation	2	1	1
Dry mouth	2	N	
Nausea	1	N	
Difficulty to swallow	1	N	
Bad taste in mouth	1	N	

Key

A Number of presenting symptoms and side effects at commencement of treatment.

B Number of patients showing improvement after 12 weekly treatments and twice-daily home use.

C Number of patients maintaining improvement after 6 monthly treatments and once-daily home use.

N = No record of end result

** = One said sleep improved

*** = One did not record result

Dr. Stretch to design a trial on the exact lines required for research to be acceptable by the scientific community.

I would like to thank all the therapists and Parkinson's Disease sufferers who took part in this stage of the project, which shows an overall improvement rate of eighty percent at the completion of the project and an improvement result of ninety percent during Stage One. A few of these, of course, could be a placebo effect. However, this would still leave an improvement rate of approximately fifty percent, and the results so far have been well worth it from the perspective of the researchers and those who have benefited.

Project Two Report

The aim of Part Two was to ascertain whether the use of essential oils at home (without massage by a therapist) would provide any benefits to sufferers of Parkinson's Disease. Participants were given pure essential oils (as in Project One) to use in the bath once or twice a week, and the same oils in a lotion to be applied once a day. Although a lotion base was supplied to avoid getting oil on clothes, participants were given the choice of a vegetable oil base should they prefer it. Previous tests have shown there is no difference in effect when using straight vegetable oil, or emulsified vegetable oil and water, as a base for the essential oils. After three months the participants were asked to try the lotion every other day for a further six months to see if any improvements were maintained.

The objective was to provide a less expensive yet effective treatment for those who could not afford to have continuous aromatherapy massage treatments.

Twenty people began the project, but eight gave up because they could not keep up the regularity of treatment and recording of results.

Of the remaining twelve, one discontinued treatment after three months when she had a mastectomy, but her comments about those months included: balance much better; depression no longer a problem; increased self-confidence and positive outlook (which was noticed by her doctor).

Another, who experienced stress from the daily application and having to get oil off clothes (this person chose to have a vegetable oil base, unfortunately) gave up after three months of showing improvement. A third, who gave no specific comments other than "deriving benefit from it," had his medication changed in the fourth month, thus making future comments uncertain.

The nine people who completed the project were taking the following medication: Selegiline [7], Madopar [6], Artane [2], Sinemet [2], Prothiaden [1, for side

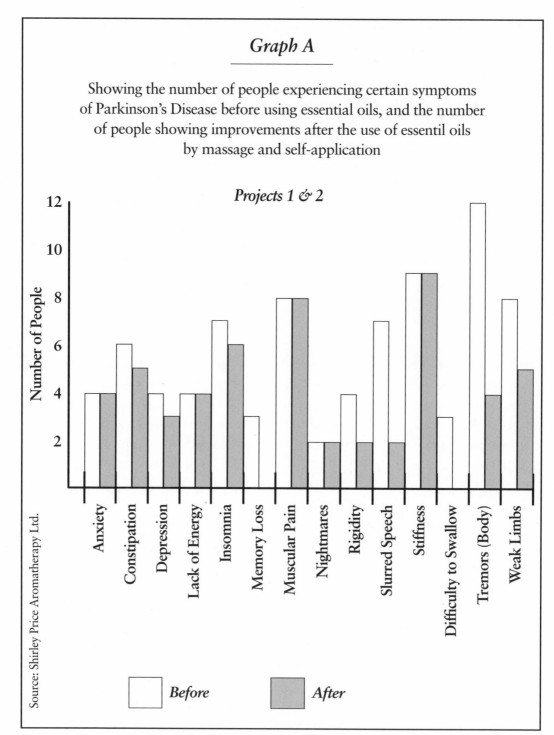

Graph A

Showing the number of people experiencing certain symptoms
of Parkinson's Disease before using essential oils, and the number
of people showing improvements after the use of essentil oils
by massage and self-application

Projects 1 & 2

Number of People

Anxiety • Constipation • Depression • Lack of Energy • Insomnia • Memory Loss • Muscular Pain • Nightmares • Rigidity • Slurred Speech • Stiffness • Difficulty to Swallow • Tremors (Body) • Weak Limbs

Source: Shirley Price Aromatherapy Ltd.

☐ *Before*   ▨ *After*

effects]. Some individuals were also taking medication for arthritis, high blood pressure, and heart problems.

Symptoms presented by more than one person: weakness in limbs [6], tremors [5], muscle and joint pain [4], stiffness [4], anxiety [2], constipation [2], cramp [2], depression [2], difficulty swallowing [2], insomnia [2], rigidity [2], slurred speech [2].

Singly presented symptoms: involuntary twitching, low energy, memory loss, nightmares, staggering, vertigo, weepiness.

Two participants felt better when applying lotion every day than on alternate days; there was no comment from the other seven.

The following areas showed improvement: muscle pain [4], stiffness [4], strengthened movement [3], anxiety [2], constipation [2], depression [2], tremors [2].

Singly presented improvements: nightmares, cramps, insomnia, involuntary twitching, low energy, staggering, weepiness.

The neurologist noticed the improvement of one participant, and suggested reducing his Artane and finally stopping the medication altogether.

Summary

Essential oils without professional massage appear to give relief in the same areas as those noticed in the project where professional massage with essential oils was given on a regular basis.

In Project Two, aching and stiffness, bizarre dreams, constipation, tension, twitching and weepiness were reduced in all presenting these symptoms.

- Two felt the improvement was limited.
- One with rigidity and balance problems walked better at first, but experienced no overall improvement.

The graph presents only those symptoms that were portrayed by clients in both Project One and Project Two.

Project Three Report

The aim of the third project was to ascertain if the massage with unscented oil were as beneficial to Parkinson's Disease sufferers as the massage using essential oils proved to be. It is extremely difficult to run a double-blind test in aromatherapy, as one can imagine, and unfortunately this necessitated being untruthful to the therapists. Therapists on Project Three queried the oil sent to them, because of its lack of aroma, and had to be told an untruth—that the essential oils were present in a very low concentration, in order to make a comparison with Project One, which used oils at normal concentration. Bland, unscented vegetable oils were used in exactly the same way as in Project One: twelve weeks of weekly massage, followed by six months of monthly massage, and application of the bland lotion or vegetable oil containing no essential oils at home daily.

Twelve people began the project, eight carrying it through to completion. Of the four who ceased, two had their routine broken by visits to hospital. Two did not continue to apply the oil at home, although one said that the treatments by the therapist had helped her to cope better, and that her joints felt looser; the other felt she had had fewer aches and pains this winter, so benefit was obviously gained from the massage.

The eight people finishing the project were taking the following medication between them: Madopar [6], Sinemet [4], Selegiline [3] Dizipal [1], Eldepryl [1]. Three were on medication for arthritis, kidneys, and muscular pain respectively and one was on no medication at all.

Symptoms presented: tremors [6], muscular pain [5], constipation [3], insomnia [3], low energy [3], rigidity [3], slow movement [3], slurred speech [3], cramps [2], stiffness [2], memory loss [1].

There did not appear to be sufficient difference in effect between weekly and monthly treatments; the general improvements, though not long-lasting, were in: muscular pain [3], insomnia [2], slow movement [2], stiffness [1], constipation [1], cramp [1], tremors [1].

Summary

Four people found the therapist treatment relaxing, and reported feeling better afterwards, although the effects were not lasting; two found the treatment relaxing, but felt no other noticeable change; two felt brighter in themselves and in their general health.

This project, without essential oils, was carried out to be a direct comparison with Project One, which included essential oils. Massage alone obviously presents improvements. However, as the graph shows, more permanent improvements were effected in Part One of the project, showing the value of the addition of essential oils.

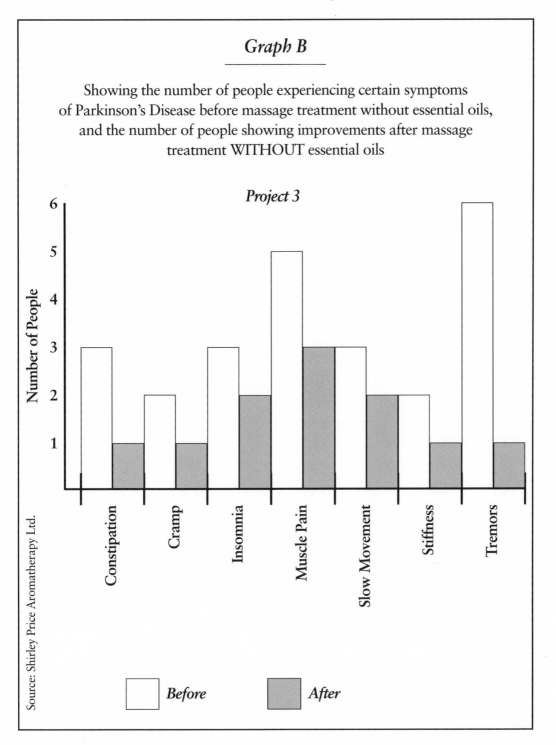

Graph B

Showing the number of people experiencing certain symptoms of Parkinson's Disease before massage treatment without essential oils, and the number of people showing improvements after massage treatment WITHOUT essential oils

Project 3

Source: Shirley Price Aromatherapy Ltd.

Before   *After*

Conclusions

1. Massage without essential oils, although beneficial on several points, scored the lowest in lasting effects. The use of essential oils, with or without massage, had almost equal benefits.
2. A perceived extra benefit of Part One (massage with essential oils) over Part Two (essential oils without massage) would probably be the complete relaxation of the body for the rest of that day, and possibly more than one day, and improved circulation, though this was not mentioned.
3. As Part Two gave similar results to Part One, the choice of the client rests on the cost. It would be worth asking the doctor if there were any chance of professional treatment being covered by the health plan. Possibly treatment once a fortnight may give similar results to once a week. It was found on the whole, however, that once a month was insufficient.

Cost of Treatment

The cost of private treatment by an aromatherapist varies from area to area and ranges from £15–30 for a treatment taking ninety minutes. For the initial consultation, add another twenty to forty minutes onto the time for the first visit, and oils that would still need to be used at home. The cost of essential oils to carry out the project completely at home works out at approximately £12 a month; perhaps £17 a month if a lotion base is chosen.

First published in *The Aromatherapist,* Vol.1, No.1., Shirley Price Aromatherapy Limited. Hinckley, England.

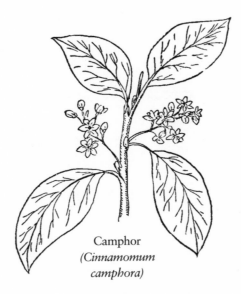

Camphor
*(Cinnamomum
camphora)*

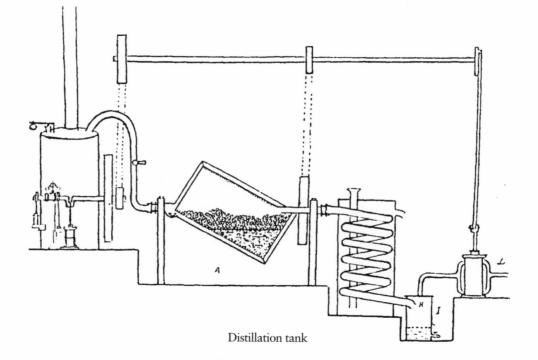

Distillation tank

VI

Business and Research

30

Bringing Credibility to the Aromatherapy Industry

Susan Earle interviews Marianne Griffeth

Marianne Griffeth

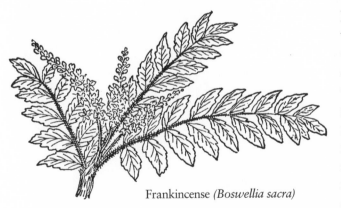

Frankincense *(Boswellia sacra)*

Before becoming involved with essential oils, *Marianne Griffeth* managed a sales organization in the gift industry. During that time, she gained extensive experience in marketing, sales, management, and product development while representing over fifty different manufacturing companies.

For the last seven years, she has gained a knowledge of the personal care industry while studying chemistry, herbalism, and aromatherapy. As president of Prima Fleur Botanicals, Inc., she is the chief formulator and product-development consultant. She lives in San Anselmo with her husband, Ron, her son, Brendan, and her new daughter, Gabrielle. Prima Fleur Botanicals is a family-owned and operated business.

*P*rima Fleur Botanicals is an essential-oil importer, wholesaler, and distributor as well as a product formulator and manufacturer. With a strong dedication to therapeutic quality and a commitment to client and consumer education, Prima Fleur and the woman behind the company, Marianne Griffeth, have not only increased consumer access to high-quality essential oils but have also changed the direction of the aromatherapy industry.

I have had the pleasure of working with Ms. Griffeth and this wonderful company, and was delighted that she could take some time to discuss her accomplishments and future goals, as well as her valuable experiences in the aromatherapy industry. (SE)

What is an essential oil wholesaler and distributor? What is their role and responsibility in aromatherapy?

Prima Fleur is a direct importer and distributor. We import almost all of our oils from distillers. Domestic oils such as peppermint and citrus oils are also purchased directly from producers. We supply our oils in bulk to manufacturers, therapists, and others who sell to retailers. In some cases we sell in bulk directly to retailers who have aromatherapy bars.

We established this company to fill a gap between European distillers of therapeutic-quality oils and the American market. Many of the existing American distributors catered to the fragrance and flavor industries. The few who specialized in high-quality oils also had their own retail lines, and selling essential oils in bulk was only a second endeavor.

When you began your business, your goal was to cater to this particular market of aromatherapy practitioners, or people who wanted to use quality essential oils in beauty care products, and to open the market for these high quality oils. In what ways has that goal changed?

Initially I thought we would be able to compete with the bigger companies that had been established here, and I found that the interest in therapeutic quality oils is smaller than I had hoped it would be. When we created a product, we found that the companies wanted to keep the cost of ingredients as low as possible, so that the money paid by the customer goes back to the company rather than for ingredients or packaging. Therefore, using cheaper low-grade or synthetic oils is preferable to many large companies.

Instead of focusing on larger, existing companies, we are now working with many new companies that are more open to the concepts of aromatherapy and the values that must follow. We have some really wonderful customers. Most of them are quite knowledgeable when it comes to essential oils and other botanical products. They serve an important function in educating the customers. Isn't it always the upstarts in any industry who initiate changes, bring creativity, and stimulate excitement? These are the pioneers.

Have you found, in creating this market, that you've had to do a lot of education?

This is one of our favorite services. We are constantly answering questions about the oils. People are so eager to learn. We also refer people to books and classes. I truly believe in giving people the whole picture, and as much as possible giving them the tools to sell their products. When they are confident and feel the passion that comes with the business, that is carried through to everything they do. The more you know of the truth, the more difficult it is to compromise. I know it's difficult to change profit margins, but the risk is a good one and has proven to be rewarding for those who have taken it.

I imagine it would be tempting to try and get something cheaper and of lesser quality, if that's what is in demand. How do you keep from supplying those oils as well, since that's what people seem to want?

In order to avoid this problem, we have accepted the fact that we need to work with slim profit margins. There are many factors we have to consider when pricing our oils, including the exchange rate, which is very unpredictable. Even though the exchange rates go up and down, we try to keep our prices very steady and reasonable, so they will be more attractive as raw materials competing with lower-grade oils and synthetics.

It's my choice to build a company that will flourish with the increased appreciation of quality. I often compare this industry to the wine industry in California. Originally, there were a few large companies that sold average wines. They were no competition for the European wines. Now, there is a proliferation of smaller, high-quality vintners who have created the market by educating and exposing their customers to better grades of wines.

I have been in business a long time. I know you have to define who you are, and stick to that. If you lose that direction, you neutralize your effect. It's hard not to compromise in this business. There is such a lure from the potential BIG customers who don't want to pay for quality. You can waste a lot of time with these people at least, it never works for me. It could work for them if they would take the chance and not compromise quality. We have one customer who gave us carte blanche to develop a line, and now they have the most beautiful, successful line of products. They can be proud of each ingredient. They came to us with a belief in quality, confidence in themselves, and respect for their customers.

Every time I am presented with the problem of not being able to satisfy a customer, I look at the oils that we have and think about the people who produce them, and it's impossible to abandon those principles. It's as if the oils are little people looking at me with hopeful faces, saying, "You've got to promote us. . . . You've got to get people to appreciate us." It's almost like a family.

The tremendous sincerity of our producers is another reason not to compromise. They know that there are a lot of people who adulterate oils, that the oils change hands three or four times, and in between they've lost control over the quality and what actually goes on in the market. When they find someone who really appreciates their quality, they are so excited. The United States market is golden to many foreign businesses. I'm always amazed at the enthusiasm of foreign producers when we tell them we want to import directly to the American market.

Our beautiful Roman Chamomile is produced by a fifth-generation farmer in Italy. When he sold to the French, they would label the oil as coming from France, and this marvelous producer and distiller became invisible. Until he sold to Prima Fleur, this Roman Chamomile was never recognized as coming from Italy. This producer was unable to experience the personal and national pride that comes from having a product on the international market that is considered to be of outstanding quality. The farmers and companies I'm working with have been producing quality for a long time, for the most part. They don't compromise, so why should I?

Have you ever had any trouble with a producer? Have you ever had to let go
of a producer because they weren't willing to maintain your standards?

I haven't had problems with producers. The only time I've ever had that problem was with another distributor. I've had to send things back twice in about three-and-a-half years. That's not a bad record, especially since we can't always go to the places we are buying from and actually see the product ourselves. We do have to try to get to know the people as much as possible, even if just by phone and fax. Beyond that, there's not much you can do. Most of the time what we get is the good quality we expect. We have developed some very special relationships with the producers we work with, because we both appreciate quality.

You have a special relationship with your producer in Madagascar. Can you talk about that?

I have a partner who is from Madagascar, and he helps facilitate the purchase of essential oils from Madagascar. Madagascar is an island-continent with a wealth of geological and cultural diversity. It has rainforests, deserts, and mountains.

The people of Madagascar have been trying to change their government from socialism to democracy. The transition has been peaceful but disruptive to the economy. By-passing the French distributors and selling directly to the U.S. market gives them a little extra profit, and the opportunity to learn more about business and industry here.

The chairman of the Bank of Madagascar and the ambassador to the U.S. have been very helpful in our work with Madagascar. We hope to build the demand for their exquisite oils, including the Ravensaras, Calophyllum, Ginger, and Geranium de Madagascar, which is an appellation given to a beautiful new Geranium that is now being produced with stalks from the Reunion Bourbon Geranium. It's a lovely, pale-green, soft, rose-scented Geranium.

We have a similar arrangement with producers of hydrosol in California. You hear many people talking about saving their rainforest, which is very important, but it's important to save our own environments as well. The Aromatic Plant Project was put together by Jeanne Rose to create native-grown hydrosols for the United States industry, and is producing marvelous, fresh, organic hydrosols while supporting the organic farming industry in California. These are produced under the trade-marked name of Organic · · California-Grown, California- Distilled®.

So far we've been able to offer Lavender, Rose Geranium, and Lemon Verbena. We are looking for the right clients to work with us to develop this industry. Next year we are producing over 3,000 gallons of California hydrosols. Jeanne is carefully selecting the producers, and helping them select the right plants to give us the best quality product. We're all learning a great deal in the process. It is truly an art to marry the best varieties of plants with the best geography, climate, and distiller.

It's obvious that you feel a lot of inspiration in working with these oils to benefit the producers, the industry, and the consumer. What are some of the rewards you've found for yourself?

I really enjoy working with businesses, especially new businesses, in developing products and concepts and helping them with marketing and even packaging. One of the most exciting areas of this business is taking something from the level of a producer who makes a great vegetable oil, like the *Calophyllum inophyllum* from Madagascar, that very few people in this country have ever heard of, and that even fewer use, showing it to someone and getting them excited about it. It's amazing to watch how the same oil used by the Malagasay becomes a product here. Through our creative efforts, a wonderful raw material becomes a product with a package. There is something so satisfying in selling a product that is "true." The beauty is in its performance.

The satisfaction comes from building a business where there is joy. Our business is never dull. It's quite stressful, but there is joy in what we do. We face some exciting challenges in manufacturing products with ingredients that aren't common. I'm from a family of artists, and I compare this to working with the most magnificent colors to create a painting. Creating a blend that's a symphony of scent, where each component is at its optimum, contributing the highest values it can achieve—that's a thrill.

It's the nature of our business to work with new projects all the time. The reward is in seeing someone take a risk, rise to the challenge, and succeed. We are in there too, trying to give them all those things they need to get there.

So you're not only serving as a distributor or manufacturer, but also as a consultant?

Along with providing high quality wholesale oils and ingredients, we also do formulation. If a company wants to create a line of products, they tell us what they want, and we create and manufacture the formulas. We also source and purchase the packaging. If a company wants to have a hand and body lotion, a bath salt, and a cream, we can develop a formula exclusively for them. A company may want an natural babycare line, or a spa may want an exclusive, high quality line of products sold under the spa's name. We work with them to decide what ingredients to use, based on their theme and identity, and use those ingredients to make a formula. We make a small batch of samples for the company to review, and choose a final formula. We give the client a price for the product that includes all aspects of the product design including creating the formula, putting the raw materials together, bottling, labeling, putting it in a box and shipping it to them.

We give a little bit more than other custom manufacturers because we also help with education. It's very important, when using high-quality natural raw materials, that the client, who will be selling the product knows how the ingredients act therapeutically, and is familiar with the background of the ingredients, because it helps develop a marketing approach. Our goal is always to help the client market the products. That helps us too. We want to see the products succeed.

Why is a CO_2 preferable in some cases to an essential oil? What is the benefit of a native-grown hydrosol over an aromatic water? With this educational information included in the marketing, it serves the purpose of not simply selling a product, but also informing the consumer. The consumer becomes actively involved in supporting quality, supporting our clients' high standards, and supporting the dedication and hard work of our suppliers all over the world.

There are many people who have just picked up an aromatherapy book for the first time, who have put together a couple of blends or cosmetic treatments, who are motivated, love the oils, and want to start a business. What would be your advice to someone just starting out with aromatherapy, who wants to make it a greater part of their life by starting a business?

The oils seem to drive people to quit their jobs and do whatever they have to do to have them in their lives full-time!

Once you have developed the heart of your business, the creative part, and the financial part, you've got to bring them together. There's a saying: "You are always judged by your own worst effort." If that means everything you do when you are developing a line of products, everything in that line has to be the best. Move at a steady pace, piece by piece, and don't be so eager to get it out there that proper attention is not given to the product. Starting a business can take years.

I come in contact with a lot of people in this new industry of aromatherapy that have a concept of something they want to do that's going to make money. Whether it's making products or using essential oils in a health care practice, developing a sense of being a businessperson is where I see many people getting frustrated or wasting time and money.

In all businesses, there are basic practicalities that you must be familiar with. There are tools available, often free of charge, that you can use to start a businesses.

I strongly recommend going to the library, talking to friends who have businesses, attending small business association meetings, taking classes, going to trade shows, making use of all the resources available.

It's important to approach your business in a very practical way, so that you don't waste your time and get defeated before your start. Give yourself some time limits and some goals, write a business plan, know how much money you need, whom you are and are not going to involve, the classes you are going to take, and where you are going to be in a year.

It's important to not get discouraged. The time that is spent learning and observing is all very important and critical time. Never give up, keeping your goal in mind and approaching it practically, step by step.

How much time did you spend before Prima Fleur was started—planning and thinking about it?

I began planning my own business after I left the gift industry, where I had worked for ten years. I wanted to develop a line of personal care products, including those for skin care. My grandmother, Eulla Allen, worked for Edgar Cayce for many years. She also had learned from the Native American Okanogans of Eastern Washington, where she lived as a young woman. She homesteaded a farm in a desolate region, and had three babies and an errant and ultimately absent husband. She was forced to work with nature. She taught me a great deal about the importance of knowing how to use plants to heal. Much of what we do comes from our ancestry. I always knew I would work in the area of healing with natural energy forms.

From my early planning to the time I actually formed a business was about seven years. I abandoned the idea of having my own skin care line when I started looking for quality raw materials and began to establish business relationships with producers. I saw a tremendous need for therapeutic-quality essential oils. I knew that there would eventually be many more companies producing personal care products. The industry was beginning to fractionate into various niches such as the salon industry, the natural products or health food industry, as it used to be called, or the bath and boutique industry.

What is the most difficult part of managing Prima Fleur?

Juggling so many things in the air all the time is the most difficult part of managing a company. There is so much business, and there are so many opportunities, that I have to be careful to stay focused and not try to take too many things on at once. Even if a client hasn't paid me, if I've committed to working with them, to helping them with their products, then it's important that I keep my workload manageable so that I can provide them with outstanding service. If I know I don't really have the time to take on their account, I need to tell them to go elsewhere.

It would be easy to scoop everything up and say, "I want all this business," but frankly it's impossible to do all the business that is potentially there. I have to really stay focused and be very clear about how much time I have to do things. I enjoy every account, and the biggest challenge is to know when I have reached a maximum workload and will not be able to take on any other accounts until the schedule opens a bit.*

Do you think that because you're a woman you run or manage your business differently from businesses that you've been involved with or have worked with in the past?

My husband and I both run the business, so I think there's a good balance of male and female energy there. It may be because I'm a woman, or it may just be my personal approach, but, I tend to want everybody to be doing what they do best. I am a boss, that's for sure, but I can't just look at people as employees. I see them as people. I want to get to know them, and I'm not afraid to bring them into my life. I have a very strong respect for people who do a good job at anything, no matter what level of work it is. This isn't something that men don't do, but I may tend to get a little closer than a man might get, and perhaps give people a little extra room to develop and maximize their talents.

Do you think that helps your business?

I think it serves us in that we have longevity of employees, and people are willing to put up with more because they feel that they have a place that's going to grow with them, and because we work really closely as a team. When I'm able to reward people, I do it. I don't think anybody in business should ever forget that they may have had the original concept but the people who work there are the ones that really make it happen. It's the person who answers the phone, and their

---

* What Ms. Griffeth does not tell you in her answer is that, when this interview was taken, she had a new baby. Out of dedication to Prima Fleur and to Ms. Griffeth, her staff pulled together and worked with her throughout her pregnancy. Her newborn daughter is very lucky to be surrounded by Prima Fleur's beautiful essential oils and dedicated employees, who love what they are doing and whom they are working for.

attitude, the person who puts the products together in a box, packing it a certain way, that present your image.

It's not something that you can control by being a boss or by dictating what the chores are. When you respect people, it benefits the business. Even if their job is to come in and clean the place up, you let them know that the job they're doing is very important and that you really appreciate it. Then that employee is going to make a contribution; they're going to help you.

More and more people are starting aromatherapy businesses or lines, or incor-porating aromatherapy into their current business. What are the things that those businesses and practitioners should know when dealing with a wholesale, distributor, or manufacturer of quality essential oils?

There are many different approaches to aromatherapy, and you can't rely on other people to hand you knowledge. There are some very good books, and it's important to do research and talk to many different people, not just study with one teacher, or read one book. Gather information from the numerous sources available, and make choices as to whom you want to believe and what you want to do as far as quality is concerned. You can recognize the differences in quality of essential oils simply by working with them.

Reliability is also a factor. When you order an oil or a product, how long does it take to get it? Does the company you're working with try to keep things in stock all the time? Is the company you're working with really geared to service you, or are you just a secondary customer to them? You want to work with people to whom you are important, and who are willing to provide education and support.

It's important to remember you're providing a product that will affect the buyer in a physiological and emotional way. It's a very serious business in that re-gard. Anybody who's a massage therapist or an aesthetician has to be very particu-lar about the quality of the ingredients they're using, and they have to know that the company they're working with understands their position and is able to pro-vide for them.

What are your upcoming challenges and new goals? What's next?

We'll be continuing to develop the manufacturing. There are two parts to the business: the manufacturing and the importing. They work together, certainly, be-cause many times we can provide essential oils to use in manufacturing that we get directly from producers, so we aren't going through another middle-man, which keeps the pricing very good for those oils.

Every time we get to a point where we start to get comfortable, we push ourselves a little more and take on new challenges—and then we're not comfortable any more. I don't know if I'll ever be comfortable. I want to keep expanding the manufacturing part of Prima Fleur, to develop unique products using different combinations of botanicals.

We are sourcing products other than essential oils, such as hydrosols and herbal infusions, that we use in formulations to work with the essential oils to achieve wonderful effects and to make the item a little more unique. Essential oils are still a good premier raw material in any product. I think of them as the crown jewel of any product. But the other raw materials have to be beautiful too, or the integrity of the whole product is brought down. There's the scientific part of manufacturing, and the intuitive part, which are equally valuable. You can see people's reactions when they use products that have potency directly from nature. It's reaffirming.

We've been working on ways to develop our smaller accounts and to make our services more available to a wider range of clients. We've developed a stock line of products that are available to people who want to repackage them. Most of the products are "blank," which means they don't have essential oils in them yet, so people can customize them. If they have five gallons of lotion, they can put their own blend in it, or the customer can buy a blend and add it themselves. This is something many people seem to want. We have a hand and body lotion, bath salt base, two different cleansers, a moisturizing cream, shampoo and bath and shower gel we created to start with. *[A 1% solution is 99 gallons of product + 1 gallon essential oil. -Ed.]*

Several accounts have used this service to create an "aromatherapy bar," which really is a great idea. These accounts have been very successful in selling pure essential oils, and their customers seem to prefer the essential oils over synthetic fragrances. Many of our "aromatherapy bar" clients started by offering fragrances and essential oils, and found that the essential oils were making more money for them. Customers will drive for miles to come to them, because pure essential oils just aren't available everywhere else. This is a really great way for people to get to use the essential oils, because they can buy the base lotion or shampoo and customize it and use a different blend according to their needs. Developing this type of business is not especially difficult. It helps to have a background in aromatherapy or to have taken some classes, since the store owner does end up doing a lot of consumer education.

We can also use these high quality basics as a starting point to customize products by adding herbal infusions or essential oils, without having to formulate a whole new product for the client. This is a good option for smaller businesses that want good quality customized products but can't afford to have them specifically formulated.

Our stock line is geared to service the "aromatherapy bar" clients as well as aestheticians and massage therapists who need these products in large quantities.

What are some of the most important lessons you've learned from owning your own business in the aromatherapy field?

Many of the lessons I've learned were things I knew intellectually, that I would have told other people if I were advising them in starting a business, but that I hadn't experienced them myself. The most difficult times have been when I've had other people involved in my business, and those relationships turned from dreams into nightmares. That is very disappointing and distracting. I've had to find my own direction again after getting distracted because someone else's goals conflicted with mine.

I have always believed, and now I've experienced, that you have to follow your own heart's path and not let yourself get distracted. I'm stronger now in my conviction of following my own path. It doesn't matter if market trends or anything else is telling you that what you're doing is wrong; you just don't buy into it. I've learned that if I do what I believe in and follow my own heart, it will be right. I have faith in that.

31

Endometriosis, Infertility, and Aromatherapy

Valerie Ann Worwood

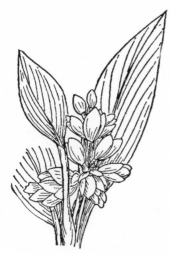

Cardamom
(Elettaria cardamomum)

Valerie Ann Worwood has been a clinical aromatherapist for many years, gaining much of her early experience in Europe, particularly in Switzerland, where the use of essential oils and herbal remedies is very much a part of life and medical practice.

Ms. Worwood has been writing since 1986 and is the author of *The Complete Book of Essential Oils and Aromatherapy* , *Aromantics* , and *The Fragrant Mind*. She has contributed to many other books, and her work has been widely reported, as well as speaking at many international conferences and appearing widely in the media all over the world.

Ms. Worwood has been awarded a degree as Doctor of Medicine (Medicina Alternativa) by the Open International University for Complementary Medicine, Sri Lanka. She was the first chair of the Research Committee of the International Federation of Aromatherapists, which awarded her a fellowship in 1994 for her contribution to aromatherapy. She was a founding committee member of the Aromatherapy Organisation Council, and is also currently a member of the International Society of Professional Aromatherapists.

I have for many years been treating women with endometriosis, a painful condition that is on the increase and is said to affect over ten percent of women throughout the Western world. In 1990, I wrote an article called "Silently Bleeding Tears" for the *Journal of Aromatherapy*, Vol. 2, No. 4, outlining the work I had been doing in this special field, listing the oils to use and other treatment details. I have been pleased in the intervening years to learn that other therapists have been able to replicate my procedures with success.

Endometriosis is a unique disease in which tissue naturally occurring in the uterus develops in another site. Such implants are most often found (ninety-five percent) in or around the abdominal cavity—the intestines, peritoneum, rectum, and reproductive organs. Implants also rarely occur in such unlikely places as the cheeks, elbows, and neck.

This abnormally-located tissue undergoes the same periodic changes as the endometrium, the lining tissue within the uterus, and responds to the hormonal surge of each menstrual cycle by enlarging and bleeding. Bleeding from the pelvic endomentrial implants spills into the peritoneal cavity. This bleeding contributes to the progression of the disease, leading to scar tissue and adhesions onto which new implants can seed themselves. The bladder and the intestines are often bound together, or to the uterus, by adhesions.

Lesions can develop, similar to cysts, which can rupture and lead to the characteristic chocolate-like blood that typifies endometriosis. Affected areas may have clusters of bluish-black areas that resemble blood-blisters. The black areas are known as "powder burns" or "chocolate cysts." Their size varies from that of a pin-head to that of a grapefruit.

Endometriosis is often misdiagnosed as pelvic inflammatory disease, diverticulitis, hernia, ectopic pregnancy, ovarian cysts, and cancer. The most frequently encountered symptoms include pelvic pain, painful sexual intercourse (dysparunia), heavy menstrual flow, vaginal discharge, swelling of the joints, muscle weakness, pain in the left rib-cage, and diarrhea. The Fallopian tubes can become blocked, leading to infertility, another common symptom of endometriosis. Endometrial tissue close to the gastrointestinal tract can cause constipation, rectal bleeding, and painful defecation during menstruation, symptoms sometimes mistaken for irritable bowel syndrome. Adhesions on the bladder cause pain and frequency of urination.

The continual abdominal pain characteristic of endometriosis is caused by the reaction of the peritoneum to localised bleeding, irritation, and inflammation. The most common symptom of endometriosis is painful periods, although there is no direct correlation between the severity of the disease, which is revealed by a surgical procedure called laparoscopy, and the degree of pain experienced. Indeed, many women do not experience pain, and only discover they have endometriosis when they are unable to conceive. Psychologically, endometriosis can have a devastating effect on a woman's sexuality and self-esteem, as it affects her sexual response, menstrual cycle and, possibly, fertility. Many women report their relationships become strained to the point of break-up.

Although endometriosis affects so many women, even in some cases those as young as nine years of age, the cause of the disease is still unknown. Several theories have emerged over the years, but none have been conclusively proven. Environmental factors are thought to be involved, as the U.S. Endometriosis Protection Agency has found a close association between the levels of dioxin found in the bodies of sufferers and the severity of their disease. Other theories include those relating to retrograde menstruation, and those maintaining that endometriosis is an auto-immune disease. Conventional treatments, including hysterectomy and other less absolute surgical procedures, have not in some cases proven very successful.

In 1991, I initiated a research trial with volunteer members of The International Federation of Aromatherapists, and thanks to the generosity of certain essential oil companies. The trial was based on my previous work with endometriosis. Initially, twenty-five full members of the IFA and fifty endometriosis patients were involved in the trial. The women presenting with endometriosis were members of the British Endometriosis Society, and had the full consent of their gynæcologist or general practitioner to take part in the trial.

The trial was carried out on the "cross-over" basis, and followed all usual research procedures. At the end of the trial, eighty-five percent reported an improved lifestyle; eighty percent said they experienced overall benefits; and sixty-five percent reported feeling less pain. The trial involved the use of specialist body-work techniques. At no time did the therapists know the essential oils used in the massage oil, and no other treatments such as counseling or nutritional advice could be given. In normal aromatherapy practice, this would not be the case, and other useful adjuncts could be employed. The full report of this trial will be published in 1996. I am hoping to replicate the trial in America and Australia with members of the appropriate associations in due course.

Among the essential oils I have found to be particularly useful in the treatment of endometriosis in everyday practice are often those that are classically used in the treatment of gynecological problems. These include Geranium *(Pelargonium graveolens)*, Cypress *(Cupressus sempervirens)*, Clary Sage *(Salvia sclarea)*, Angel-ica *(Angelica archangelica)*, Parsley *(Petroselinum sativum)*, Fennel *(Foeniculum vulgare dulce)*, Oregano *(Origanum vulgare)*, Rose Otto *(Rosa damascena)*, Ro-man Chamomile *(Chamamælum nobile)*, and Marjoram *(Origanum majorana)*. Although one nonpracticing commentator has suggested that certain of these oils, being estrogenic, may exacerbate the condition, this assertion is contradicted by the experience of successful and repeatable hands-on therapy.

Aromatherapy treatment for endometriosis should involve twice-weekly visits for a period of six weeks, and once-weekly thereafter—up to at least three months. Dietary changes could be suggested, and exercise such as swimming, yoga, and walking recommended. There should ideally be no sexual intercourse during the initial six-week treatment period. No tampons should be used, and nutritional supplements such as Evening Primrose oil, vitamin B6, Vitamin B complex, and Selenium could also be recommended. Lymphatic drainage must be avoided in the early stages due to the remote possibility of endometrial cells being spread to other parts of the body.

Gentle stress-reducing aromatherapy techniques appear to have no significant effect on the condition, but specialist neuromuscular and deep tissue massage designed to be used on women with endometriosis can be very helpful. However, massage is contraindicated over any painful areas, or those areas known to be problematic. The choice of oils used in any individual treatment would depend in very great part on the history of the particular woman presenting, on her current condition, and other factors including medication and the woman's emotional and physical health, both past and present.

Editor's Note: Ms. Worwood gives some very interesting information regarding endome-triosis in *The Complete Book of Essential Oils & Aromatherapy,* pages 237-239. Her cold and hot sitz bath lists these oils for the hot part of the bath cycle: Geranium, 10 drops; Rose Maroc, 5 drops; Cypress, 2 drops; Nutmeg, 10 drops; and Clary Sage, 8 drops. Use 9 drops of this mixture per bath.

Infertility

As someone who has treated endometriosis for many years I am very familiar with the heart-breaking pain of infertility, one of the possible side effects of endometrio-sis. For many reasons, aromatherapy is an exciting treatment for infertility, espe-cially in those cases where the usual diagnostic tests have not been able to provide an explanation for the problem. For further information on this subject, please refer to pages 167–173 of *Aromantics,* and pages 227–229 of *The Complete Book of Essential Oils and Aromatherapy.* This book also lists certain essential oils to help infertility in women and men, as follows:

Essential oils to help female infertility:
Cypress, Geranium, Clary Sage, Fennel Seed, Thyme, Roman Chamomile, Nutmeg, and Coriander

Tonic oils for the uterus and ovaries are:
Moroccan Rose, Bulgarian Rose, Melissa, and Geranium.

Essential oils to help male infertility:
Thyme, Basil, Cumin, Cedarwood, Sage, Vetivert, Clary Sage, and Angelica.

32

Integration of Botanical Remedies and Kinesiology

Anne Hall

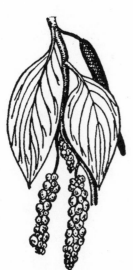

Black pepper,
Piper nigrum

Anne Hall, S.K. is a member of the Touch For Health (TFH) Instructors Association, the National Association of Holistic Aromatherapy (NAHA), the Flower Essence Society, and a facilitator for Three In One Concepts, and serves on the board of directors of the International Association of Specialized Kinesiologists (IASK).

She is an associate of The Natural Healing Network, Mystic Valley Better Life Center, and runs her own business, Balances Skill & Support Center, travels to teach her work, and produces aromatic products for professional and private use.

Her background is with Dr. Ron Barnes of New Zealand, who comes from a long line of Romany medicine women in Europe; Jeanne Rose, Jessica Bear, N.D., Ph.D., and Dr. John Thie, among others.

She created Integration with Botanical Emotional Remedies to encourage the use of aromatherapy, pure essential oils, and flower essences as adjunctive tools for natural healers and established health professionals. Her work has been approved for certification by the International Association of Specialized Kinesiologists. She also lectures at conferences, and travels to teach in Italy, Switzerland, and Germany.

*M*y approach to aromatherapy is as a supplement to an established healing modality, rather than as a therapy that stands alone. Over time, I have developed a background that allows me to use aromatherapy synergistically with kinesiology and the concepts of Touch for Health and Three in One Concepts healing modalities. Use of these therapies in conjunction with aromatherapy allows me to increase the effectiveness of my healing work for maximum benefit to the mental and physical condition of the client.

Kinesiology

The healing techniques I use, called Touch for Health and Three in One Concepts, involve kinesiology, a noninvasive muscle-monitoring skill that indicates stress in the system by a muscle weakening when the body's signals are interrupted. The information comes from the source (self) and is used to help identify the cause of "dis-ease" that hinders living at full potential.

The storage of memories in the cells of our brain and body, combined with genetic imprinting, creates patterns that are subject to interruption under stress. Our life-force or vital chi "wave" is disrupted, and this is reflected in our muscular system. Unhealthy behavior, poor muscle reaction, loss of energy to our organs, and distressed thinking patterns are signs that our inner transmission system has become temporarily confused. Repeated stress and our subsequent reaction can cause the confusion to become ingrained. What began as a temporary reaction to a stress becomes the norm, resulting in "dis-ease" and imbalance in our everyday response to the world around us. Kinesiology attempts to determine the imbalance or interruption in the chi wave through muscle testing, so that the stress can be relieved, and the body's response can return to the active, rather than the reactive, state.

Kinesiology is a skill. It takes practice to master the process so that the information is accurate. The most important part of the art is being able to muscle test with no expectation of the outcome. If the kinesiologist prejudges or misinterprets the client's response, the purpose is defeated. Our objective is to serve as facilitators to help clients recognize their involvement with their problem and take responsibility for their return to better health. They are the only ones qualified to judge and utilize the data that is gathered. We can only share information with them to help their interpretation, assist them with kinesiology techniques, and support them while they integrate necessary changes.

It is important to help clients appreciate their personality, see their behavior patterns, assimilate their belief system, know their expectations of themselves, and comprehend how they interpret stress, either emotionally or physically. If the problem is physical, I determine which meridian energy line in the body is holding the condition, and work from there. Pain is an expression of an imbalance within the individual's entire being.

To begin treatment, I muscle test a client's selected indicator muscle, until we get an interruption in the circuit. I then show the client where the indicator responded, on charts such as the Behavioral Barometer produced by Touch for Health and the Three in One Wheel of Emotions. The client reads the information, and interprets what it means to him or her personally, and we discuss alternative ways to perceive what has been learned using essential oils and other healing tools.

Use of Flower Essences with Aromas

Flower essences are a valuable companion to essential oils. Their effectiveness does not come from the biochemical action of physical constituents as with pure essential oils, but rather from vibrational or subtle energetic properties.

Essences are blooms taken at their peak spiritual development, imprinted in pure spring water, and bottled with a touch of brandy as a preservative. They do not carry a fragrance but impart an energy frequency which can be traced in the bloodstream and measured on electromagnetic scanning devices such as MRI and EEG. They can be used by placing drops on the tongue, in water for sipping, rubbed on the palms, face, and neck, or diluted and sprayed in the air around the body. My objective is to help clients and students find their "sovereign personality" with the use of the Wheel of Emotions, a chart developed by Jessica Bear, N.D., Ph.D.

Dr. Bear has researched the work of Dr. Edward Bach, who developed the Bach flower remedies, as well as ancient writings of the world's religions, to understand the spiritual gifts of plants. According to her healing concepts, there are twelve personality types in the Bach remedies. Each vibrates with one of the original essences. The vibrational frequency of the chosen flower essence supports the positive aspects of the personality. I use Bach flower remedies to support the positive aspects needed for the client to overcome the fault that causes imbalance.

Integration of Therapies

Here I will give a prototype according to the Wheel of Emotions of one personality, and an aroma blend of essential oils that I would choose:

1. *Muscle Testing.* Through muscle testing and the use of the Wheel of Emotions chart, I have found that my client is predominately a Clematis-type personality.

2. *Description According to Wheel of Emotions.* A Clematis-type personality is a mediator by character. When in an unbalanced state, they seem to be indifferent, and are unable to materialize their ideas. Melancholy and idealistic, with only a half-hearted interest in their present circumstances, they seem to be homesick for another part of themselves that they can't reach.

Physical aches become too large, in their mind, to deal with, taking minor pain to the extreme and showing signs of hypochondria. They may have a tendency toward addictions for escape. Anxiety, fear, and suspicion can separate their reason when they are ill.

They are sensitive to the energy around them, and easily become overwhelmed by the expectations of others. This leads to withdrawal and avoidance of present circumstances. They tend to live in the future or another world, to be daydreamers with impractical visions.

Brain fatigue and patterns of procrastination can be major issues. They dread starting a new project, but will become interested until they have resolved the problem, then often quitting before completion. They love to solve puzzles.

Intellectually, they become easily confused and lose normal reasoning power due to scattered thoughts. Forgetfulness and mistakes lead to a lack of ability in self-expression.

Their behavior reflects anxiety, inner agitation, and a general nervousness that may lead to insomnia and pacing.

The virtues that we would like to access for this type are: focus, embodiment, inspiration in practical life, alert presence, grounded energy, a deep sense of responsibility, and an ability to respond to present circumstances. When in balance, this type can be very creative, steadfast, efficient, loving and supportive of the people around them.

3. *Treatment.* Treatment includes use of the appropriate Bach flower remedy along with the use of appropriate essential oils. My selections of aromas also address the

physical traits of weakness with the Clematis personality: Lavender *(Lavendula angustifolia)* for lungs and respiratory weakness; Juniper *(Juniperus communis)* for glandular systems and infections; and Rosemary *(Rosemarinus officinalis)* as a cardiotonic for the heart. Rosemary is also indicated as a vasodilator and stimulant for the adrenocortical glands. Rosemary has a calming influence, and works with Lavender to stimulate vital energy for poor memory, confusion, mental fatigue and strain. Lavender is indicated for depression and anxiety, and works well with Juniper for insomnia and nervousness.

Aromas as Triggers

My particular interest has been in the effects of different fragrances/odors on the brain as triggers for the memory and emotions.

Denial of the truth is always a large part of any problem, and I use aromas to gain an advantage. Aromas bring the person very dramatically into the present, while calling up memories or images from the past that are relevant to the issue being dealt with. The pathway of smell makes direct connection with the limbic system which is known to be concerned with motivating behavior, memory, and emotion. Sometimes the mere hint of an odor can trigger instant and vivid recall of a scene from the past, and revive emotions connected with it.

Smell also contributes to the bonding action in the reformation of thought and response by triggering a series of nerve impulses. Helping a person accept the past, release the negative energy of it, and focus on what is happening to them right now can bring about the most profound changes, allowing a shift which might otherwise have taken longer to initiate.

The hypothalamus can be thought of as a "mind/body laboratory." It takes thought/emotion impulses from the storage banks in the brain and transforms them into the chemicals we need for response. The chemicals that are thus formed determine our perceptions. People with chronic depression are often told they have a "chemical imbalance," and synthetic drugs are prescribed which are claimed to restore chemical balance within the brain. Scent molecules diffuse across nerve junctions or synapses in the brain, and are thought to attach to and alter the receptor sites on the membranes they affect, temporarily distorting the molecular structure. The normal polarized electrical wave passing over the receptor site is altered. This disturbs the electrical arrangement of neighboring molecules, and ions can pass freely in all directions.

I have found that when clients use well-chosen essential oil blends by inhalation during their session, they have a shorter integration time and more far-reaching results. My theory is that the "charge" from an emotional imprint in the brain has been lifted, giving the client a new perspective.

It is impractical to blend the appropriate essential oils during a client's session, so I have researched and pre-blended formulas that address each category of personality, meridian energy line, and behavior trait. I refrain from using a diffusor, as it leaves lingering molecules in the air that may not be compatible with the needs of the next client. I simply keep the blends on hand, to be inhaled when needed.

Essential oils are wonderful healing tools whose power we are just beginning to understand. I have found them invaluable as a part of an integrated healing modality, and am always encouraged and intrigued by the various ways healers of all backgrounds have found to incorporate these precious volatile substances into their practice.

33

Percutaneous Confusion

or the Evidence on Cutaneous Absorption of Essential Oils

Sylla Sheppard-Hanger

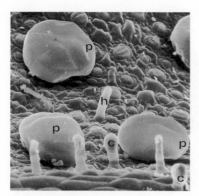

Essential oil glands of
Mentha x piperita
p: peltate trichome
c: capitate trichome
h: non secretory hair
magnification x 600

Courtesy of Professor
Massimo Maffei,
Department of Plant
Biology, University
of Turin, Italy

Sylla Sheppard-Hanger combines twenty years of
experience and personal research into the practice
of aromatherapy and the power of essential oils.
In 1993 she completed the Medicinal and Aromatic
Plant Program at Purdue University.

She was a founding member of the American
Aromatherapy Association (1988), and served two
terms on the board of directors. As the founder and
director of the Atlantic Institute of Aromatherapy in
Tampa, Florida, Sylla developed comprehensive aromatherapy educational programs that are presented
throughout the USA. She is the author of *The Aromatherapy Practitioner Correspondence Course and
of the Aromatherapy Practitioner Reference Manual.*

Sylla volunteers her time and aromatic skills
with women's (abuse/recovery) groups, and consults
for private-label aromatherapy companies. She also
maintains a private aromatherapy practice as a
licensed massage therapist and cosmetologist in
Tampa, Florida.

hether or not essential oils penetrate the skin and are absorbed into the bloodstream is a very confusing issue, and there are two schools of thought. One maintains that very little or no essential oil is absorbed, while the other presents evidence that essential-oil molecules appear in the bloodstream after application to the skin. Most aromatherapy sources say that the skin readily absorbs essential oils, and that the oils are eventually carried to the bloodstream, indicating that external application of essential oils is a means in which significant volumes of oils can enter the body.

Oils are believed to be easily absorbed not only because the skin is the largest organ of the body and the molecular structure of essential oils is very small, but also because some essential oils are extremely lipophilic in nature, suggesting tremendous penetration capabilities for a wide range of treatments. Research has proven the penetration ability of several drugs now administered in the form of patches, and it is assumed that essential oils are also freely absorbed into the bloodstream in the same way.

However, by investigating a wide range of dermatological literature, one also finds evidence to support the opposite case—that most essential oils are *not* freely absorbed into the bloodstream. Very few essential oil constituents, naturally occurring or synthetic, are shown to be absorbed through the skin into the bloodstream. In some cases, the complete or whole essential oil, neat or diluted, has not been detected at all in the bloodstream after application. Most chemical constituents are absorbed into the circulation in reasonably significant amounts via nasal membranes and lungs, if the concentration in the atmosphere is at an appreciable level. The unknown, complex mechanism of skin permeability cannot fit completely into the theoretical generalizations current in modern science.

Human skin has evolved as a highly effective barrier, and tends to absorb a small number of water-soluble plant chemicals. Theoretical models of how the skin is constructed and of how absorption should work assumes that essential oils can pass through this tough barrier. For many years, aromatherapy articles have claimed that it is "most unlikely" that any essential oils "fail to reach the bloodstream," with liberal use of operative words such as "may" and "probable," and very convincing evidence based on the current theoretical model of skin. But skin absorption of essential oils, neat or in dilution, has yet to be definitively shown.

Little evidence shows that the skin will readily admit lipid-soluble portions of plants. Few constituents present in essential oils are readily absorbed by the skin, and most of the constituents that are absorbed, with a few exceptions, are well-documented as causing adverse dermal and systemic reactions. Many of those that are absorbed, such as chamzulene, have beneficial skin-healing qualities. This seems to indicate that a wide range of essential-oil chemicals are alien to the immune system when taken into the body via the skin.

It is widely assumed that substances with low molecular weight will penetrate the skin. Essential oils and their naturally occurring constituents are mostly in the range of 100 to 300 amu (molecular weight). On the other hand, molecular weight may have little to do with absorption, as sex hormones can penetrate under occlusion (when covered), and they are far larger than several of the fragrance chemicals mentioned later as not being absorbed. It is also said that, due to their lipophilic nature, some essential oils and vegetal oils have a good penetration ability (10), thereby allowing easy passage into the bloodstream and through the blood–brain barrier, and that they also have an affinity to lipid-rich organs or structures such as the central nervous system. Experiments seem to show a correlation between decreased water-solubility (increased lipophilicity) and increased efficacy of some constituents of essential oils. In addition, it is said that due to this lipophilic nature, essential oils are soluble in fat, and some "fat-dissolving" oils (those high in ketones) are said to be able to induce "neuro"-toxicity, dissolving the myelin sheath around nerves.

If essential oils managed to get into living cells in sufficient quantity to dissolve the fat, then they would certainly also kill the cells. The test of putting a drop of Thuja *(Thuja plicata, T. occidentalis or Arbor vitae)* essential oil on chicken fat and seeing it dissolve is not considered proof that essential oils penetrate the skin to enter the blood stream, and cannot at all be compared to aromatherapy use any more than watching a drop of Lavender *(Lavandula angustifolia)* essential oil eat a hole in a styrofoam cup. Normally in aromatherapy treatments, the oils are not used in this concentration, nor does one intentionally ingest massive quantities.

The absorption of medications on patches and Garlic oil applied to the feet, which is then detected on the breath, is also inconclusive evidence of penetration through the skin. Application of occluded, concentrated medication chemicals cannot be compared to essential oil application by massage. Garlic has a chemical composition totally different from any other essential oil. Because of its fantastic volatility, inhalation is impossible to avoid (most people have to leave the room when a bottle is opened); therefore, the oil is detected on the breath for hours afterwards because of the inhaled essential oil, not because of dermal application.

Another consideration is that a carrier is usually used for skin application. The molecules of vegetal oils are much larger than essential oils and, in spite of their lipophilic nature, are unable to pass through the skin into the bloodstream (1, 1a). Tests showed topical application of Safflower and Evening Primrose oils applied to highly permeable skin of pre-term infants did not decrease fatty acid deficiency; they found no evidence at all of transdermal absorption of fatty acids. The theoretical model most often used is that skin is relatively permeable to fat-soluble molecules, and relatively impermeable to water and salts. It is thought that, because sebum seeps between cells and because cell membranes have a lipid bilayer, fat-soluble molecules can pass through the skin. Most carrier oils and the essential oils added to them, however, have been found to reside only in the outer, dead layer of skin, the *stratum corneum*, without penetrating into the bloodstream (5,11). Because of this reservoir effect in the outer skin layers, the emollient qualities of vegetal oils cannot be denied. Therefore they are highly suitable as carriers for essential oils. The viscosity or degree of saturation of the carrier plays a part in the ability and rate of penetration (4). Viscous, heavy fats such as lard and wool fat seem to retard absorption. Almond and Olive oil are mono-unsaturates, and have been shown to penetrate the outer layer of guinea pig abdominal skin slowly, while Linseed, rich in polyunsaturates, penetrated rapidly (8).

Dermatological Studies

Because sensitization reactions have been experienced, it seems that some chemical constituents of essential oils must pass into the skin. However, it is very difficult to find substantial scientific evidence that the absorption is of pharmacological significance, and that the amount absorbed causes systemic reactions, such as diuretic effects, which would result from penetration into the bloodstream. The whole oil does not appear to be absorbed into circulation through the skin at all.

The main reference sources cited as evidence for theoretical skin absorption have several areas of uncertainty in methodology: a single synthetic chemical is used as a model for an essential oil; the synthetic substance is diluted in ethyl alcohol; the concentrated substance is used under occlusion; testing with an essential oil is done for main constituents only, instead of the hundreds found in an essential oil; and test procedures do not include prevention of inhalation.

Synthetic Fragrance Chemical Studies

Many single synthetic fragrance chemicals have been shown to penetrate the skin (3), and most of these cause allergic or sensitizing reactions. Benzoic acid, found in Benzoin *(Styrax benzoin)*, is well known to be readily absorbed, and has been used to test variability of absorption over the body.

The inner forearms and back were found to be the best sites for absorption. Benzyl acetate, found in Jasmine *(Jasminum officinale)*, has been recovered from urine twenty-four hours after neat application, and both Jasmine absolute and synthetic Jasmine have been shown to produce irritation reactions. Benzyl benzoate, found in Ylang-Ylang *(Cananga odorata)*, and benzyl alcohol, up to thirty percent of Peru Balsam *(Myroxylon balsamum)*, were absorbed within twenty-four hours. Cinnamic alcohol, found in Cinnamon leaf *(Cinnamomum zeylanicum)*, and Benzoin, cinnamic acid from Cinnamon bark, both severe sensitizing agents, and safrole, a carcinogen found in Sassafras *(Sassafras albidum)*, are also absorbed. Cinnamic aldehyde, found in Cassia *(Cinnamomum cassia)*, and in Cinnamon bark was absorbed well following neat application, and is not advised due to strong sensitizing potential. Methyl salicylate, found in Sweet Birch *(Betula lenta)* and Wintergreen *(Gaultheria fragrantissima* or *procumbens)*, is very freely absorbed, especially in the presence of water; therefore cautious, highly diluted, local use only is imperative with applications of these oils. The ease of absorption of the above constituents may be the reason they are irritants or sensitizers.

Tests *in vitro* on isolated chemicals mentioned previously are unreliable compared to the whole oil and compared to *in vivo* situations. Care should be taken when using oils that contain these chemicals in significant quantities. *In vitro* studies on human breast tissue and foreskin and animal skin showed that benzyl acetate was rapidly absorbed, creating a reservoir in the *stratum corneum,* or upper dead cell layer (4, 5, 6, 11), as mentioned previously. This seems to indicate that, although carriers may decrease fragrance material volatility, a major proportion of essential oils applied to the skin may leave by evaporation rather than passage through the skin.

A recent paper by Sharon Hotchkiss (1994) indicates that the kinetics of absorption from the skin into the systemic circulation may be so slow that skin desquamation (sloughing) may remove the *stratum corneum* reservoir layers before further systemic absorption occurs.

The chemicals tested in fragrance studies are often synthesized, and are not from natural sources. In addition to the synthetic chemicals mentioned previously, the following have been shown to be absorbed through animal skin (human skin is far less permeable): camphor, d-carvone, coumarin, p-cymene, d-limonene. Across isolated human skin, only three percent of d-limonene is absorbed, while in rats six percent is absorbed.

Some chemicals often considered the "active" components in the most important essential oils are shown not to be absorbed:

linalool (within two hours of application)
d-pulegone, found in Pennyroyal *(Mentha pulegium)*
carvacrol, found in Thyme *(Thymus)* and Mint *(Mentha)* species
eugenol and isoeugenol, found in Clove and Cinnamon
menthyl benzoate, found in Clove, Tuberose, and Ylang-Ylang
fenchone, found in Anise, Fennel, some Lavenders
geraniol, found in Geranium and Palmarosa (3)

The finding of linalool within the bloodstream within two hours of application is interesting, as Buchbauer showed linalool and linalyl acetate in the bloodstream within twenty minutes after massage application of the whole oil of Lavender *(Lavandula angustifolia)*, whereas the single synthetic chemical was shown *not* to be absorbed after two hours.

Many of the skin permeability tests used occlusion, a method whereby a concentrated synthetic chemical is applied to the skin and covered for a period of time. Carriers include ethyl alcohol, which is a major ingredient in perfumes and has been shown to enhance percutaneous absorption. A recent study showed seventy-five percent of fragrance in ethyl alcohol was absorbed through the skin when occluded, regardless of the fragrance, as opposed to uncovered, in which only four percent was absorbed (4). The tests also used isolated synthetic aroma chemicals such as benzyl acetate as the prototype molecule for essential oils (4, 5), which cannot compare to using the whole essential oils in dilution and uncovered.

Some of the dermatological tests may be unreliable with reference to humans as they were, unfortunately, conducted on animal skin. Leading dermatologists acknowledge that human skin is far less permeable than animal skin. Most importantly, no studies found on skin absorption of essential oils used a mask and outside air supply to prevent absorption into the bloodstream from inhaling the volatile components, with the exception of the following experiment with Pine oil.

In a test with a massive dose (over 150 mls) of Pine oil in hot bath water (combining heat and humidity, which is known to increase terpene absorption), and using a nose clip to prevent nasal inhalation, a-pinene and camphene were both absorbed in possibly significant amounts. Both chemicals were found to be excreted in the urine up to twenty-four hours later (2). No doubt the test assistant probably also excreted the same chemicals, considering the concentration of Pine oil that must have been in the air. Other studies by the same group showed terpene (from ointments and baths) resorption through skin without inhalation. In addition, a group at the Munich Institute of Balneology and Climatology proved that terpenes permeate the skin a hundred times faster than water, indicating the increased permeability of terpenes with water. While this study inhibited nasal breathing, it failed to state how the subjects breathed, as there was no mention of oxygen apparatus in methodology.

The findings of Buchbauer and his group using Lavender *(Lavandula angustifolia)* essential oil are so far the most appropriate for aromatherapy comparison purposes, although, since inhalation was not prevented, the results seem inconclusive. The essential oil was diluted to two percent and applied to human skin; only the main constituents, linalool and linalyl acetate, were detected in the bloodstream. After a ten-minute massage on a male adult stomach area, traces of linalyl acetate and linalool showed within five minutes in the blood, with maximum concentration in twenty minutes and elimination within ninety minutes. Test methodology did not indicate if other constituents were detected or tested for (7). Again, no breathing apparatus was used to prevent lung absorption; thereby, the experiment did not satisfy the question of skin absorption of whole essential oils.

In addition, because the skin is an important site of metabolism of drugs and solvents, essential oil chemicals may be changed before even the permeable constituents can enter. Essential oils may undergo molecular transformation by specialized skin enzymes (P450s) and esterases. (8) Benzyl acetate (Jasmine) is broken down very effectively by esterase enzymes in the skin.

Increasing Permeability

Increasing the permeability of the skin is possible and can be achieved by several means. It must be remembered that increased permeability can also mean increased skin reactions such as irritation and sensitization. Reactions may occur with any essential oil, especially on hypersensitive or atopic persons, including those suffering from hay fever, allergic rhinitis, eczema, asthma, wool or animal intolerance, or anyone with a family history of these conditions. Caution is needed when using essential oils, especially the known irritating or sensitizing oils, when any of the following conditions are present, which have been shown to increase permeability of the skin (3, 8):

- *Increased skin temperature.* Occurs before, during, or after exercise, or sauna.
- *Increased environmental temperature.* These can occur from outside climate and weather, room, massage therapists' hands, or bath water.
- *Humidity and presence of water.* In water, the normally water-resistant skin becomes hydrated, thus more permeable; caution is advised in hot, humid climates, or hot water.
- *Addition of detergent, soaps, and lipid solvents.* These have been shown to increase permeability by disrupting the skin's natural lipid barrier.
- *Diseased, damaged, or abraded skin.* Broken skin absorbs more easily; thus irritation, and sensitization reactions are much more likely to occur in infections, open wounds, eczema, or psoriasis-type conditions.
- *Occlusion.* Covering the area after application aids penetration by preventing evaporation.

In addition, certain areas of the body appear more permeable to small molecules than others. The tough outer barrier, the *stratum corneum,* is a lipid-rich layer of keratinized cells that acts as the primary barrier to most percutaneous compounds, and as a storage depot (11). Palmar (palm) and plantar (sole) regions may slow permeability due to their thickness but appear to be one of the most permeable areas, as well as thin-skinned areas including the scrotum, forehead, armpits, and scalp. Areas rich in hair follicles and sweat glands, such as the face, neck, shoulders, arms, legs, and the backs of the hands, appear more permeable (8). Good to excellent penetration and often irritation have been observed in the mucus membranes of the mouth, nose, pharynx, gastrointestinal tract, and rectum (12).

Conclusion

The important question remains whether sufficient quantities of essential oil enter the body through the skin to have beneficial pharmacological effects.

In spite of the lack of conclusive evidence, aromatherapy works! It is the method of administration that is in question. Certainly essential oil therapy works symptomatically by external application on superficial skin layers with antiseptic, anti-inflammatory, and other beneficial properties. The complexity of effects during an aromatherapy massage in which when essential oils are inhaled, combined with the added benefits of touch and the placebo effects of client-therapist interaction, provides excellent results. More importantly, in some cases, essential oils can have an effect via direct inhalation, regardless of the application method.

Since essential oils are highly volatile, they do enter the bloodstream very quickly through respiration, if the amount in the air is appreciable. This has been demonstrated many times by blood tests, brainwave studies, and brain CAT-scans. It may be, therefore, that many of the actions claimed for essential oils are due to inhalation or internal ingestions of essential oil, rather than to skin application through aromatherapy massage.

It still remains to be shown conclusively that whole essential oils penetrate the skin into the bloodstream, although single constituents may do so. Of the few constituents that may penetrate the skin, besides being mostly irritant and sensitizing, the amounts needed to cause systemic pharmacological actions remains to be determined. Further scientific research is needed.

What permits one substance or another to penetrate human skin is much more complex than lipophilicity or molecular size, and does not fit comfortably into the theoretical models thus far created by science. By not questioning the evidence, we are not considering the very large number of variables likely to affect the safety and efficacy of any treatment with essential oils. As fragrance compounds do possess a distinct pharmacological efficacy beside their fine odor, the biological activity and pharmacological aspects of essential oils must be compared to that of drugs, and should be investigated more thoroughly.

References

(1)   Lee, E., Gibson, R., Zimmer, K. 1985. Application of Oil in Prevention of Fatty-Acid Deficiency in Pre-Term Infants. *Food & Chemical Toxicology* 28:27–28.

(1a) Lee, E., Gibson, R., Zimmer, K. 1993. Archives of Disease in Childhood 68: 29–31.

(2)   Rommelt, et al. 1974. Percutaneous Absorption of Essential Oil and Fragrance Compounds. *Munch Med Wochenschr,* 116:537.

(2a) Rommelt, et al. 1988. Z. Phytotherapie. 9:14.

(3)   Watt, M., 1994. Plant Aromatics, A Data & Reference Manual on Essential Oils and Aromatic Plant Extracts.

(3a) Watt, M. 1994–95. personal communication.

(4)   Bronaugh, et al., 1990. *In vivo* percutaneous absorption of fragrance ingredients in rhesus monkey and humans. *Food & Chemical Toxicology* (28) 5: 369–373.

(5) Hotchkiss, et. al. 1990. Percutaneous absorption of benzyl acetate through rat skin in vitro. Validation of an *in vitro* model against in vivo data. *Food & Chemical Toxicology* 28 (6): 443–447.

(6) Hotchkiss, et al. 1992. Percutaneous absorption of benzyl acetate through rat skin *in vitro*. Effect of vehicle and occlusion. *Food & Chemical Toxicology* 30 (2): 145–143.

(7) Buchbaer, J. G., Jirovetz, Firtzer. 1992. *Percutaneous Absorption of Chemists*. Jan–Feb 49–54.

(8) Balacs, T., 1992. Dermal Crossing. *International Journal of Aromatherapy* (4) 2: 23–25.

(9) Hanger, Sylla Sheppard, Lisin, G., Watt, M., Moyler, D. (eds.) 1995. Cutaneous absorption of Essential Oils. *The Aromatherapy Practitioner Reference Manual* 1:34–37.

(10) Buchbauer, G. 1993. Molecular Interaction. *International Journal of Aromatherapy* (5) 1:211–14.

(11) Scott, Miselnicky, J. Lichtin, Sakr, Bronaugh. 1988. Influence of Solubility, Protein Binding and Reservoir Formation. *Journal of the Society of Cosmetic Chemists* 39: 169–172, June.

(12) Su, K.S.E. and Campaniaie, K.M. 1985. *Transnasal Systemic Medications*. Yie W. Chien, Ed., Amsterdam; Elsevier Science Publications, p. 139.

34

Scientific Research Validates Psychological Benefits of Fragrance

Annette Green

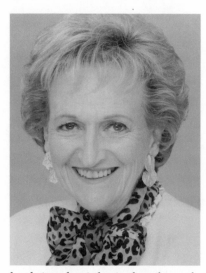

Annette Green is recognized in the world of fragrance and science as one of the first olfactory activists and futurists. Ms. Green is president and secretary of the board of directors of the charitable, tax-exempt Olfactory Research Fund, which is the only organization in the world dedicated to funding studies in universities and hospitals on the sense of smell and the beneficial effects of fragrance. Since the creation of the Fund, the study of the positive effects of fragrance on behavior has made a giant leap into the consciousness of the scientific research community.

Today, in universities and hospitals around the world, the olfactory system is being studied for both its physiological and psychological effects. Through the science of Aroma-Chology (the term coined by Ms. Green), we are learning how the sense of smell influences our responses to stress, sleep, relaxation, social relationships, and performance.

Ms. Green is also the president of The Fragrance Foundation, a nonprofit, educational arm of the international fragrance industry.

Introduction

*A*s a long-time fragrance historian, my fascination with aromatherapy began early in my career and remains to this day. In the late sixties, I became aware of the interest in aromatherapy, particularly in Europe. I began to follow sensory trails in the United States, in the hope that I would discover more about the role of aromatherapy in the United States.

It was on one of these investigations that I found my way to the home and aromatherapy studio of Jeanne Rose. Her knowledge, integrity, and creativity excited me. We became friends, and I followed her career steps as she did mine. In the seventies, I invited her to speak at one of my industry seminars. My goal was to help the members of the industry begin to understand the growing interest in aromatherapy. Ms. Rose was, despite the loss of her notes, an inspiration.

I traveled to London and had the pleasure and privilege to meet with one of the world's great aromatherapists, Madame Micheline Arcier. We spent hours talking, and I was treated to an aromatherapy massage and facial. I listened as customers and devotees visited Madame Arcier's salon. Each was knowledgeable and totally committed to the use of her products to achieve a whole range of psychological and physiological effects.

In the intervening years, as we know, many Americans have embraced the concepts of aromatherapy, and more and more practitioners are entering the field.

The Olfactory Research Fund

My interest in aromatherapy led me to focus on the lack of scientific substantiation of the claims aromatherapists were making. It seemed to me that we were quickly moving into a time when the public was demanding products and service that must be backed by facts. I was convinced that claims of promised results without science were unacceptable.

Much of the sensory revolution that we find ourselves in the midst of today had its real beginnings in 1982, when the board of directors of The Fragrance Foundation, a nonprofit educational arm of the fragrance industry, voted unanimously to support the creation of a charitable, tax-exempt organization dedicated to the study of the sense of smell and the psychological roles odors play in our lives.

The organization, which became known as the Olfactory Research Fund, has spearheaded unparalleled interest in olfaction. The Fund grants scholarships, sponsors scientific research, and promotes the study of the olfactory arts and sciences.

In addition, the Fund sponsors meetings, lectures, and symposia, and creates programs and exhibits for libraries, art galleries, and museums to promote and stimulate the study and understanding of the sense of smell and fragrance.

Olfactory research, including much of the Fund-supported research, concentrates on the beneficial behavioral effects of fragrance, and demonstrates the growing recognition of the interrelationship between fragrance technology research and psychology, which I coined "Aroma-Chology" in 1986.

Several of the research projects recently funded by the Olfactory Research Fund will take us a step further toward understanding how the sense of smell can significantly improve our lives.

Olfactory Research and its Implications

The results of Aroma-Chology research promise new methods of care for the medical profession. Researchers at the prestigious Memorial Sloan-Kettering Cancer Center in New York have found that fragrance can be used to reduce the anxiety and distress that patients experience during magnetic-resonance imaging (MRI), a widely used medical procedure. In a preliminary study, conducted by Drs. William H. Redd and Sharon Manne of the Center's Psychiatry Service, patients who were exposed to a fragrance while undergoing MRI experienced approximately sixty-three percent less overall anxiety. The fragrance used in the study was Heliotropin, a sweet, vanilla-like scent.

These and other breakthrough findings in Aroma-Chology are also inspiring businesses and entrepreneurs with new ideas. Research verifying that certain fragrance ingredients and blends can promote relaxation and relieve stress while others stimulate and energize is certain to spawn vast new marketing opportunities. Already, more and more people are using fragrance to help them sleep and reduce stress, in addition to energizing themselves and improving social relationships.

The fragrance industry has moved in lockstep with the romantic lure of fragrance for a millennium. Now, because of the new scientific discoveries, fragrance is being perceived from a much broader perspective, and will increasingly find its way into designs for both personal and public environments.

Looking into the future, technology will make it possible to have calming sensory enclosures in homes, complete with relaxing and refreshing fragrance choices, computer-driven interior designs, and paintings with built-in sound, light, and scent systems, which may be changed at the touch of a button. Odors, sounds, and tactile devices will be programmed to recreate nature. Living spaces will be sculptural and mobile. Outer-space colors, shapes, and sounds will be the inspiration for art, music, and fashion.

Interior design is also being transformed by the sensory revolution inspired by a group of designers in Milan who are convinced that design has moved beyond form. The greatest influence for the future, they believe, will be sensory. In fact, The Fragrance Foundation sponsored an exhibition in 1992 at the Peter Joseph Galleries in New York to introduce Thomas Hucker's Milan-inspired furniture designs, which are based on sensory interaction incorporating fragrance, sound, temperature, and texture. Hucker worked with International Flavors and Fragrances, which had developed the AromaCote SYMBOL 212\f "Symbol" technology—a water-based, nontoxic polymer with control-release systems, which allows fragrances to be "painted" directly onto wood and other compatible materials.

In a recent Olfactory Research Fund seminar, it was reported by Dr. Clifford Bragdon, vice president for Advanced Technologies at the National Aviation and Transportation Center at Dowling College in New York, that environmental spaces of tomorrow should incorporate all the senses and, most importantly, the sense of smell. Dr. Bragdon remarks that, "Clearly, sensory planning is growing as a discipline, since it addresses health, safety, comfort, and enjoyment issues. The sense of smell is central to the entire subject matter. There are many applications of aroma to sensory planning that can be found at the micro to macro levels of our environment: Cockpit/Crew resource Management; Medical Environments; Corporate Environments; Commercial Shopping; Hotel and Resort Properties; Theme Parks . . . The use of aroma in the built environment [which Dr. Bragdon describes as the portion of the biosphere that supports the human population, including both outdoor and indoor spaces] will prove to enhance behavior, create a more positive environment that translates into improved health and welfare for the population as a whole." An article appeared in the *New York Times* on April 22, 1995 as a result of this meeting, during which Dr. Bragdon and I made an olfactory tour of New York City.

Olfactory Research and The Future

Aroma-Chology research has emerged as a therapeutic force, offering everyone the opportunity to select fragrances and fragrance-enhanced products to achieve a variety of health and psychological benefits.

As life expectancy increases, people will not only be more concerned about their outer aging signs, but also about learning the techniques for keeping all of their senses at peak performance. For the next fifty years, top futurists predict, much labor will be replaced by automation, contributing to a growing leisure class around the world. Meanwhile, life expectancy will rise to nearly one hundred years. If these forecasts do indeed come true, certainly the role of the senses and fragrance will become increasingly important.

The sense of smell is the least understood and least appreciated of all our senses, and may well become the key to unlocking many of the body's and the brain's most penetrating mysteries. At a Fragrance Foundation symposium, Gary Beauchamp, director and president of Monell Chemical Senses Center, remarked, "Literally, you have some of your brain out in the nose, and what's remarkable about this part of the brain is that it regenerates. . . . If we understood how that worked, it might well be that we could understand ways to make other parts of the brain regenerate, which might be the most fundamental of all biomedical achievements in the twenty-first century."

The study of the sense of smell will present future opportunities for fragrance and other sensory innovations that will take us far beyond the present technology.

We have learned that the sense of smell is interrelated with the sense of well-being. The success of many of the lifestyle breakthroughs that will benefit all of us in the remainder of the 1990s and beyond will depend on how effectively industry and the scientific communities interrelate with each other to master the future and reap the enormous opportunities of the emerging world of fragrances.

In the years ahead, I believe there will be a coming together of aromatherapists and Aroma-Chologists based on the scientific knowledge being generated by the Olfactory Research Fund. The results should take us a million miles from where we are now, giving new meaning and dynamics to the self-care of the body and mind.

Sections of this article excerpted from: Green, A. (1993, March-April). "The Fragrance Revolution . . . The Nose Goes to New Lengths." *The Futurist*, pp. 13-17.

35

Performing a Consultation

Ann Berwick

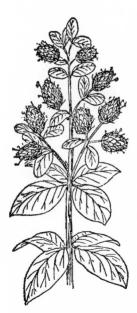

Sweet Marjoram
(Origanum majorana)

Ann Berwick earned a Bachelor of Science degree in Sociology from the Polytechnic of North London, but found this did not answer all her questions about the meaning of the human experience. This led her to read widely in spiritual areas, and to further study at the Faculty of Astrological Studies in London.

Her interest in astrology and tarot was accompanied by an interest in herbs and natural healing. After receiving a facial using essential oils, she knew this was an area she wanted to explore. The London School of Aromatherapy provided the training she needed. She eventually bought a natural health clinic in St. Albans, just outside of London, where she specialized in aromatherapy, massage, and skin care.

When she returned to the United States in 1989, she founded Quintessence Aromatherapy, which offers quality essential oils and aromatherapy training. She also works as a massage therapist and æsthetician, teaching at a local massage school, and writing.

Ann Berwick was instrumental in establishing the National Association for Holistic Aromatherapy and is the author of *Holistic Aromatherapy*.

In this chapter we will examine the process of conducting an aromatherapy consultation and determining an individual blend. We will then discuss the issues involved in setting yourself up as an aromatherapy consultant, professional ethics, and what it means to be a practicing aromatherapist.

Once you have internalized the information presented in this and other books, and have an intimate knowledge of the oils through living, working, and learning with them, you will know which oils will be appropriate in various situations without having to go through the process of listing, cross-referencing, eliminating, and so forth. However, no matter how extensive your knowledge of aromatherapy is or may become, it is always important to spend some time in consultation with each client before you mix the oils. There are many issues that you must consider, and many things that you can observe if you take the time with each person. The consultation is designed to get a complete physical, mental, emotional, and spiritual picture of the person before you. This picture will help you to choose a range of oils that will be appropriate for this particular person at this particular time.

You will be amazed at how much your clients will progress if they are using the right oils in the right way. At times the rate of change will seem miraculously rapid, but in other cases you will need to persevere to see any real change. Be observant, encourage them to be observant, and please develop the habit of keeping records of the oils you use and the results you get. This should also be done by your client, as his or her perceptions will be different from yours.

Please note that if the oils are doing their job, change will occur, and each time you see the client you probably will need to go through the process again. Don't make up one blend that is used without change; you will need to adjust it from time to time. Furthermore, it is not advisable to use one oil continuously in excess for an extended period. The properties of the oils overlap enough that you can and should change them regularly.

Before the client arrives, make sure your room or office is attractive, clean, and cheerful. Use color and lighting to create the atmosphere you wish to convey; flowers are always a nice addition. You might have a burner on with an appropriate oil, or you may choose to spray the room with an aromatherapy air spray. Prepare yourself for the consultation by centering, calming, cleansing, and protecting yourself. Everyone has their own method for doing this, through breathing, repeating a mantra, or imagining cleansing images, such as a waterfall, or protecting images, such as a white light, surrounding oneself. You owe it to yourself and your client to do this. Soft music may be appropriate, and you may wish to take the phone off the hook.

I think that the way that you dress is important. When I first arrived in the United States from England, I was shocked to see massage therapists working in T shirts and jogging pants, as I was trained to always wear a professional-looking white uniform. Although America is more informal, and we cannot represent ourselves as medical persons, I do think it is important to look professional when we are working with clients, particularly if we want aromatherapy eventually to be recognized as a profession. People will have more confidence in what you have to offer if you look the part and conduct yourself accordingly.

I normally set aside about thirty minutes for a consultation. If you are not going to give a treatment such as a massage at this time, thirty minutes is usually enough to go through the consultation process and help the client choose oils that would be appropriate. Charge a consultation fee that is comparable with those charged by other health professionals in your area.

Remember that you can choose whom you see. Do not be pressured into working with someone if you feel instinctively wary of the person, or if it is not convenient for you to see them at that particular time. Don't be afraid to say "No," and don't be bullied into doing a consultation by telephone, or making up oils for someone you have never seen. You will regret it, and could end up in trouble.

You must see the person before you can choose appropriate oils. I get letters from people asking what oils would be good for their eczema, for example, and I always reply that I work only through personal consultation, as each case is individual, and each person will need a unique blend of oils.

You may think Chamomile would be great for eczema, and send a big bottle of it through the mail. What if that person is allergic to Chamomile and the rash gets worse? Also, you do not know who you are dealing with. If the person is not serious enough to make an appointment to see you, he or she is not serious enough about changing his or her situation or state of health. Use your time and energy wisely and professionally; if you respect yourself, others will respect you. Many of you will wonder why I am saying all of this. It seems obvious, and if you are already a therapist you will know it already. I know all of it too, but I still get drawn into situations I don't want, forget to take time to prepare myself adequately for a consultation, take on others' burdens, fail to say "No" when I should, and so on, so there is no harm in reminding ourselves of these things.

The Consultation

Let's say that the client has arrived and you are ready to begin. First you will record your client's name, address, phone number, occupation, marital status, and date of birth on your form. Many practitioners have a questionnaire that clients fill out themselves, but I have always found that by going through the questionnaire with them I get far more information than if they merely tick boxes or write comments without elaborating or giving me any more insight into their character.

I like to have the date of birth rather than age, because some people object to giving their age, and asking for birthdate does not seem so threatening. Also, because I have observed some truth in astrology, it lets me know what birth sign they are. This often correlates with the type of oils they like; for example, earth types often like the heavier earthy or woody oils, while fire types like the hotter oils. Even if you get only an idea of the element, it is useful and gives you another little insight into their character.

The client's marital status can give you clues to his or her emotional state; the occupation can tell you about his or her educational background, lifestyle, and self image. Sometimes you can also get some idea of his or her personality type and psychological profile.

I would then ask about the client's medical history, specifically about any of the conditions that would contraindicate the use of certain oils, for example, epilepsy or pregnancy. Asking what type of treatment he or she has received in the past also tells you about his or her attitude toward health, and openness to what you have to offer.

If the client is presently receiving treatment from another practitioner, it is important that you not interfere with that process. If you have any doubt, you should contact the practitioner and discuss what you are proposing. If still in doubt, keep away, and ask the client to come back after the treatment is finished. Of course, it is important to ask what he or she hopes to work on with you, and why he or she is here today. Why a person chooses aromatherapy is often illuminating too. How did he or she find out about you? What does he or she know about the oils?

You can then go on to explain how the oils are believed to work, how many levels he or she can work on at once, and the different ways in which the oils can be used. This gives you an opening to explore the deeper dimensions of the problem, if this is appropriate. For example, if the problem is recurrent migraines, you could go into the nature of the headaches, their frequency, how long the condition has been occurring, and what medication your client may be taking for the pain.

You could then go on to look at physical causes such as diet or PMS, and then psychological and emotional factors like pressure from the boss at work or a husband who is having an affair.

All of the factors involved will determine which blend of oils you finally choose. You will also need to take into account the relative importance of each factor to the client. In the end, dealing with her fears and sense of betrayal because of her husband's affair, and recovering her own sexual self-confidence, may be more important for your client to work on with the oils than the actual migraines, although of course the oils also can help with the physical pain. This is where the individual blend is crucial in holistic aromatherapy. While we are helping with the headache, we are also helping to rebalance the whole person on many levels. If this is not done, the headaches will come back, no matter how many painkillers she takes. Of course, the beauty of the oils is that without consciously blending for all of these levels, a single oil will often do this anyway. For example, Lavender would help the pain both physically and emotionally.

Alternatively, if your client replies that the problem is depression and apathy, you may want to ask questions that will help to determine on what other levels this is operating. For example, Mr. Jones may be cold physically, he may be constipated, and may suffer indigestion. You could use oils to warm both body and spirit, selecting them by the three-column blending method described in *Holistic Aromatherapy*.

Sometimes you will simply want to use the oils on a physical level, such as making a facial blend for a mature dry skin, and will use one oil as an antiwrinkle aid, one for broken capillaries, and one as a sebum balancer. However, factors such as diet and hormonal balance will still come into play.

You may also blend for purely spiritual purposes, for example, creating a blend that will deepen breathing, open the third eye, and calm the mind. One day someone may ask you to create a personal perfume; in this case your three columns might be concerned with picking top, middle, and base notes.

Thus, the reason why a person is consulting you will determine your next set of questions. I recommend having a set of questions covering the main body systems, and a set covering all types of stress. You don't have to ask everything; just use what is appropriate.

Once you have concluded your questionnaire, have your client sign a disclaimer assuming full responsibility for using the oils. This will protect you, particularly since it is illegal for us as unlicensed practitioners to prescribe, diagnose, or treat any medical condition. We cannot say, "This Chamomile oil will help your eczema," or "I want you to apply this Rosemary to the area of your liver three times a day," or "It sounds like your have exhausted adrenal glands."

Once you have determined which oils you think would be applicable, the best thing to do is to present them to the client, and let him or her choose the ones he or she feels most drawn to. You don't have to explain in detail why you have chosen them, although you can refer to the commonly accepted use of each oil: "Chamomile has been traditionally used as an anti-inflammatory oil," or to what an authority says: "Tisserand speaks of Tea Tree as a booster of the immune system." You could also refer to research: "There has just been a study by Australian scientists showed that Tea Tree to be effective against candida in eighty-five percent of cases." You can also refer to your own experience: "I found Tea Tree very useful when I had candida." Do not say, "I want you to use this Tea Tree three times a day as a treatment for your candida."

Having made the blend, you can give it to your client with a list of accepted means of using the oils and instructions for how much oil to use for each, so that he or she has general instructions for use. Do not write on the bottle, "Add eight drops of Rosemary oil to your bath twice a day." Your sheet might say, "The recommended amount of essential oil to use in a bath is six to eight drops."

If you approach your consultation and the administering of the oils in this way, you will not be accused of practicing medicine without a license, and if you have your clients sign the disclaimer, thus taking responsibility for their own health, you are merely acting as an advisor or consultant.

It is best to call yourself an aromatherapist or aromatherapy consultant. As yet, there is no licensing or regulation of aromatherapy or the use of oils in the United States. We can use them because they appear on the list of GRAS (generally recognized as safe) food additives published by the U.S. Food and Drug Administration (FDA). As of this writing, the FDA has no plans to interfere with the use of oils for psychological purposes, and will approach other aromatherapeutic uses on a case-by-case basis. If drug-like claims are made openly, this could attract unwanted attention, so we must be very careful about how we represent ourselves as practitioners. The National Association for Holistic Aromatherapy is studying the establishment of training and professional standards for all of us. It is much better that we regulate ourselves rather than have strict regulations imposed on us.

If you are already a massage therapist, cosmetologist, acupuncturist, chiropractor, physician, registered nurse, or any other licensed professional, you can use the oils within your established practice. Licensing requirements differ widely from state to state, so if you wish to do hands-on work, or massage, and do not have a license, it is important that you determine your local requirements. Please check with your local authorities and comply with the regulations for the area in which you live.

Ethics

The subject of ethics is a complicated issue—everyone has their own values. However, I believe that it is very important for us to have our own code of ethics as aromatherapy practitioners. One of the most important considerations is to work within your own limits. Do not pretend to know more than you do, and use the oils in a responsible, humble way. Do not underestimate their power, and let them teach you about themselves by using them with respect, restraint, and subtlety. The National Association for Holistic Aromatherapy (NAHA) publishes a Code of Ethics for practitioners and teachers.

Too often I have seen the oils overused, overblended, and causing damage through the neglect of the people using them. Use them gently, with pride in your craft, and they will work wonders for you.

If we are to be holistic practitioners, we should respect the laws of nature, observe her patterns, and attempt to live in harmony with the Earth. I hope you will strive to avoid excess commercialism and exploitation of aromatherapy and the essential oils. These remedies are not merely another product to be sold; they contain the life force itself. Be as simple and honest as possible in all of your dealings, and when recommending the oils to others, always err on the side of caution and restraint.

Practice what you preach, use the oils in your personal life, and try to speak from personal experience. Question everything until you have internalized the knowledge, and know what is true from your own experience and inner work. Strive for the very highest standards in your training and practice. Continue asking questions and growing in your knowledge. The more I use the oils, the more they teach me; if you let them, they will show you far more than any book, course, or teacher ever could.

Excerpted from *Holistic Aromatherapy* by Ann Berwick, Llewellyn Publications, P.O. Box 64383, St. Paul, MN 55164.

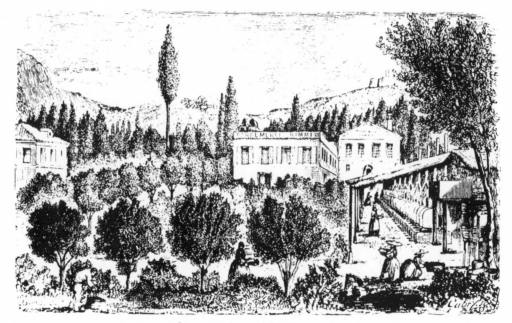

A flower garden and distillery at Nice

VII

A Student's Project

36

Aromatherapy: Making Sense of Scents

Meg Seiter

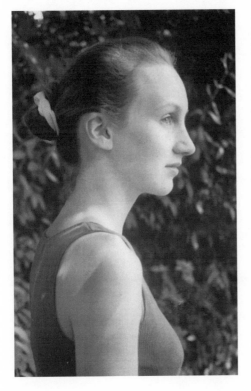

In 1995, high-school sophomore *Meg Seiter* pursued her interests in aromatherapy and behavioral science through a science fair project. Peers were eager to participate in her experiment, and curious about the results. Many wanted to know if they had felt the "right" emotion.

Meg lives in a small suburb north of Boston. Her other interests include playing tennis, writing, playing the piano, and having endless phone conversations.

The editors were delighted by such a complete and sophisticated experiment by this high-school student. We hope that her interest in aromatherapy will persevere, as she would certainly be a credit to the art and science of aromatherapy.

The following article is a student project in Behavioral Science by a sixteen-year-old tenth grade student at Hamilton-Wenham Regional High School, South Hamilton, Massachusetts.

Project Summary

Purpose

*T*he purpose of my experiment was to find out whether the effects of aromatherapy are only alternative-medicine hype; specifically, does an essential oil used in aromatherapy change a person's mood only because the person using it is told it will produce a specific emotional effect?

Procedure

I tested 120 human subjects, asking them to inhale the scent of a drop of essential oil on a perfume blotter for a period of five minutes. During the five-minute testing period, the subjects were asked to fill out a feedback sheet on which they identified from a list of nine possible emotions the one which most closely matched the way were feeling. When testing the control group, I made no mention of the particular effect traditionally associationed with the oil being tested. When testing members of the variable group, I selected a false effect of the oil being tested, and told the subjects that it was a true effect of the oil. I used two different essential oils. I tested each adult with one of the two oils, and I tested each student twice, each time using one of the two oils. In total, I performed 197 tests.

Conclusion

Based on the data I gathered from the feedback sheets, I conclude that aromatherapy's effect is not a placebo. The most common reaction to each oil was the effect traditionally attributed to the oil. This was true in both the control and the variable groups despite suggestion provided to the contrary.

Question

Are the effects of aromatherapy no more than alternative-medicine hype; specifically, are the emotional changes associated with aromatherapy produced by the power of suggestion, or by the essential oils themselves?

Hypothesis

An essential oil produces a specific emotional effect strong enough to be identified, and strong enough to override a suggested false effect.

Aromatherapy

Aromatherapy is defined most simply as "the ancient art of healing by scent."[1] However, behind this simple phrase is a complex system in which essential oils are extracted from plants and used to heal and maintain the human body and mind.

In modern society, we spend hours each day trying to scrub away and conceal every trace of human scent with synthetic odors. Baby-powder-scented deodorant, pine-scented air fresheners, floral perfumes, spicy aftershaves, and fruity shampoos mask the messages our bodies send out each day. While the rest of the animal kingdom is using scent as a critical means of communication, we are covering the scents that transmit messages, and are hindering our sense of receptive smell with incredible handicaps.

The human nose, despite all obstacles, is still a phenomenal instrument that receives millions of messages each day—messages that affect us both physiologically and psychologically. Most people are unaware of the immense power of scents to heal and maintain us, both emotionally and physically, through a practice called aromatherapy.

Essential Oils

The complex process of extracting essential oils from plants begins in the chloroplasts of plants, where these aromatic properties are formed. The oils combine with glucose to create glucosides, which are transported throughout the plant. This distribution is similar to the distribution of nutrients through the human bloodstream. "Essential oils are the high-grade fuel of plants, and by taking them into our bodies, we ingest the best of the goodness plants have to offer."[2]

Essential oils are similar to hormones. In flowering plants, they assist in the fertilization process by attracting pollinating insects. Essential oils also catalyze and control biochemical reactions, distribute messages among cells in response to stressful situations, and regulate the production and renewal of cells. When the sun's heat causes essential oils to evaporate from a plant's surface, a protective shield of scent surrounds the plant, defending it against parasites and infection by bacteria or fungi.

In order to take essential oils into our bodies, we must extract them from the plant so that we receive them in their most concentrated, potent form. The essence is the most delicate and elusive part of a plant. It is also more potent than the plant as a whole, and has a much more dramatic effect on the body than the complete plant.

Because various plants and essential oils are different, there are several methods of extraction. The first is steam distillation, which begins with small pieces of plant material mixed with water in a container. This mixture is heated, and the oil droplets are extracted by the steam and carried through a tube cooled by cold water. This causes the steam and oil droplets to condense into a receptacle. Because essential oils are not soluble in water, they either float on top of the water or sink to the bottom, depending on their density. The oil is then collected.

A second method of extraction is the cold-press method, used primarily for citrus fruits. If one were to examine the skin of an orange or a lemon, one could see the small glands in which essential oils are stored. Until 1930, essential oils of citrus fruits were extracted by pressing the peel into a sponge. Today cold-pressing is used. The skin of the citrus fruit is shredded and mixed with water. Then the oil is extracted by pressure.

One of the more recent methods is extraction by chemical solvents. The process begins with a salve-like solid, called a concrete, which is treated with alcohol to separate a plant wax from the essential oil. A solvent is then added, such as hexane, petroleum benzine, or ether, which is then extracted by vacuum distillation, leaving behind the pure essential oil.

Extraction is a very detailed process in which mistakes can be made easily. If the steam distillation process is not completed, important substances will be missing—substances that make essential oils therapeutically effective. If any heat is applied during the cold-press process, the delicate oil will be destroyed, and if there are any pesticides on the skin of the fruit, these are be transfered to the essential oil. Because the solvents used in the chemical solvent method are highly toxic, even tiny amounts can cause allergic reactions and weaken the human immune system. The concentration of leftover solvent in an essential oil should be no higher than five parts per million. Because of these risks, it is important to purchase oils from reputable suppliers. The purity and quality of essential oils are incredibly important, and influence their effectiveness.

"Reconstitutions," "nature identicals," "isolates," "perfume compounds," and "aromas" are not the same thing as essential oils. Manufacturers of synthetic oils very often have convincing and misleading labels. Even manufacturers of essential oils are often guilty of adulteration; the scents of expensive oils are replicated by combinations of other less expensive oils, but sold under the same name. Although the two will smell almost identical, the therapeutic effects will not be those of the plant being imitated. Some essential oils are diluted in carrier bases to make a small amount of essential oil go farther.

One way to tell if oils are, in fact, pure essential oils, is to examine the prices. Some oils are dramatically more expensive than others due to the rarity of the plant they were extracted from, or the difficulty of extraction. If many different oils are all being sold at the same price, it is a sign that they are likely not pure. Health food stores are usually a good source of essential oils, as well as reputable wholesale distributors. Beauty and perfume shops are more likely to carry adulterated or "fake" oils.

Once pure oils have been purchased, careful storage is imperative in securing the quality of the oils. They should be stored in air tight bottles made of brown or dark-colored glass to protect them from light. The oils should also be kept away from heat and moisture. Without proper preservation, oils will be subject to oxidation, polymerization (compounds with different properties form from the original), and resinification (the oil dries out and thickens).

Bottles of essential oils are seldom dated, so it is important to find a reputable supplier who has not had the oils sitting around for months. Most oils' potency and effectiveness fades over time, while some, such as sandalwood and patchouli, ripen over time. The average therapeutic life of an essential oil is two years.

The science of chemistry has enabled us to break essential oils into their component parts for identification and separation. The chemical composition of essential oils is complex, commonly containing alcohol, ketones, terpenes, aldehydes, and esters. Dr. Taylor of the University of Texas at Austin has demonstrated that essential oils contain "more previously unexamined compounds than all the chemists in the world could analyze in a thousand years."[3]

"The component parts of essential oils—the vitamins, hormones, antiseptics, and antibiotics they contain—account, to an extent, for their curative action; but these constituents do not entirely explain their success in beauty and health care. The first modern scientist to practice aromatherapy, Gattefossé, was the first to demonstrate that 'the whole is greater than the sum of its parts.' Essential oils work holistically. The complex, global structure of an essence working as a whole will always be far more effective than the individual components of an essence applied separately. This is why synthetic oils that have the exact same chemical components as an essential oil fail to provide the same results."[4]

History

Many things will be reborn which have been long forgotten. —Horace

Humans have known the power of aromatic plants since prehistoric times. During the Neolithic Period, about 6000-9000 years ago, humans extracted fatty oils from plants such as olives by pressing them. They used these oils to keep their hair manageable, as protection against the sun, and in their cooking. Many historians speculate that their cuisine entailed many aromatic herbs, and it is likely that scented oils were first used during this period of time.

Many ancient civilizations utilized the powers of aromatic oils in daily life. In ancient Egypt, the first aroma therapists began their sophisticated practices. Many of these were priests who used the oils in religious rituals. In Heliopolis, a city established for the worship of the Sun God, Ra, incense was burned three times a day. As the day progressed, the complexity of the incense would increase, and by sunset a mixture of raisins blended with thirteen aromatic oils would fill the air. This blend was named *kyphi*.

The Egyptians practiced fumigation, a practice in which ailing person sat in a tiny room full of fragrant smoke. Evil spirits were believed to manifest themselves in the form of nervous conditions, and fumigation was said to combat these evil spirits. Cones of scent, made of animal fat infused with aromatic plants and placed in head-dresses, were another means of warding off evil spirits. The cones of scent would melt in the warm atmosphere, and the scent would be released thorughout the day.

The importance of scented oils to the ancient Egyptians can be found in many burial tombs, where alabaster vessels of aromatic oils have been discovered. These vessels date back to 3000 B.C. The Egyptians believed that a person remained in the earthly body in the afterlife, and valued preservation of beauty for this reason. They bathed frequently with aromatic oils, often followed by a fragrant massage. Cedarwood oil, a favorite of the ancient Egyptians, was used in mummification, and the dead were buried with their most cherished oils.

In ancient India, sandalwood oil was a favorite. Temples in India were built entirely of sandalwood, which created a permanent fragrance. Vedic texts and the Kama Sutra hold references to the use of essential oils. These writings date back several thousand years. The earliest written evidence that perfumes were common is in the Ramayana, an Indian epic from 2000 B.C. Aroma therapy is still practiced in modern India, both religiously and in hospitals.

In 2000 B.C., Emperor Kwang-Ti of China wrote about the healing powers of pomegranate, opium, and rhubarb. He classified remedies and illnesses into yin and yang. The yin was a "feminine" power, associated with wetness, darkness, passivity, and cold. Yang, the "male" power, was associated with dryness, light, motion, and heat. Chinese healers strove to restore a balance of yin and yang in patients. Exotic essences such as jasmine and cinnamon originated in China.

The pantheistic religious beliefs of the ancient Greeks ascribed divinity to all plants, and plant essences were seen as pure spirit. Many myths involved Gods on sweet-smelling clouds, and perfume was said to be heaven-sent, carried to Earth by the nymphs of Aphrodite, the goddess of love.

The Romans practiced more elaborate uses of oils than the Greeks. Several major cities had "perfume districts" and the unguentarii, Roman perfumers, always had many customers. Public baths, where one could soak in aromatic waters and receive a fragrant massage, were the center of cultural life. The Romans' use of essential oils was widespread; they used them on their bodies, their hair, furniture, clothes, walls of their homes, and even flags.

After the fall of Rome, the Romans fled to Constantinople, and the Byzantine empire became awash with fragrance. The science of chemistry was rapidly growing in Arabia, and the process of distillation was discovered by an Arabian philosopher, Avicenna. The Crusades brought essential oils to Europe, where people who worked with the oils were the only ones to gain immunity to the plagues.

In the twelfth century, the first perfume-manufacturing units were started, and by 1202, France had become defined as the aromatics center of Europe. During the fourteenth and fifteenth centuries, information about the medicinal properties of essential oils was recorded and distributed, brimming with recipes for health and beauty aids.

During the sixteenth century, William Turner, an herbalist commonly called the "father of botany," classified herbs and illnesses in terms of hot and cold. He created "hot" remedies to heal "cold" illnesses, and vice-versa. Between 1500 and 1730, perhaps 114 essential oils had been identified.

During the 1800s, more sophisticated synthetic drugs displaced herbal medicine. Although apothecaries no longer carried essential oils as a part of their regular inventory, the European perfume industry was always well-stocked with natural oils. There was steady growth in this industry, and the south of France became a major area of cultivation and extraction.

In the twentieth century, aromatherapy has seen a rebirth. In the early part of the 1900s, René-Maurice Gattefossé carried out scientific studies of the therapeutic properties of essential oils. He wrote ". . . in my personal experience, after a laboratory explosion covered me with burning substances which I extinguished by rolling on a grassy lawn, my hands were covered with a rapidly changing gangrene. Just one rinse with Lavender oil stopped the gasification of the tissues. This treatment was followed by profuse sweating and healing began the next day. (July 1910) . . . " Gattefossé devoted his life to the study of essential oils, and coined the term "aromatherapy."

After Gattefossé, Dr. Jean Valnet of France used essential oils to treat war injuries during World War I. In 1964, he wrote *l'Aromathérapie, Traitement des Maladies Par Les Essences des Plants*. Valnet was especially interested in spreading knowledge of aromatherapy to physicians, and today more than one thousand French physicians use essential oils in their practice.

The Sense of Smell

Smell is a potent wizard that transports us across thousands of miles and all the years we have lived. —Helen Keller

In order to understand how aromatherapy works, it is important to become familiar with the sense of smell.

A polluted atmosphere and a heavily mucus-producing diet are two factors that abuse our sense of smell. Humans are classified as microsomatics, animals with a poor sense of smell. But despite many obstacles, and despite the fact that humans, compared with many other animals, are dramatically less dependent on their sense of smell for survival, the human nose is still an incredible instrument which cannot be duplicated, even in today's highly technological society.

Humans breathe about 23,000 times each day, and with each breath we carry fragrant molecules into our noses. Our olfactory systems are constantly receiving messages.

In *A Natural History of the Senses,* Diane Ackerman says, "Smell is the most direct of all our senses. When I hold a Violet to my nose and inhale, odor molecules float back into the nasal cavity behind the bridge of the nose, where they are absorbed by the cilia. Five million of these cells [line the olfactory epithelium and send] impulses to the brain's olfactory bulb or smell center. Such cells are unique to the nose. If you destroy a neuron in the brain, it's finished forever; it won't regrow. If you damage neurons in your eyes or ears, both organs will be irreparably damaged. But the neurons in the nose are replaced about every thirty days and, unlike any other neurons in the body, they stick right out and wave in the air current."[5]

There is a complex series of events which must occur for us to perceive an aroma. First, we cannot detect a scent unless there are odor molecules in the air. An object volatile enough to release odor molecules is known as an olficient. When humans inhale, the odor molecules given off by the olficient are swept into the nasal cavity, where they hit the olfactory epithelium. It takes only eight odor molecules to trigger an impulse in a nerve ending, but forty nerve endings must be stimulated before we can consciously perceive a scent.[6]

Once the odor stimuli cause impulses in the olfactory nerves, the impulses travel to the opposite end of the olfactory nerve, located in the limbic system of the brain. "From the limbic system in the brain, memory and emotion are affected as well as the intellectual processes and the cortex. Here, the hypothalamus, which is responsible for the integration of many basic mechanisms and behavioral patterns . . . absorbs the tiny molecules of oil. The hypothalamus appears to be the single most important control area for the regulation of the human internal environment. It is the location of short- and long-term memory. The inhalation of essential oils stimulates this area, and this is why we say that 'scent is the most memoristic of the senses.' The hypothalamus also has an effect on aggression control, and affects the pituitary and adrenal glands. Via the pituitary glands, the sexual glands are affected, which is why scent can be an aphrodisiac."[7]

One of the challenges when dealing with the sense of smell is the difficulty we face in finding words to match scents; olfaction is known as the mute sense. This is because the links are weak between the smell and language centers of the brain.

When describing a scent, we use one of four methods of description. We use emotive adjectives (pleasant, disgusting), vocabulary associated with other senses (sweet, sharp), cross-definition ("it smells like a Rose"), and tautological statements ("Sandalwood has a woodsy scent").

Because of this scent-language barrier, scent classification has puzzled scientists for years. Hans Henning was one of the first scientists to attempt scent classification. He grouped scents into spicy, flowery, fruity, resinous, putrid, and burnt. However, experimentation in objective classification has led to no positive results. Another source lists the basic categories of scent as minty (Peppermint), floral (Roses), ethereal (Pears), musky (musk), resinous (Camphor), foul (rotten eggs), and acrid (smoke). There is no unanimously agreed-upon system of classification.

How Does Aromatherapy Work?

The simplest form of aromatherapy is direct inhalation of an essential oil. Each molecule of essential oil has a specific shape, which fits into a specific place on the olfactory epithelium, like a key in a lock. Once the essential oil "unlocks" the door, a chemical message is transmitted to the limbic system. Odor stimuli in the limbic system release neurotransmitters—messages from the brain to the body saying such things as "calm down," "cheer up," or "produce more white blood cells to fight this infection!"

If inhaled through the mouth, the essential oil will enter the bloodstream in the lungs, from which it will travel throughout the body. Inside organs, "the powerful vitamins and enzymes contained in essential oils are processed."[8]

While traveling throughout the human body, the main function of essential oils is to assist the body in helping itself. When using synthetic drugs, we develop a dependence because the drug is doing the work for us. When using essential oils, one never builds a tolerance or dependence because essential oils remind the body to do the work itself, and help it to do so. This strengthens the immune system, increasing the health of the entire being. As Michael A. Weiner wrote in *Maximum Immunity*, "the age of antibiotics is fast coming to a close. Because of their great numbers, viruses and bacteria have quickly evolved resistant strains for almost every major man-made pharmaceutical. Positive, preventative health is becoming more and more important."

Essential oils don't act as an "on/off switch" that stimulates or sedates, as synthetic medicines do. Essential oils normalize and establish balance, and are sensitive to specific body chemistry.

Each essential oil is unique and has an affinity with specific parts of the body and mind, but their similarity lies in their ability to stimulate the production of leukocytes. In this way, essential oils are natural, risk-free antibiotics. Essential oils fight infection because of their highly acidic pH and antiseptic agents.

Once essential oils have done their jobs, they leave the body via exhalation, through pores in the skin, or with other waste products through the bladder.

The Sweet Smell of (Future) Success

"Sniff your way to health and happiness?" asks Joan Duncan Oliver in *Health*. "Maybe not, but even those who dismiss the claims for aromatherapy admit that . . . oils scented with the essences of flowers, fruits, stalks, roots, or bark can [lead to] a terrific 'in-body' experience. The relaxing results have convinced many that using such oils for psychological and medical treatments is a healing art for the nineties: a fragrant, noninvasive, all-natural means to help achieve well-being."[9]

Many people believe aromatherapy is going to continue to catch on very rapidly. To see this, one needs only to look at aromatherapy's popularity in Japan. The Shimizu construction company in Tokyo developed "aromatherapeutic environmental fragrancing [in which] air-conditioning ducts hidden among the ceiling tiles . . . release a mixture of eight therapeutic 'aroma chemicals.' As of October [1992], eighty companies in Japan were using Shimizu systems."[10] Even in the United States, many store owners fill their stores with specific scents aimed at putting customers in better moods, encouraging them to spend money more easily.

Annette Green, president of the Fragrance Foundation and vice- president of the Olfactory Research Fund in New York, believes that "technology will make it possible, in the very near future, to have calming sensory enclosures in every home, complete with relaxing and refreshing fragrance choices, computer-driven interior designs, and paintings with built-in sound, light, and scent systems, which may be changed at the touch of a button."[11]

Ms. Green also speculates about "a 'smart' cocktail dress that senses when its wearer is attracted to someone across the room and begins to emit an alluring scent. Alternatively, the fabric might emit a foul repellant to ward off Mr. Wrong."[12]

The possibilities are limitless.

Project Materials

197 chemically pure perfume blotters
197 feedback sheets
120 human subjects
   1 15 ml. bottle Orange oil *(Citrus aurantium)*

1 10 ml. bottle Nutmeg oil *(Myristica fragrans)*

1 10 ml. bottle Spikenard oil *(Nardostachys jatamansi)*

1 empty 15 ml. bottle with lid

1 dropper spout

1 dropper

Procedure

I. Creating the synergy:
   1. Combine 40 drops Orange oil and 2 drops Nutmeg oil in empty 15 ml. bottle.
   2. Put dropper spout into mouth of 15-ml. bottle.
   3. Screw lid onto 15-ml. bottle.
   4. Shake to blend.

II. Testing human subjects:
   1. Read instructions (Control Group Instructions for control group, Variable Group Instructions for variable group) aloud to subjects.
   2. Hand out one feedback sheet to each person.
   3. Count out number of blotters needed for testing group.
   4. Line up blotters together in a group.
   5. Using dropper, distribute Spikenard Oil over blotters. Make sure oil is visible on each blotter.
   6. Hand out one blotter to each subject.
   7. Begin timing as soon as the last person receives a blotter.
   8. At the end of five minutes, collect sheets and blotters.
   9. Repeat steps 1-8 with Orange/Nutmeg synergy on a separate day.
   10. Repeat steps 1-9 with other classes and adult groups.

Control Group Instructions

I said the following to control group subjects:

For my science fair project, I'm testing the effects of aromatherapy on emotions. Aromatherapy is the ancient method of healing the body and mind by inhaling the scents of essential oils. Essential oils are extracted from plants and bottled immediately. Nothing is added or taken away; what you are smelling is the scent of the substance exactly as it smelled when released by the plant before extraction.

My experiment procedure is to have you inhale the scent for five minutes and then fill out a feedback sheet for me.

Try to maintain your normal breathing rhythm. It isn't necessary to breathe harder or more often to get the effects of the scent. In fact, if you interrupt your normal breathing rhythm, your body might react by yawning. This could lead you to believe that the scent of the oil made you tired, even if it didn't.

Variable Group Instructions

I said the following to variable group subjects:

For my science fair project, I'm testing the effects of aromatherapy on emotions. Aromatherapy is the ancient method of healing the body and mind by inhaling the scents of essential oils. Essential oils are extracted from plants and bottled immediately. Nothing is added or taken away; what you are smelling is the scent of the substance exactly as it smelled when released by the plant before extraction.

Spikenard oil: This oil is reported to make humans feel energetic and excited.

Orange/Nutmeg oil: This oil is reported to make humans distracted and unfocused.

My experiment procedure is to have you inhale the scent for five minutes and then fill out a feedback sheet for me.

Try to maintain your normal breathing rhythm. It isn't necessary to breathe harder or more often to get the effects of the scent. In fact, if you interrupt your normal breathing rhythm, your body might react by yawning. This could lead you to believe that the scent of the oil made you tired, even if it didn't.

Aromatherapy Project Questionnaire

Name: _____

Age: _____ Sex: M / F

Time tested: _____ AM / PM

Scent: _____

Do you have a cold or stuffy nose? Y / N

Which of the following most closely matches your feelings after inhaling the scent?

1. happy, pleased   6. tired, sluggish

2. sad, downcast   7. energetic, excited

3. calm, peaceful   8. distractible, unfocused

4. angry, irritable   9. alert, focused

5. stressed, overwhelmed

What color is the scent? _____

What music do you hear? _____

_____

Have you ever smelled this scent before? _____

Can you identify the scent? _____ If yes, what is it? _____

What comes to mind when you perceive this scent? (a picture, memory, etc.)

_____

_____

_____

Did you feel a change in emotions? Y / N

The original project incorporated charts to show the results of the above proce-
dure. The following is a summary of the original charts.

Results: Spikenard Oil

Calm and peaceful feelings are traditionally associated with Spikenard oil. The
control group was given no suggestion as to the effects of Spikenard oil, while the
variable group was told, "This oil is reported to make humans feel energetic and
excited." Of the control group, forty-seven percent claimed feeling calm and
peaceful, while sixty-five percent of the variable group felt calm and peaceful. Of
both groups, the traditional effects of Spikenard were reported more often among
females than males. Forty-seven percent of females in the control group and thirty-
nine percent of females in the variable group reported feeling calm and peaceful,
while forty-three percent of males in the control group only twenty-nine percent of
males in the variable group reported feeling calm and peaceful. Of the variable
group, only twelve percent chose the suggested false attribute of feeling energetic
and excited. An outstanding number of respondents associated the color green
with Spikenard. Brown was the second most-often associated color.

Results: Orange/Nutmeg Synergy

The traditional effect of the Orange/Nutmeg synergy is happy or excited. The control group was not given a suggestion as to the effects of the synergy, while the
variable group was told the oil was ". . . reported to make humans feel distracted
and unfocused." Forty-seven percent of the control group claimed that this aroma
made them feel happy or excited, and forty percent of the variable group had this
reaction. Only thirteen percent of the variable group chose the suggested false
effect of feeling distracted and unfocused. Females were more likely to choose the
traditionally associated attribute in each group. Forty-seven percent of females in
the control group and thirty-nine percent of females in the variable group chose
happy or excited as the emotion associated with the oil. Forty-four percent of
males in the control group and twenty-nine percent of males in the variable group
felt happy or excited. Orange was the color most often associated with this oil,
with Yellow being the second most-often associated color.

A Student's Project

The following descriptions are excerpts from student's answers to the "Aromatherapy Project Questionnaire."

Spikenard
What Comes to Mind When You Perceive This Scent?

. . . a bottle of mentholatum in my bathroom when I was little. . . raking leaves in the backyard near the woods. . . Vick's Vaporub. . . a cedar closet. . . a flower shop. . . my barn in summer. . . a field of marigolds and wildflowers. . . a dirty locker-room. . . riding my bike in the rain. . . a horse stable. . . buying my mom bath soaps at Christmas. . . pine trees in Alaska—I love it!. . . cutting down Christmas trees with my family. . . marijuana. . . buying patchouli. . . my grandparent's house. . . a bright red store in Martha's Vineyard that sold weird new-age clothing. . . a Grateful Dead concert. . . a Buddhist temple in Hong Kong. . . a vague memory of my grandfather—maybe something he had? wore? a room?. . . canoeing and fishing in a lake deep in the woods. . . the Church of the Advent in Boston. . . incense. . . a quiet, peaceful forest. . . a window. . . sawdust. . . spaghetti sauce and a good friend. . . a bottle of tile cleaner. . . walking in the woods, camping, early morning, nature, clean. . . a college-friend's room. . . a sunny room in my grandmother's house that had several plants on a wall. . . Kali's room. . . a winter day in a warm house by the fire. . . buying shrubs at the Ann and Hope Garden Center. . . childhood memory—a very general feeling of evening in the house in which I grew up. . . a photobook I just read on sequoias and redwoods. . . Nyquil. . . tea-time at the nursing home. . . a big psychedelically swirled peace train coming to take me to the land of dandelions. . . the Muppets. . . nothing. . . the Pyramid Book Store in Salem smells just like this, where all the candles and rocks and strange perfumes are. . . . something from Nature's Elements. . . a rotating spice rack. . . Eucalyptamint. . . peppermint. . . dust in an old wooden attic. . . a haystack. . . herbal tea. . . a spring day, playing outside in the dirt. . . my greenhouse. . . dark black storm clouds. . . an Indian marketplace, like in Aladdin. . . a memory from when I was thirteen. . . the dentist's office. . . the Boston Museum of Science. . . sitting in a field of orange wildflowers, surrounded by pine trees, lying on my back listening to music. . . a cool, clear lake, with a blue sky framed by a green tree line. . . a day when my dog and I went swimming in a swamp and then delivered newspapers. . . the garden at my grandfather's house. . . a Chinese garden. . . the hamsters I had when I was younger. . . camp last summer. . . the ocean. . . sunsets. . . a girl at a concert. . .

Orange-Nutmeg Synergy
What Comes to Mind When You Perceive This Scent?

looking at the back yard of a country home. . . an orange container. . . freshness and energy. . . Citra-solv. . . eating fruit. . . eating oranges with kids in the kitchen. . . Florida orange groves across from my grandparents' winter home. . . candy. . . drinking lemonade in the summer. . . spring or summertime, lemonade, blue skies, beautiful weather, cool breeze, sunshine, blonde-haired girls. . . a pomander ball in a bowl of lemons—yum!. . . a lollipop. . . summer picnics; makes me feel thirsty. . . everything is bright!. . . a sunny orchard of orange and lemon trees with odoriferous emanations. . . church. . . loud music. . . California—my aunt has fresh citrus trees in her yard. . . half-time during basketball games, when we refuel with water and oranges. . . juice squirting into my eyes as I cut into oranges. . . swimming in summer. . . peeling an orange for early morning breakfast. . . watching Melissa getting her thrills out of peeling her orange at lunch. . . jazzy music, a modern jazz quartet—kind of perky but not too much in the horn section. . . a beach. . . oh, man, it's a full moon, I'm in a field of lotus plants, a shovel floats past my head, ah, it's shovelin' me out, ahhhhh. . . tangerines. . . lemon Ricolas. . . noise. . . tropical island. . . high-tension wire, auto races played in fast-forward. . . Lemon Pledge. . . classical musical instruments. . . cough drops. . . being in my grandparents' backyard under an orange tree, eating lemon sherbet. . . limes. . . drying and stringing oranges at Christmas-time. . . tennis balls. . . someone playing vibes. . . grapefruit. . . cooking. . . a lime-green lollipop. . . clementines. . . Florida orange-juice commercials. . . Disney World—the ride with all of the vegetables running around. . . apple pie. . . a disco. . . happy xylophone music, like in the Violent Femmes. . . the lemon loaf my mother makes at Christmas. . . eating an orange and getting the white part of the peel under my fingernails, and being able to smell it all day because of it. . .

Conclusion

Based on the data I gathered from the feedback sheets, I conclude that my hypothesis was supported: The effects of aromatherapy seem to be more than alternative-medicine hype. The emotional changes associated with aromatherapy are produced by the oils themselves, and not by the power of suggestion. The essential oils I used—Spikenard oil and a synergy of Orange oil and Nutmeg oil—had strong emotional effects that overrode suggested false effects, and the most common reaction to each oil was the effect traditionally associated with the oil. This was true in the control group, where I made no mention of the particular effect associated with the oil being tested, and also in the variable group, where I selected a false effect of the oil being tested and told the subjects that it was a true effect.

From this experiment, I have learned firsthand some of the difficulties intrinsic to gathering data from humans. The variability in responses both fascinated and frustrated me. What fascinated me was how much I learned about individuals based on the images they shared in response to the scents. What frustrated me was that subjects often left one or more questions unanswered.

Each human I tested was a potential source of error. Variables such as memories connected to scents, moods, head colds, and fatigue all had the capability of affecting the subjects' perceptions. Because my project depended on their self-perceived emotional reactions, possible errors were inherent in the project from the beginning.

If I were to repeat my experiment, I would do additional study of the effects of different essential oils before selecting oils to use in my testing. The oils I used were recommended to me by an aromatherapy professional. I took her recommendations and researched them, but another time I would make my selection based more fully on my own research. In particular, I am interested in researching the oils known for their ability to create feelings of bliss and euphoria.

References

1. Victor Blevi and Gretchen Sween. *Aromatherapy.* New York: Avon Books, 1993.
2. Valerie Ann Worwood. *The Complete Book of Essential Oils and Aromatherapy.* San Rafael: New World Library, 1991.
3. Blevi and Sween: 20
4. Ibid.
5. Diane Ackerman. *A Natural History of the Senses.* New York: Random House, 1990: 10.
6. Ackerman: 16.
7. Jeanne Rose. *The Aromatherapy Book: Applications & Inhalations.* Berkeley: North Atlantic Books, 1992: 189-190.
8. Blevi and Sween: 19.
9. Joan Duncan Oliver. "Making Sense of Scent," *Health.* Nov. 1989: 53.
10. Mary Roach, "Scents and Science," *Vogue.* Nov. 1992: 208.
11. "Sweet Future for the Fragrance Industry," *USA Today.* June 1993: 15.
12. Ibid.

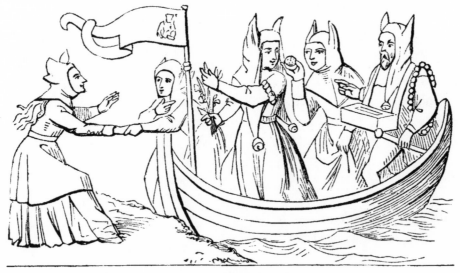

The boat of foolish smells

A List of the Essential Oils
and Their Correct Latin Binomials

abs = absolute
bd = bud
bk = bark
berr = berries
flw = flower

hb = herb
lvs = leaf or leaves
ndl = needle
pl = peel
pds = pods

rs = resin
rt = root or rhizome
sd = seed
wd = wood
weed = weed

Ambrette *(Hibiscus abelmoschus)* sd
Angelica *(Angelica archangelica)* rt
Anise *(Pimpinella anisum)* sd

Basil *(Ocimum basilicum)* hb
Bergamot *(Citrus bergamia)* pl
Black Sage *(Salvia mellifera)* hb

Cajeput *(Melaleuca minor* aka. *M. leucadendron)* lvs
Camphor (is always synthetic)
Caraway *(Carum carvi)* sd
Cardamom *(Elettaria cardamomum)* sd
Carrot *(Daucus carota)* sd
Cedar oil comes from a variety of woods, needles, and bark. Know what you
      want, as some are skin irritants and/or toxic.
    Cedarwood *(Cedrus atlantica)* wd
    Cedarwood *(Cedrus libani)* wd
    Cedarwood *(Thuja occidentalis)* wd
    Cedarwood *(Juniperus virginiana)* wd or ndl

Celery *(Apium graveolens)* sd

Chamomiles can be either of the Roman, German or Moroccan type.

    Chamomile *(Chamamaelum nobile)* flw from the perennial Roman type.

    Chamomile *(Matricaria recutita)* flw from the annual Hungarian type.

    Chamomile *(Chamamaelum mixtum)* flw from the annual Moroccan type

Cinnamon *(Cinnamomum zeylanicum)* bk

Citrus oils have many confusing names, these are the current correct ones.

    Citrus aurantifolia var. *limetta* is Lime peel oil

    Citrus aurantium var. *amara* lvs is Orange petitgrain or leaf oil

    Citrus aurantium var. *bergamia* is Bergamot peel oil

    Citrus aurantium bigarade is Orange flower oil or Neroli

    Citrus limonum is Lime peel oil

    Citrus paradisi is Grapefruit peel oil and comes in pink or white

    Citrus reticulata, green is Tangerine peel oil

    Citrus reticulata, red is Mandarin peel oil

    Citrus sinensis is Sweet Orange peel oil

Clary Sage *(Salvia sclarea)* lf

Clove *(Eugenia caryophyllata)* bd

Copal *(Bursera spp.)* rs

Coriander *(Coriandrum sativum)* sd

Cumin *(Cuminum cyminum)* sd

Dill *(Anethum graveolens)* sd or weed

Eucalyptus *(Eucalyptus globulus)* lvs

Fennel *(Foeniculum vulgare)* sd

Frankincense *(Boswellia carterii)* rs

Geranium *(Pelargonium graveolens)* lvs & flw

German Chamomile *(Matricaria recutita)* flw

Ginger *(Zingiber officinale)* rt

Honeysuckle *(Lonicera caprifolium)* abs from flw

Hyssop *(Hyssopus officinalis)* hb

Jasmine *(Jasminum officinale)* abs from flw

Juniper *(Juniperus virginiana)* wd (sometimes called Cedarwood)

Lavender *(Lavandula angustifolia* or *Lavandula x intermedia)* flw & tops
Lavender *(Lavandula spp.)* flw & tops
Lemon *(Citrus limon)* pl
Lemongrass *(Cymbopogon citratus)* rt
Lemon Verbena *(Aloysia triphylla)* lvs
Lotus *(Nymphaea lotus* or *Zizyphus lotus)* flw
Lovage *(Levisticum officinale)* rt

Mandarin *(Citrus reticulata)* pl
Marjoram *(Origanum majorana)* hb
Melissa *(Melissa offcinalis)* hb
Mountain Sage *(Artemisia californica)* hb
Mugwort *(Artemisia herba alba)* hb
Mugwort *(Artemisia vulgaris)* hb
Myrrh *(Commiphora molmol)* rs
Myrrh *(Commiphora myrrha)* rs

Neroli *(Citrus aurantium)* flw from Bitter Orange
Neroli *(Citrus bigarade)* flw
Neroli *(Citrus reticulata)* flw
Neroli *(Citrus sinensis)* flw from Sweet Orange
Nutmeg *(Myristica fragrans)* sd

Orange *(Citrus aurantium spp. aurantium)* pl
Orange *(Citrus sinensis)* pl from Sweet Orange
Orange-flower absolute *(Citrus aurantium)* abs from flw
Oregano *(Oreganum compactum)* hb
Oregano *(Oreganum vulgare)* hb

Palmarosa *(Cymbopogon martinii* var. *motia)* lvs & overground parts
Patchouli *(Pogostemon patchouli)* lvs & hb
Pennyroyal *(Mentha pulegium)* hb
Pepper, Black *(Piper nigrum)* berr
Peppermint *(Mentha x piperita)* hb
Petitgrain *(Citrus aurantium amara)* lvs
Pine Geranium *(Pelargonium graveolens pinus)* lvs

Rosemary *(Rosmarinus officinalis)* hb
Rose *(Rosa damascena)* flw
Rosewood *(Aniba spp.)* wd

Sage *(Salvia officinalis* or *Salvia lavandulifolia)* hb
Sandalwood *(Santalum album)* wd
Savory *(Satureia hortense* or *S. montana)*
Scotch Pine *(Pinus sylvestris)* ndl
Spearmint *(Mentha viridas)* hb

Tangerine *(Citrus reticulata)* pl
Tansy oil comes from a perennial which is toxic, as well as an annual called Blue
        Tansy which is used in skin care. Be wary!
    Tansy *(Tanaceum annuum)* flw from an annual plant
    Tansy *(Tanacetum vulgare)* flw & tops from perennial plant
Tarragon *(Artemisia dracunculus)* hb
Tea Tree *(Melaleuca alternifolia)* lvs
Thuja *(Thuja occidentalis)* wd (also called Cedarwood, but this one is TOXIC.)
Thyme *(Thymus vulgaris)* hb
Tuberose *(Polianthes tuberosa)* abs from flw

Vanilla *(Vanilla planifolia)* pds
Vetiver *(Andropogon zizanioides)* rt

Wintergreen *(Gaultheria procumbens)* lvs (generally methyl salicylate is used)

Yarrow *(Achillea millefolium)* flw
Ylang-Ylang *(Cananga odorata)* flw

Sources for Everything

Essential Oils & Oil Products

Benzoin is available from the following:

Melanie Templer, P.O. Box 81, Ubud, Gianyar, Bali, Indonesia, Fax 62 361 975 162.

Fleur, Pembroke Studios, Pembroke Road, Muswell Hill, London, N10 2JE, UK.

Fragrant Earth, P.O. Box 182, Taunton, Somerset, TA1 35D, UK.

Saffron Oils, Belmont House, Newport, Saffron Walden, Essex, CB11 3RF, UK.

Jasmine sambac concrete is a pure Jasmine, and is available from Leydet Aromatics, P.O. Box 2354, Fair Oaks, CA 95624.

Lavender and Lavandin essential oils are available from Shirley Price Aromatherapy, Essentia House, Upper Bond St., Hinckley, Leics., LE10 IRS, England.

Lavender Lane, 6715 Donerail Dr., Sacramento, CA 95842 has Turkey red oil.

Leila Castle, Amrita Aromatics, P.O. Box 302, Point Reyes Station, CA 94956, Tel. 415-663-1954 for information about custom blends, Goddess Perfume Oils.

Prima Fleur Botanicals, 1201-R Andersen Dr., San Rafael, CA 94901. Prima Fleur sells wholesale essential oils. Their oils are of the best on the market, and Ms. Griffeth is dedicated to providing absolutely pure and unadulterated essential oils. If you are not able to purchase the oils in wholesale quantities, ask them for a provider of therapeutic quality essential oils in your area.

Resinous oils are available from Industrial Aromatics, 184 Furnace Dock Rd., Peekskill, NY 10566.

Santa Fe Fragrance, P.O. Box 282, Santa Fe, N.M. 87504, Tel. 505-473-1717. Pure essential oils, aromatherapy blends and colognes. Christine Malcolm, owner.

Products & Companies

Aromaland, Route 20, Box 29, Santa Fe, NM 87505. Essential oils, diffusing lamps, electric diffusors, reference cards and more.

Balances Skill & Support Center, 2800 Accomac, St. Louis, MO 63104, Tel. 314-776-6103. Aromatic Kits for Behavioral Barometer and Fourteen Touch For Health Meridians.

Essence Aromatherapy, P.O. Box 2119, Durango, CO 81302, Tel. 800-283-0244, phone/fax 970-247-0959. Aromatherapy candles in sacred shapes for transformation, anoints, dream pillows, bath salts, massage oils, etc. Ixchel S. Leigh, owner.

Essentiel Elements, 2415 Third Street #235, San Francisco, CA 94107, Tel. 415-621-9881. Mineral Bath Salts for the Foot Bath.

FES Flower Essences. Balancing Essentials, J. Bear, Ph.D., N.D., 348 Deauville St., Las Vegas, NV 89106, Tel. 702-598-0727.

Hauschka Cosmetics, 59-C North Street, Hatfield, MA 01038, Tel. 800-247-9907. Bath Concentrates for facial compresses and foot bath.

Herb Products, 11012 Magnolia Blvd., North Hollywood, CA 91601. Herbs, oils and other items. Reasonable prices, wonderful company.

Magick Botanicals, 3412 W. MacArthur, Suite K. Santa Ana, CA 92704, Tel. 800-237-0674. Clay for facial masks.

Opie Gems, 57 East Street, Ilminster, Somerset, TA19 OAW, UK. Crystals.

Oshadhi, 32422-C Alipaz. San Juan Capistrano, CA 92675. Massage oils, elixir and silky powder from Hauschka.

Jeanne Rose Aromatherapy, 219 Carl St., San Francisco, CA 94117, Tel. 415-564-6785, Fax 415-564-6799. First Aid Kits containing therapeutic-quality essential oils for a variety of uses. A source for pure essential oils as well. *The Aromatherapy Book: Applications & Inhalations, The Herbal Body Book,* and *The Aromatherapy Studies Course*™ all include instructions for building a home still. Mail-order only.

Mountain Rose Herbs, PO Box 2000 Redway, CA 95560. Herbs, books, oils and bottles to package your own products and original medicinal-tea blends.

Oak Valley Herb Farm, 14648 Pear Tree Lane, Nevada City, CA 95959. Essential oils, herb products.

Oil Lady Aromatherapy, Candace Welsh, 674 11th Street North, Naples, FL 33940, Tel. 941-263-3451, Fax 941-263-0898. Complete Medicine Tin.

Original Swiss Aromatics, P.O. Box 8642, San Rafael, CA 94903. Essential oils, base ingredients, cosmetics.

Prima Fleur Botanicals, 1201-R Andersen Dr., San Rafael, CA 94901, Tel. 415-455-0957 and Woodspirits Soaps, 1920 Apple Rd., St. Paris, OH 43072. Organic California-distilled Hydrosols® and soaps.

Purely Natural Body Care, 4717 S.E. Belmont, Portland, OR 97215, Tel. 800-669-1863. Since 1975 Alexandra Avery, owner of this company, has provided high-quality aromatherapy skin-care products.

Shirley Price Aromatherapy, Training Department, Essentia House, Upper Bond Street, Hinckley, Leics., LE10 1RS, UK.

Simplers Botanical Co., P.O. Box 39, Forestville, CA 95436. Hydrosols, essential oils, carrier oils, herbal extracts.

Tisserand Aromatherapy, P.O. Box 750428, Petaluma, CA 94975, Tel. 707-769-5120. The "Aroma Stream" diffusor.

Woodspirits Soap Works, 1920 Apple Road, St. Paris, OH 43072, Tel. 513-663-4327. Fine hand-made soaps and hydrosols.

Zia Cosmetics. For a catalog of Zia's products and a supplier in your area, contact Zia Cosmetics, Tel. 800-334-SKIN.

Knowledge

Aromatherapy Practitioner Reference Manual, two volumes by Sylla Sheppard-Hanger, is available from Atlantic Institute of Aromatherapy, 16018 Saddlestring Dr., Tampa, FL 33618, Tel. and Fax 813-265-2222.

The Aromatherapy Quarterly is the longest-running magazine in the aromatherapy world, with readers in over fifty countries. It is a valuable educational resource. For subscription information in the U.S. call 415-663-9159, or write to Box 421, Inverness, CA 94937-0421. In the UK, write to 5, Ranelagh Ave., Barnes, London SW13 OBY, UD, Fax: 011-44-181-392-1691.

Aromatherapy Studies Course™ and Herbal Studies Course™, see Jeanne Rose in product list for address.

Aroma Research Institute of America (ARIA), P.O. Box 282, Santa Fe, NM 87504. Encourages and assists the research and development of new agricultural projects that produce aromatics as well as researches and educates about the senses of smell and taste.

Charts—*Chakra Chart* and *Angel Chart* designed by Tricia Davis, includes info on oils and crystals. Contact: Healing Art, P.O. Box 16, Totnes, Devon, TQ9 5UY, UK.

Chicago Museum of Art, Chicago, IL. Display of a miniaturized version of the embalming art.

The Compendium of Olfactory Research is available through the Olfactory Research Fund. Please write to 145 East 32nd St., New York, NY 10016 for further information.

"The Fragrance Revolution . . . The Nose Goes to New Lengths." *The Futurist* is available through The World Future Society, 7910 Woodmont Ave., Bethesda, MD 20814, Tel. 800-989-8274.

Hydrosols—For a packet of information about hydrosols send $3 and stamped, self-addressed envelope to NAHA, P.O. Box 17622, Boulder, CO 80308.

Updates as to the Organic · · California-Grown, California-Distilled® project, as well as updated information regarding hydrosols subscribe to AROMAtherapy 2037 Newsletter, 219 Carl St., San Francisco, CA 94117.

NAHA, P.O. Box 17622, Boulder, CO 80308. Write for Scentsitivity quarterly and membership. Also provides a list of aromatherapy certification courses, information about certification, and a Code of Ethics for practitioners and teachers.

Pacific Institute of Aromatherapy, P.O. Box 6723, San Rafael, CA 94903. Correspondence course, seminars, retreats. Course includes aromatherapy chemistry. Taught by Kurt Schnaubelt.

Latin binomials from *The Plant Book* by D.J. Mabberly published by Cambridge University, 1989.

Workshops. Caroline Wyndham and Simon Alleguen regularly offer crystal courses at Introductory, Intermediate and Advanced levels. Also occasional one-day or weekend seminars at several venues in the Southwest of England. For information send SASE for details to Earthheart, Mapleton House, West Street, Ashburton, Devon, TQ13 7DU.

Bibliography

A

Ackerman, Diane. *A Natural History of the Senses.* New York: Random House, 1990.

Adler, Jerry. "What Kind of Therapy Smells?" *Newsweek,* March 2, 1987: 62.

Albertus, Frater. *Alchemist's Handbook.* York Beach: Samuel Weiser, Inc., 1974.

Alternative Medicine: The Definitive Guide. Pullyap, ID: Future Medicine Publishing, 1993.

Arcier, Micheline. *Aromatherapy.* London: Hamlyn, 1990.

Arctander, Steffen. *Perfume and Flavor Materials of Natural Origin.* Elizabeth, NJ: Steffen Arctander, 1960.

"Aromacology: The Psychic Effects of Fragrances." *The Futurist,* Sept./Oct. 1990: 49-50.

The Aromatherapist. Essentia House, Upper Bond Street, Hinckley, Leics. LE10 1RS, UK, all issues.

Asre, S. *Chemical Composition and Anti-microbial Activity of Some Essential Oils.* M.Sc. Thesis. Macquarie University, 1994.

Austin, Hallie Iglehart. *The Heart of the Goddess.* Berkeley:Wingbow Press, 1990.

Avery, Gilbert (editor). *Compendium of Olfactory Research . . . Explorations in Aroma-Chology: Investing the Sense of Smell and Human Response to Odors.* Olfactory Research Fund, Ltd. and Kendall/Hunt Publishing Co., 1995.

B

Bailey, Liberty Hyde and Ethel Zoe Bailey. Hortus Third. New York: MacMillan Publishing Co., 1976.

Bauer, Garbe & Surburg. *Common Fragrance and Flavor Materials.* Germany: VCH, 1990.

340

Berwick Ann. "Aromatherapy and Flower Essences." *Scentsitivity,* Volume 4, No. 1: 3-4, 1993.

Bianchini, Francesco. *Health Plants of the World.* New York: Newsweek Books, 1977.

Black, Pamela J. "No One's Sniffing at Aroma Research Now." *Business Week,* December 23, 1991: 82-83.

Blevi, Victor and Gretchen Sween. *Aromatherapy.* New York: Avon Books, 1993.

Branson, Ann Sela. *Soap: Making It, Enjoying It.* New York: Workman Publishing Company, 1975.

Britton, Lord and Hon. Addison Brown. *An Illustrated Flora of the Northern United States and Canada, Vol. II.* New York: Dover Publications, 1970.

Brunschwygk, Hieronymus. *Small Book of Distallacyon.* 1527.

Buchbauer, G., W. Jager, L. Jirovetz, J. Ilmeberger, and H. Dietrich. *24th International Symposium on Essential Oils,* Berlin, 1993.

Butterfield, John and Jim Sexton. "New Remedies for Old Ills." *USA Today Weekend,* December 1994: 4-22.

C

Carper, Jean. *The Food Pharmacy.* New York: Bantam Books, 1988.

Cavitch, Susan Miller. *The Natural Soap Book: Making Herbal and Vegetable-Based Soaps.* Pownal,VT: Storey Publications, 1995.

Chopra, Depak. *Creating Health.* Boston: Houghton-Mifflin Co., 1987.

"Common Scents," *Dateline NBC.* WBZ-TV, Boston. 16 Dec. 1994.

Croutier, Alev Lyle. *Taking the Waters: Spirit, Art, Sensuality.* New York: Abbevilee Press, 1992.

Culpeper, N. *Culpeper's Complete Herbal.* London: W. Foulsham & Co., 1824.

Cunningham, Scott. *Magical Aromatherapy.* St. Paul: Llewellyn Publications, Inc., 1989.

D

Davis, Patricia. *Aromatherapy: an A-Z.* Saffron Walden, UK: C.W. Daniel, 1988.

_____. *Subtle Aromatherapy.* Saffron Walden, UK: C.W. Daniel, 1991.

Donato, Giuseppe & Monique Seefried. *The Fragrant Past: Perfumes of Cleopatra and Julius Caesar.* Italy: Instituto Poligrafico E Zecca Dello Stato, 1989.

Dorland, Wayne E. *The Flavors and Fragrance Industry.* WED Co., 1977.

Downer, John. *Supersense: Perception in the Animal World.* New York: Henry Holt, 1988.

Duraffourd, Paul. *The Best of Health Thanks to Essential Oils.* La Vie Claire, 94520 Perigny, 1984.

Dye, Jane. *Aromatherapy for Women & Children: Pregnancy & Childbirth*. Essex, UK: The C.W. Daniel Co., Ltd., 1992.

E

Edwards, Victoria and Dorothy Ganie. "In Search of the Ultimate Anti-Depressant." *Scentsitivity*, Autumn 1992:2.

Edwards, Victoria. "Spikenard. . . The Annointing Oil." *Scentsitivity*, Summer 1993.

Ehrenreich, Barbara & Deirdre English. *For Her Own Good*. Garden City, NJ: Anchor Press/Doubleday, 1978.

Eisner, Thomas. "Rare Mint Patch Makes Ideal Picnic Spot." *Science News*, January 20, 1990.

Engen, Trygg. *The Perception of Odors*. New York: Academic Press, 1982.

F

Fawcett, Margaret. *Aromatherapy for Pregnancy & Childbirth*. Brisbane, Australia: Element, 1993.

Firth, Grace. *Secrets of the Still*. McLean, VA: EPM Publications, 1983.

Fischer-Rizzi, Suzanne. *Complete Aromatherapy Handbook*. New York: Sterling Publishing Co., 1990.

Franchomme, P. and Docteur D. Pénoël. *L'Aromatherapie Exactement*. Limoges, France: Roger Jollois Editeur, 1990.

Franchomme, P. *Phytoguide No. 1: Aromatherapy, Advanced Therapy for Infectious Illnesses*. La Courtete, France: International Phytomedical Foundation, 1985.

G

Gattefossé, René-Maurice. *Gattefossé's Aromatherapy*. Essex, UK: C.W. Daniel, 1993. (First published in France in 1937.)

Genders, Roy. *Perfume Through the Ages*. New York: Putnam, 1972.

Gibbons, Boyd. "Smell, The Intimate Sense." *National Geographic*, September, 1986.

Gibbons, Euell. *Stalking the Healthful Herbs*. New York: David McKay Company, 1966.

Gilbert Avery N. and Charles J. Wysocki. "The Smell Survey Results." *National Geographic*, 1987.

Gimbutas, Marija. *The Language of the Goddess*. San Francisco: Harper & Row, 1989.

Grayson, Jane. *The Fragrant Year*. London: Thorsons, 1993.

Green, Annette. "The Fragrance Revolution. . . The Nose Goes to New Lengths." *The Futurist*, March-April 1993: 13-17.

Griffen, Katherine. "A Whiff of Things to Come." *Health,* Nov./Dec. 1992:34-36.

Griggs, Barbara. *Green Pharmacy: A History of Herbal Medicine.* New York: Viking Press, 1981.

Guenther, Ernest, Ph.D. *The Essential Oils.* Malabar: Krieger Publishing Co., 1976. (original edition 1952) (in six volumes)

Gumbel, G. *Principles of Holistic Skin Therapy with Herbal Essences.* Heidelberg, Germany: Haug, 1986.

H

Hoffman, D. *The Holistic Herbal.* Forris, Scotland: The Findhorn Press, 1983.

Holy Bible, Exodus 30, 22.

Howes, David. "New Guinea: An Olfactory Ethnography." *Dragoco Report,* 1992: 71-81.

Hunter, Jeff. "Ways With Peppermint." *Countryside & Small Stock Journal,* May/June 1991.

J

Juneman, Monika. *Enchanting Scents.* Wilmot: Lotus Light Publ., 1988.

Junius, Manfred M. *The Practical Handbook of Plant Alchemy.* Rochester, NY: Healing Arts Press, 1979.

K

Kallan, Carla. "Probing the Power of Common Scents." *Prevention,* October 1991.

Karagulla, S. and D. van Gelder Kunz. *The Chakras and the Human Energy Fields.* Wheaton, IL: Quest Books, Theosophical Publishing House, 1989.

Kaufman, William I. *Perfume.* New York: E.P. Dutton, 1974.

Kennett, Frances. *History of Perfume.* London: Harrap, 1975.

Kerenyi, Karl. *Goddesses of the Sun and Moon.* Dallas: Spring Publications, Inc., 1979.

Keville, Kathi, Ed. *The American Herb Association Quarterly.* Vols. 7:1-10:1. Nevada City, CA: The American Herb Association, 1988-1994.

Kindscher, Kelly. *Medicinal Wild Plants of the Prairie.* Kansas City, Kansas: University Press of Kansas, 1992.

L

Landing, James E. *American Essence: History of the Peppermint & Spearmint Industry in the U.S.* Kalamazoo, MI: Kalamazoo Public Museum, 1969.

Lavabre, Marcel. *Aromatherapy Workbook.* Rochester: Healing Arts Press, 1990.

Lawless, Julia. *The Encyclopedia of Essential Oils.* Rockport: Element Books, 1992.

———. *Aromatherapy and the Mind.* San Francisco: Thorsons, 1994.

Lawrence, B. Monographs on Essential Oils. *Perfumer and Flavourist.* Carol Stream: Allured Publishing. 1975-94.

LeGuerer, Annick. Scent: *The Mysterious and Essential Powers of Smell.* New York: Turtle Bay Books, 1992.

Leigh, (Ixchel) Susan. "Aromatherapy: Making Good Scents." *Mothering Magazine.* Santa Fe, 1991.

———. "Nurturing During Pregnancy With Aromatherapy." *Another View Magazine.* Van Nuys, 1991.

Leuang, Albery Y. *Encyclopedia of Common Natural Ingredients Used in Food, Drugs and Cosmetics.* New York: Wiley-Intersceince, 1983.

Lewis, Walter H. "Notes on Economic Plants." *Economic Botany,* 1992: 426-430.

Loughran, Joni. "Aromatherapy." *Mothering,* Summer 1988: 29-30.

M

McKenzie, Dan MD. *Aromatics and the Soul.* New York: Paul B. Hoeber, Inc., 1923.

Mabberley, D.J. *The Plant Book.* Cambridge: Cambridge University Press, corrected reprint, 1989.

Manniche. *An Ancient Egyptian Herbal.* London: British Museum Publications, 1989.

Maury, Marguerite. *Marguerite Maury's Guide to Aromatherapy, the Secret of Life and Youth.* London: Mac-Donald, 1964.

Marinell, Giovanni. *The Ornamentation of Ladies.* 1562

Meyer, Scott. "Garden Apothecary: Grow These Herbs for Relief Outside Your Door." *Organic Gardening,* January, 1990.

Miller, Alan and Iona. *The Magical and Ritual Use of Perfumes.* Rochester, NY: Inner Traditions, 1990.

Millspaugh, Charles F. *American Medicinal Plants.* New York: Dover Publications, 1974.

Mindell, Earl. *Earl Mindell's Herb Bible.* New York: Simon & Schuster, 1992.

Mookerjee, Ajit. *Kali: The Feminine Force.* New York: Destiny Books, 1988.

Morris, Edwin T. *Fragrance: The Story of Perfume from Cleopatra to Chanel.* New York: Charles Scribner's, 1984.

O

Ogle, Jane. "Exploring Scent Therapy." *The New York Times Magazine,* November 17, 1985: 115.

Oliver, Joan Duncan. "Making Sense of Scent." *Health,* November 1989: 51-65.

Olson, Cynthia. *Australian Tea Tree Oil Guide.* Fountain Hills: Kali Press, 1992.

Original Swiss Aromatics—Professional Price List. San Rafael: n.p., 1994.

P

Palaiseul, Jean. *Grandmother's Secrets: Her Green Guide to Health from Plants.* New York: G.P. Putnam's Sons, 1973.

Paris, Ginette. *Pagan Meditations.* Dallas: Spring Publications, Inc., 1986.

Parry, Ernest J. *Parry's Cyclopedia of Perfumery.* Philadelphia: P. Blakison's Son & Co., 1925. (in two volumes)

Parsons, Pamela. "Chamomile." *The Aromatic Thymes,* Spring 1994:2.

Parvati, Jeannine. *Hygieia: A Woman's Herbal.* Monroe, UT: Freestone Publishing, 1978.

Piesse, G.W. Septimus. *The Art of Perfumery: Odors of Plants.* Philadelphia: Presley Blakiston, 1880.

Pool, Lawrence J. *Nature's Masterpiece: The Brain and How it Works.* New York: Walker and Co., 1987.

Poucher. *Perfumes, Cosmetics and Soaps.* New York: Chapman and Hall, 1976.

Price, Shirley. *Shirley Price's Aromatherapy Workbook: Understanding Essential Oils from Plant to Bottle.* San Francisco: Thorsons, 1993.

_____. *Practical Aromatherapy: How to Use Essential Oils to Restore Vitality.* Wellingborough: Thorsons, 1987.

_____. *Aromatherapy for Common Ailments.* New York: Fireside, 1991.

R

Raphael, Anna. "Ahhh! Aromatherapy." *Delicious,* December 1994: 47.

Rich and Wilson. *The Cambridge Economic History of Europe.* Cambridge: Cambridge University Publishers, 1967.

Rimmel, Eugene. *Book of Perfumes.* London: Chapman and Hall, 1865.

Roach, Mary. "Scents and Science." *Vogue,* November 1992: 208, 212.

Rodale's Illustrated Encyclopedia of Herbs. New York: Rodale Press, 1987.

Rombough, Lon J. "Grow a Multitude of Mints." *Organic Gardening,* March 1993.

Rowett, H. *Basic Anatomy and Physiology.* London: John Murray, 1959.

Rose, Jeanne. *Aromatherapy 2037.* San Francisco: The Herbal Rose Report, Summer 1992.

_____. *The Aromatherapy Book: Applications & Inhalations.* Berkeley: North Atlantic Books, 1992, 1994.

_____. *Aromatherapy Studies Course.* San Francisco: Herbal Studies Library, 1994.

_____. "Culinary Aromatherapy." *Aromatherapy 2037.* San Francisco: The Herbal Rose Report, Winter 1994-1995: 10-11.

_____. *Guide to [225] Essential Oils.* San Francisco: Herbal Studies Library, 1993. (third edition)

_____. *Guide to [325] Essential Oils*. San Francisco: Herbal Studies Library, 1994.

_____. *Herbal Studies Course, Chapter 32*. San Francsico: Herbal Studies Library, 1988.

_____. *Herbs & Aromatherapy for the Reproductive System*. Berkeley: Frog Ltd, 1994.

_____. *Herbs & Things: Jeanne Rose's Herbal*. New York: Workman, 1972.

_____. *Jeanne Rose's Herbal Body Book*. New York: Grosset and Dunlap, 1976.

_____. *Jeanne Rose's Modern Herbal*. New York: Putnam Publishing Group, 1987.

_____. *Kitchen Cosmetics*. Berkeley: North Atlantic Books, 1990.

Ryman, Danielle. *Aromatherapy: The Complete Guide to Plant and Flower Essences for Health and Beauty*. New York: Bantam Books, 1993.

S

Sagarin, Edward. *The Science and Art of Perfumery*. New York: McGraw Hill, 1945.

Sanderson, H., J. Harrison, S. Price. *Aromatherapy for People with Learning Difficulties*. London: Hands On Publishing, 1990.

Schiller, Carol. "Essential Oils for Body and Mind." *Mothering,* Spring 1993: 56-61.

Schnaubelt, Kurt. *Pacific Institute of Aromatherapy Correspondence Course, Part I*. San Rafael, CA: Pacific Institute of Aromatherapy, 1986.

The Secrets of Master Alexis the Piedmontese, 1615 edition.

Sellar, Wanda. *Directory of Essential Oils*. Essex, UK: C.W. Daniel Co., 1992.

Sinclar, Brett Jason. *Alternative Health Care Resources*. West Nyack: Parker Publishing, 1992.

Straley, Carol. "Aromatherapy." *Parents,* Nov. 1986: 193-196.

Stone, Judith. "Scents and Sensibility." *Discover,* December 1989: 26-31.

Sudworth, George B. *Forest Trees of the Pacific Slope*. New York: Dover Publications, 1967.

"Sweet Future for the Fragrance Industry." *USA Today,* June 1993: 15.

T

Theophrastus. *In Enquiry Into Plants*. 2 vols. (4th century B.C.) Reprint. Sir Arthur Hort, trans. 1916.

Tisserand, Maggie. *Aromatherapy for Women*. Wellingborough: Thorson's Publishers Ltd., 1985.

Tisserand, Robert. *The Art of Aromatherapy*. Saffron Walden, UK: C.W. Daniel Co., Ltd., 1983.

_____. *Essential Oil Safety Data Manual*. Brighton, UK: The Association of Tisserand Aromatherapists, 1985.

———. *To Heal and Tend the Body.* Wilmot: Lotus Press, 1988.

Tutin, Heywood, Burges, Moore, Valentine, Walters and Webb, Editors. *Flora Europaea,* Vol. 4. Cambridge: Cambridge University Press, 1976.

V

Valnet, J. *The Practice of Aromatherapy.* Saffron Walden, UK: C.W. Daniel, 1980.

von Buddenbrock, Wolfgang. *The Senses.* Ann Arbor: University of Michigan Press, 1958.

The National Association
for Holistic Aromatherapy
(NAHA)

an educational nonprofit organization

The National Association for Holistic Aromatherapy was founded by aromatherapists and graduates of the London School of Aromatherapy whose aim was to unify and promote holistic aromatherapy in the United States. NAHA is a nonprofit educational organization incorporated in Colorado which is entirely run by its members nationwide. NAHA is an organization of hard-working, dedicated aromatherapy enthusiasts.

All levels of interest are welcome and the networking and information-exchanging tone of the association encourages interaction among health professionals, business owners, educators, researchers, writers, and aromatherapy enthusiasts. Varying levels of membership allow for a diverse membership base: Friend of Aromatherapy, Professional Member, and Donor. These members enjoy the numerous benefits associated with belonging to the only nonprofit educational organization devoted to aromatherapy in the United States that is not affiliated with any business interest. NAHA's quarterly, *Scentsitivity Quarterly,* includes the latest news and research in the aromatherapy field. The Membership Directory, published every two years, includes referrals for Professional and Donor Members. NAHA's bylaws, which include a Code of Ethics, are available to all members. In addition, all members enjoy the opportunity to participate in hosting NAHA's Conference and Trade Show—the only aromatherapy event of its kind in the United States!

Of primary importance to NAHA members is the development of aromatherapy education and certification standards. Formation of such standards would greatly increase the viability of aromatherapy as a healing art in the United States. Members at all levels of aromatherapy interest are encouraged to participate in ongoing discussion regarding this matter. Ideally, teachers will be able to use these guidelines to develop courses, and students will be able to use the guidelines to develop a program of study.

NAHA's purposes and goals are: To elevate and maintain high standards of aromatherapy education; to establish professional and ethical standards of practice; to improve public awareness regarding the benefits of aromatherapy; to provide public education and encourage dialogue among members through a quarterly newsletter; to participate in the creation and maintenance of an independent National Aromatherapy Certification Board, which will provide a forum to clarify and identify standards of national certification; to stay abreast of ongoing research regarding aromatherapy and the sense of smell; to maintain a directory of members; to provide a listing of approved aromatherapy schools and courses.

NAHA Credo

Aromatherapy is an art and a science that treats mind, body, and spirit.

The holistic approach to aromatherapy advanced by NAHA encourages the synesthesia of art and science and mind/body/spirit. As a part of nature, essential oils are both tools of a healing art and chemical components of a healing science. By application and inhalation, they affect the entire being, to promote vital health and wellness.

A firm dedication to open communication and education is the driving force of NAHA.

Essential oils are potent volatile substances with powerful healing capabilities. It is the desire of NAHA to maintain open communication, to encourage the safe and effective use of essential oils for health and wellness while providing standards of education for practitioners and for the professional use of essential oils. As with all healing tools, personal responsibility is of primary importance; yet NAHA recognizes that personal responsibility stems from proper education and the sharing of information.

NAHA is at the forefront of Aromatherapy development.

As the primary forum for dialogue, in the United States, NAHA is at the forefront of all aspects of aromatherapy development in this country. Members at all levels of aromatherapy interest are not only aware of but also involved in the latest aromatherapy developments.

Benefits of NAHA Membership Include:

1. The *Scentsitivity Quarterly.*
2. Yearly directory of members, practitioners, and aromatherapy schools.
3. Networking with other aromatherapy professionals.
4. Certificates of Donor Membership.
5. Support from the NAHA advisory board.
6. Participation in a worldwide network of aromatherapy enthusiasts of all levels.

Invitation to Join:

1. **Friend of Aromatherapy** (FA) $35.00
   - Quarterly newsletter for one year
   - Listing in Directory

2. **Professional Member** (PM) $50.00
   All of above plus. . .
   - Voting rights—can be elected to office
   - Directory referrals

3. **Donor Member** (DM) $100.00
   All of above plus. . .
   - Complimentary gift

Enclosed is a check for:

_____ $35 Friend of Aromatherapy   _____ $50 Professional Member

_____ $100 Donor Member

Name _____   Tel. _____

Address _____

City _____ State _____ Zip _____

NAHA, P.O. Box 17622, Boulder, CO 80308-7622

This book completed on April 3, 1996 at 7:15 p.m. on the night of the full moon during a full Lunar eclipse in Dawn Heyl's house on the shores of Black Lake, Couschatta, Louisiana.

—Jeanne Rose